Surgery for Morbid Obesity

Surgery for Morbid Obesity

John H. Linner

Clinical Professer of Surgery
University of Minnesota Medical School
Minneapolis, Minnesota, U.S.A.

*With Contributions by Raymond L. Drew,
James M. Gayes, Lyn Howard, John Story Jenks,
Deane C. Manolis, Joseph Milo Meland,
George L. Peltier, Charles L. Smith, and
Sheridan S. Stevens*

Illustrated by Alan Hage

With 167 Illustrations

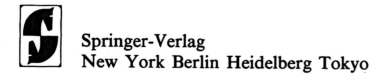

Springer-Verlag
New York Berlin Heidelberg Tokyo

John H. Linner, M.D., F.A.C.S., Clinical Professor of Surgery, University of
Minnesota Medical School, 1014 Metropolitan Medical Building,
825 South Eighth Street, Minneapolis, Minnesota 55404, U.S.A.

Illustrator: Alan Hage, 2304 Seabury Avenue,
Minneapolis, Minnesota 55406, U.S.A.

Library of Congress Cataloging in Publication Data
Main entry under title:

Surgery for morbid obesity.

Includes index.
1. Obesity—Surgery.   2. Gastrointestinal system—
Surgery.   3. Jejunoileal bypass.   I. Linner, John H.
[DNLM: 1. Obesity—Therapy.   2. Stomach—Surgery. WD 210
S9605]
RD540.S88   1984   617'.43   83–14585

Typeset by Bi-comp, Inc., York, Pennsylvania
Printed and bound by Halliday Lithograph, West Hanover, Massachusetts

9 8 7 6 5 4 3 2 1

ISBN-13: 978-1-4613-8247-8   e-ISBN-13: 978-1-4613-8245-4
DOI: 10.1007/978-1-4613-8245-4

To Evodia

Contributors

Raymond L. Drew, M.D., F.A.C.S., *Surgical Staff, Metropolitan Medical Center, Minneapolis, Minnesota, U.S.A.*

James M. Gayes, M.D., *Anesthesia Department, Metropolitan Medical Center, Minneapolis, Minnesota, U.S.A.*

Lyn Howard, M.B., M.R.C.P., *Director of Clinical Nutrition, Associate Professor of Medicine and Pediatrics, Albany Medical College, Albany, New York, U.S.A.*

John Story Jenks, M.D., Assistant Professor of Medicine, Clinical Nutrition Program, Albany Medical College; Chief, Nutrition Support Service, Albany Veterans Administration Medical Center, Albany, New York, U.S.A.

Deane C. Manolis, M.D., *Department of Psychiatry, Metropolitan Medical Center, Minneapolis, Minnesota, U.S.A.*

J. Milo Meland, M.D., *Assistant Chief, Department of Diagnostic Radiology, Metropolitan Medical Center, Minneapolis, Minnesota, U.S.A.*

George L. Peltier, M.D., F.A.C.S., *Plastic and Reconstructive Surgeon, Metropolitan Medical Center; Chief, Plastic Surgery Department, Hennepin County Medical Center; Clinical Instructor of Surgery, University of Minnesota Medical School, Minneapolis, Minnesota, U.S.A.*

Charles L. Smith, M.D., *Assistant Professor of Medicine, University of Minnesota Medical School, Minneapolis, Minnesota, U.S.A.*

Sheridan S. Stevens, M.D., F.A.C.S., *Plastic and Reconstructive Surgeon, Metropolitan Medical Center; Consulting Plastic Surgeon, Hennepin County Medical Center; Clinical Associate Professor of Surgery, University of Minnesota Medical School, Minneapolis, Minnesota, U.S.A.*

Contents

x   Contents

Preface

The surgical treatment of morbid obesity has undergone astonishing growth since its inception thirty years ago. The medical profession has long been aware of the discouraging intractability of morbid obesity to all forms of conservative management, and it is only recently that physicians have come to realize that surgery can provide very real palliation for the morbidly obese patient. Surgery does not attack the underlying etiology of morbid obesity, whatever it may be, but exerts its effect indirectly either by effecting a calorie loss through intestinal shunting, or by calorie deprivation through a radical reduction of gastric capacity.

Acceptance of bariatric surgery as a legitimate therapeutic modality has met with considerable resistance by many physicians for two principal reasons. The first relates to the rather prevalent but unjustifiable attitude both within and without the medical profession that morbid obesity is an expression of slovenliness, the result of a character defect, or a defect of the will, and that those so afflicted should not be extended the benefit of an "easy way out," but should "shape up" by rigorous diet and exercise.

The second more serious concern that has blunted enthusiasm for bariatric surgery has been the large number of late complications following jejunoileal bypass, and the high incidence of perioperative complications and revisional operations in some quarters following gastric reduction procedures. It is to these concerns that this book is addressed.

Dr. Arnold Kremen of Minneapolis, Minnesota, kindled my interest in developing a surgical approach for the treatment of morbid obesity in 1953. In a series of dog experiments in the research laboratory of the United States Veteran's Administration Hospital in Minneapolis, we studied the absorption characteristics of various lengths of jejunum and ileum, and the putative importance of the ileocecal valve. Based on these findings, in 1954 we performed what was to our knowledge the first jejunoileal bypass (JIB). The patient was a 34-year-old, white female whose maximum weight had been 385 pounds. We were unaware that two years earlier Viktor Henriksson, M.D. of Gothenburg, Sweden, had attacked the problem of morbid obesity by resecting a large segment of small intestine in an adult female patient. This case was reported during the discussion period of our paper by Philip Sanblom, M.D. at the American Surgical Association meeting in Cleveland

April 29th, 1954. Henriksson's procedure had the disadvantage of not being reversible, which limited its acceptance.

I recently learned that Dr. Richard Varco at the University of Minnesota Hospital had independently performed an end-to-end JIB for morbid obesity in a female patient at about the same time we did. This was an unpublished case. Based on Varco's initial contribution, Dr. Henry Buchwald built his extensive experience in this field.

The first patient of ours developed a bleeding duodenal ulcer two years after the JIB, necessitating a vagotomy and pyloroplasty. Several years later she bled massively again from a recurrent duodenal ulcer, and a Billroth I hemigastrectomy was required to control the bleeding. It is now known that duodenal ulcer is an infrequent complication of JIB, but at that time I was concerned that it might prove to be the rule rather than the exception, and therefore did not do another JIB until the experience accumulating at other centers could be evaluated.

Although the reported results following jejunocolic bypass operations were dismal, the experience following JIB appeared encouraging. In 1968, therefore, the JIB was reintroduced into my surgical practice. Kremen did not return to this field. Several different anatomic configurations with varying bowel lengths were tried in 173 patients between the years 1968 and 1976 in an attempt to find the most effective operation. Satisfactory weight reduction was achieved in the majority of patients, but because of the high incidence of late complications the JIB was discontinued in 1976 in favor of the gastric bypass (GBP).

Gastric reduction operations over the ensuing six years underwent a circuitous evolution in my practice, from the loop or Billroth II type of GBP to the Roux-en-Y type, to the horizontal gastroplasty (GP), then back to the Roux-en-Y GBP which has proved to be the most effective. During this time, however, it was learned that at least as important as a particular technique in achieving success was appropriate case selection, thorough patient education, and adherence to certain principles of technique.

Considerable attention has been paid to complications in this book, because it is my conviction that surgeons should not embark on this field until they have familiarized themselves with the prevention, diagnosis, and management of the potential complications. Unless they become so informed, bariatric surgery will be a harrowing experience for them, and a disaster for their patients.

Regardless of what the future holds for this subspecialty of general surgery (and it is my belief that it will occupy an important place for many years), the serendipitous consequences of bariatric surgery have been quite remarkable. It has been learned, for example, that the obese patient has an amazing ability to tolerate major surgery and general anesthesia, provided certain precautions are taken. This has resulted in the evolution of management techniques that has made surgery for the morbidly obese patient, except for the super-obese (500 plus pounds), a relatively routine event. Whereas formerly the prospect of operating on a morbidly obese patient for any reason was a frightening experience for surgeon and anesthesiologist alike, today most of these people are accepted for surgery with equanimity. Although the margin for error may at times be quite small, it is now known that the average obese patient is not an unreasonable anesthetic or surgical risk.

Another serendipitous consequence of obesity surgery has resulted from the long term complications that have followed JIB. These complications have stemmed either from malabsorption, or from the toxic effect of coliform bacteria residing within the excluded small intestine, and have provided an important field of research for investigators concerned with various aspects of malnutrition, vitamin deficiency, osteomalacia, liver failure, renal lithiasis, and immunopathies. This, of course, hardly justifies JIB, but it is fortuitous that the pathogenesis of the metabolic derangements and deficiency states that have emerged as complications of JIB has been so intensely, and profitably, studied.

The use of JIB has all but disappeared in the United States and seems currently to be confined to a few centers. This is perhaps as it should be. The JIB operation has been much like the little girl with the curl in the middle of her forehead: "when she was good she was very, very good, but when she was bad she was horrid."

Gastric reduction surgery has provided its own disenchantment among many in the medical profession, as mentioned earlier, for at least two reasons. First, it has been undertaken too lightly by some surgeons who have had no particular interest, experience, or education in this field of surgery, and on this account it has had a prohibitively high complication rate. The other disenchantment has resulted from the desire of many surgeons to develop a simple operation that requires minimum operating time, and would be attended by few, if any, complications. This salutary motive was manifested in the various gastric partitioning operations that proliferated rapidly several years ago and were heralded as the ultimate bariatric procedures. Unfortunately the failure rate in reported series with these procedures exceeded 75%, primarily because the staple lines disrupted adjacent to the channel. This was not appreciated by many surgeons around the country until the operation had received wide acceptance. Disillusionment with this and similar operations has caused their gradual decline.

The desire to simplify any operation is commendable, provided the modification is effective and the long-term failure rate is not excessive. Our efforts at simplification by adopting the horizontal gastroplasty in 1978 resulted in such a high failure rate that we returned to the more difficult, but much more effective, Roux-en-Y gastric bypass, as will be discussed in Chapter Four. Newer operations such as the vertical banded gastroplasty introduced by Dr. Edward Mason show promise but need a longer period of evaluation before their general adoption.

Even though a simpler operation such as the vertical gastroplasty or the gastric banding procedure may prove satisfactory and the procedure of choice for the majority of morbidly obese patients, there will always be a place for the gastric bypass operation in patients with a sweet tooth, and those who have failed other, simpler methods. The bariatric surgeon should familiarize himself with this operation and its complications if he wishes to undertake the surgical management of morbid obesity.

Surgery is only one aspect of a comprehensive attack on one of western man's most intractable afflictions—morbid obesity. It does provide the essential weapon in the obese patient's otherwise almost impossible battle to lose weight permanently. The remarkable enhancement in the quality of life of patients once burdened by excessive weight who achieve a normal or near normal habitus makes bariatric surgery extremely rewarding. Many previously unemployable patients obtain jobs, some women who have never had a date find themselves suddenly popular, many patients are relieved of joint pains, dyspnea, and hypertension. Diabetes and stasis dermatitis are improved. The positive ramifications are amazing.

Adherence to the principles of technique outlined herein is essential for success. A sloppy operation will fail. On the other hand, a determined hyperphagic patient can defeat the most elegant gastric reduction operation, and patients must be made to understand that to achieve the "impossible dream" they must also do their part.

The chapter on computers was included only because we thought that briefly explaining the process of adapting this material to a microcomputer would be of interest. It is certainly not a necessity in the conduct of this type of surgery, or even in evaluating the results, but it does make the analysis of comparative data, particularly for purposes of publication, infinitely simpler.

The chapter on body contour surgery is not intended to be a direction manual for general surgeons. The abdominoplasty portion may be adaptable to the surgical practice of general surgeons, but most of the other reconstructions fall within the province of the plastic surgeon. We have been impressed with the additional rehabilitation these techniques have afforded some of our patients, and we wished to have these possibilities presented in some detail. Plastic and reconstructive surgeons who have not had an opportunity to participate in the total care of this type of patient can benefit from the extensive experience represented here.

I wish to thank all the contributors to the book, Drs. Lyn Howard and John Jenks of Albany, N.Y., Drs. Deane Manolis, Charles Smith, James Gayes, Milo Meland, Raymond Drew, Sheridan Stevens, and George Peltier of Minneapolis, Minnesota, for their outstanding cooperation and expertise. A special thank you to Dr. Raymond Drew, for setting up our computer program which made the analysis of the data possible, to Ismar Cintora, M.D. and Bruce Davis, P.A., who not only assisted at surgery, but played an important role in gathering statistics, to James N. Groth, M.D. for helping to compile data, to Metropolitan Medical Center nursing, dietary, and operating room staffs for the superb care they have extended to our patients, and to Mary Walter, our office nurse, and Lillian Oquist, our secretary, who together have called and written to patients for follow-up, assisted in their instruction, and typed most of the manuscript for this book.

John H. Linner, M.D.

CHAPTER 1

Medical Aspects of Morbid Obesity

LYN HOWARD AND JOHN STORY JENKS

Morbid Obesity

In 1963 Payne and DeWind coined the term "morbid" obesity to draw attention to the life-threatening consequences of being 100%, or more than 100 lb, above average body weight.[1] Because obesity, particularly of this magnitude, has proved very resistant to medical management, radical surgical treatment seems justified.

This first chapter will attempt to provide a background against which the rationale, and potential benefits and hazards, of different types of surgical treatment can be assessed.

Definition of Morbid Obesity

Although there is general agreement[2] to accept Payne and DeWind's working definition of "morbid" obesity as 100% or 100 lb overweight, whichever is less, it must be recognized that "overweight" does not necessarily reflect excess fat[3] and there is no exact cutoff point above which obesity is acutely life threatening. A normal man or woman has a body fat content accounting for 15–20% or 20–25%, respectively, of the total body weight. A "morbidly" obese individual may have 40–70% of body weight as fat. Although percent body fat, rather than percent overweight, would provide a more precise diagnosis of morbid obesity, there are no simple techniques yet available for accurately assessing total body fat. Ultrasound techniques are being developed by the meat industry to rapidly assess the fat content of live beef cattle and something similar may soon be available for human subjects.[4] In the interim, exact measurements of human fat content involve underwater weighing[5] or dilutional techniques using fat-soluble isotopes,[6] such as propane or krypton, or the indirect measurement of total body water (D_2O)[7] and fat-free body cell mass (counting the naturally occurring ^{40}K or injecting radioactive ^{42}K).[8]

Measurements of skin-fold thickness with calipers is a simple bedside technique for assessing subcutaneous fat. If several skin-fold measurements are totaled (biceps, triceps, subscapular, and suprailiac) the reliability of this technique is increased[9] (Table 1-1). If a single site is measured, subscapular skin fold has a better correlation with other measures of fatness than the more commonly measured, triceps skin fold.[10] In severely obese men the triceps plus subscapular skin folds are greater than 52 mm and in severely obese women these combined skin-fold thicknesses are greater than 68 mm.[11] Skin-fold measurements become less reliable in older subjects because, although there is a gradual accumulation of more body fat with age, the fat is increasingly deposited in perivisceral, rather than subcutaneous sites. Recent studies indicate that morbidity (hypertension, diabetes) in obese subjects correlates more strongly with upper truncal obesity, than with lower truncal obesity.[12]

For simplicity—as in Payne and DeWind's definition—height and weight measurements are commonly used to quantitate obesity. Although such measurements provide only a fair estimate of body fat[13] they can at least be accurately and reproducibly performed, even though in morbidly obese subjects it is often necessary to use the hospital laundry scales. Probably the best guidelines for body

TABLE 1-1   The Equivalent Fat Content, as a Percentage of Body Weight, for a Range of Values for the Sum of 4 Skinfolds (Biceps, Triceps, Subscapular, and Suprailiac) of Males and Females of Different Ages

Skin-folds (mm)	Percentage Fat							
	Males				Females			
	17–29	30–39 (years)	40–49	50+	16–29	30–39 (years)	40–49	50+
15	4.8				10.5			
20	8.1	12.2	12.2	12.6	14.1	17.0	19.8	21.4
25	10.5	14.2	15.0	15.6	16.8	19.4	22.2	24.0
30	12.9	16.2	17.7	18.6	19.5	21.8	24.5	26.6
35	14.7	17.7	19.6	20.8	21.5	23.7	26.4	28.5
40	16.4	19.2	21.4	22.9	23.4	25.5	28.2	30.3
45	17.7	20.4	23.0	24.7	25.0	26.9	29.6	31.9
50	19.0	21.5	24.6	26.5	26.5	28.2	31.0	33.4
55	20.1	22.5	25.9	27.9	27.8	29.4	32.1	34.6
60	21.2	23.5	27.1	29.2	29.1	30.6	33.2	35.7
65	22.2	24.3	28.2	30.4	30.2	31.6	34.1	36.7
70	23.1	25.1	29.3	31.6	31.2	32.5	35.0	37.7
75	24.0	25.9	30.3	32.7	32.2	33.4	35.9	38.7
80	24.8	26.6	31.2	33.8	33.1	34.3	36.7	39.6
85	25.5	27.2	32.1	34.8	34.0	35.1	37.5	40.4
90	26.2	27.8	33.0	35.8	34.8	35.8	38.3	41.2
95	26.9	28.4	33.7	36.6	35.6	36.5	39.0	41.9
100	27.6	29.0	34.4	37.4	36.4	37.2	39.7	42.6
105	28.2	29.6	35.1	38.2	37.1	37.9	40.4	43.3
110	28.8	30.1	35.8	39.0	37.8	38.6	41.0	43.9
115	29.4	30.6	36.4	39.7	38.4	39.1	41.5	44.5
120	30.0	31.1	37.0	40.4	39.0	39.6	42.0	45.1
125	30.5	31.5	37.6	41.1	39.6	40.1	42.5	45.7
130	31.0	31.9	38.2	41.8	40.2	40.6	43.0	46.2
135	31.5	32.3	38.7	42.4	40.8	41.1	43.5	46.7
140	32.0	32.7	39.2	43.0	41.3	41.6	44.0	47.2
145	32.5	33.1	39.7	43.6	41.8	42.1	44.5	47.7
150	32.9	33.5	40.2	44.1	42.3	42.6	45.0	48.2
155	33.3	33.9	40.7	44.6	42.8	43.1	45.4	48.7
160	33.7	34.3	41.2	45.1	43.3	43.6	45.8	49.2
165	34.1	34.6	41.6	45.6	43.7	44.0	46.2	49.6
170	34.5	34.8	42.0	46.1	44.1	44.4	46.6	50.0
175	34.9					44.8	47.0	50.4
180	35.3					45.2	47.4	50.8
185	35.6					45.6	47.8	51.2
190	35.9					45.9	48.2	51.6
195						46.2	48.5	52.0
200						46.5	48.8	52.4
205							49.1	52.7
210							49.4	53.0

From Durnin JGVA, Womersley J: Body fat assessed from total body density. Br J Nutr 32:77–97, 1974. Used with permission from Cambridge University Press.

weight are those published by the Fogarty Conference on Obesity in 1973[14] (Table 1-2). Height and weight measurements more accurately define body fat if they are expressed as the body mass index (weight/height^2).[13]

In terms of the current definition of morbid obesity a very short person may be 100% overweight, without being 100 lb overweight (a 30-year-old woman, 57 in. tall, has an ideal body weight of 95 lb and will be "morbidly" obese at 190 lb), and a tall person may be 100 lb overweight without being 100% overweight (a 30-year-old

TABLE 1-2 Guidelines for Body Weight

Metric

Height* (m)	Men—Weight (kg)* Average	Men Acceptable		Women—Weight (kg)* Average	Women Acceptable	
1.45				4.60	42	53
1.48				46.5	42	54
1.50				47.0	43	55
1.52				48.5	44	57
1.54				49.5	44	58
1.56				50.4	45	58
1.58	55.8	51	64	51.3	46	59
1.60	57.6	52	65	52.6	48	61
1.62	58.6	53	66	54.0	49	62
1.64	59.6	54	67	55.4	50	64
1.66	60.6	55	69	56.8	51	65
1.68	61.7	56	71	58.1	52	66
1.70	63.5	58	73	60.0	53	67
1.72	65.0	59	74	61.3	55	69
1.74	66.5	60	75	62.6	56	70
1.76	68.0	62	77	64.0	58	72
1.78	69.4	64	79	65.3	59	74
1.80	71.0	65	80			
1.82	72.6	66	82			
1.84	74.2	67	84			
1.86	75.8	69	86			
1.88	77.6	71	88			
1.90	79.3	73	90			
1.92	81.0	75	93			

Nonmetric

Height* (ft, in)	Men—Weight (lb)* Average	Men Acceptable		Women—Weight (lb)* Average	Women Acceptable	
4 10				102	92	119
4 11				104	94	122
5 0				107	96	125
5 1				110	99	128
5 2	123	112	141	113	102	131
5 3	127	115	144	116	105	134
5 4	130	118	148	120	108	138
5 5	133	121	152	123	111	142
5 6	136	124	156	128	114	146
5 7	140	128	161	132	118	150
5 8	145	132	166	136	122	154
5 9	149	136	170	140	126	158
5 10	153	140	174	144	130	163
5 11	158	144	179	148	134	168
6 0	162	148	184	152	138	173
6 1	166	152	189			
6 2	171	156	194			
6 3	176	160	199			
6 4	181	164	204			

* Height without shoes; weight without clothes.
Adapted from the recommendations of the Fogarty Center Conference on Obesity, 1973. From Bray GA: Obesity in America, NIH Publication No. 79. Washington, D.C., 1979, p. 359.

man, 74 in. tall, has an ideal body weight of 190 lb and will be "morbidly" obese at 290 lb). Although these discrepancies suggest that our working definition of morbid obesity probably reflects a rather wide span of body fat content, surveys that have linked life expectancy to variations in weight show a marked acceleration of excess mortality in subjects who are greater than 50% overweight or have a body mass index of greater than 30 kg/m² or 0.043 lb/in.[2] It is reassuring that despite their differences in weight-for-height indices, both of the subjects described above meet all the criteria for an accelerated risk of mortality. Thus our current definition of morbid obesity seems to correctly identify the population who, at least statistically, are morbidly threatened by their excess weight.

Prevalence of Morbid Obesity

The exact prevalence of persons who are more than 100% or 100 lb overweight is not known. The Health and Nutrition Examination Survey measured triceps and subscapular skin fold in over 12,000 U.S. citizens between the ages of 20 and 74.[11] Using a combined skin-fold value of greater than 52 mm for men and 68 mm for women (> 95th percentile), they calculated that 4.9% of adult American men (2.8 million) and 7.2% of American women (4.5 million) are severely obese. All the subjects identified by these skin-fold measurements had a body mass index of greater than 30 kg/m², a level at which excess weight is strongly linked to excess mortality. Despite this fact, the severely obese men and women were only 37% (50 lb) and 57% (67 lb) over their desirable weight in all age groups; thus they did not meet the criteria for "morbid" obesity. This suggests that the existing definition of morbid obesity describes only extremely obese subjects and may not encompass many persons who have enhanced risk of excess mortality.

Differential Diagnosis of Obesity Syndromes

Although the overwhelming majority of obese subjects fall into the category of exogenous obesity, a number of metabolic syndromes may present with this symptom and should be considered in the medical evaluation of obese patients. Table 1-3 lists these obesity syndromes. It is worth noting that the differential diagnosis is more complex in the pediatric population, since the rare genetic syndromes and hypothalamic tumors tend to present in this age group.[11] Exogenous obesity is often not recognized in children because, while a positive caloric balance may be causing exaggerated replication of adipocyte precursors,[15] it is also a general stimulus to growth of skeletal tissues therefore obese children are usually above the 90th percen-

TABLE 1-3 Differential Diagnosis of Obesity Syndromes

Etiologic
A. Endocrine disorders
    Glucocorticoid excess, Cushing's syndrome
    Thyroid hormone deficiency
    Hypopituitarism
    Gonadal deficiency
    Hyperinsulinoma, excess exogenous insulin
      (Mauriac syndrome)
B. Genetic disorders
    Inherited predisposition to obesity
    Prader Willi/Cohen's syndrome
    Glycogen storage disease
    Laurence-Moon-Bardet-Biedl syndrome
    Morgagni-Morel syndrome (hyperostosis frontalis interna)
    Pseudo- and pseudo-pseudohypoparathyroidism
    Kleinfelter's syndrome
    Turner's syndrome
C. Hypothalamic dysfunction
    Tumors
    Inflammation
    Trauma and surgical injury
    Increased intracranial pressure
    Functional changes causing hyperinsulinemia
D. Drugs
    Phenothiazines
    Tricyclic antidepressants
    Lithium
    Corticosteroids
    Insulin
    Cyproheptadine
E. Nutritional
    In utero nutritional factors?
    Infant feeding practices?

Anatomic
A. Hypercellular and/or hypertrophic: early onset, severe obesity
B. Hypertrophic: adult onset, milder obesity

Contributing Environmental Factors
A. Physical inactivity
B. Family influence
C. Type of diet and eating pattern
D. Cultural, ethnic, socioeconomic
E. Psychologic
F. Educational

tile for both height and weight.[16] Obese children mature earlier; thus when they reach their genetically predetermined height and linear growth ceases, it may become apparent that their fat content is excessive and the earlier accelerated growth reflected excess caloric balance. Therefore in the pediatric population it is better to rely on skinfold measurements rather than just weight-for-height anthropometry. Because exogenous obesity in children is associated with accelerated linear growth, the child who is obese but short must

be diligently screened for an alternative diagnosis. The exception to this rule is the child with Klinefelter's syndrome; such boys and men are likely to be excessively tall.[17]

Very few adults with metabolic syndromes other than exogenous obesity reach a size that would be classified as morbid obesity. Even subjects with hypothalamic destruction, who have hyperinsulinemia and hyperphagia, tend to reach a new weight set point, between 250 and 350 lb.[18]

Table 1-4 summarizes the medical evaluation

TABLE 1-4 Evaluation of Obese Patients

History
A. Weight at key growth phases
   At birth
   Infancy
   Onset of adolescence
   End of adolescence (Army physical, marriage)
   Net weight gained with pregnancies
   Maximum adult weight
   Weight lost on diets, period weight loss sustained
B. Medical complications of obesity
   Known hypertension, headaches, shortness of breath, palpitations, ankle edema
   Pickwickian symptoms, narcolepsy, nocturnal apnea
   Known diabetes mellitus, polydipsia, polyuria, visual symptoms, numbness and tingling of extremities
   Known hyperlipidemia, xanthoma, pancreatitis, gallstones
   Arthritis, gout
   Menstrual irregularities, infertility
   Breast mass, rectal bleeding
C. Family history
   Parental and sibling height and weight, history of obesity or related disorders
   Relatives with genetic obese syndromes
D. Nutritional history
   Infant feeding practices
   Eating pattern during periods of weight gain and when weight stable, factors stimulating increased food intake
   24-hr dietary recall
   Dieting practices, bulimia
E. Social history and energy expenditure
   Job record
   Use of alcohol, tobacco, and other drugs
   Life style, temperature set of thermostat
   Exercise, walking, sports
   Family and social stress
F. Past medical history
   Head injuries, brain tumors
   Cholecystectomy
   Breast, uterine, bowel cancer
   Medications
   Depression

Physical Examination
A. Height and weight: refer to Table 1-2 and growth charts for children
B. Fat distribution, skin-fold thickness (Table 1-1); truncal or generalized distribution, moon facies, buffalo hump
C. Hair distribution, hirsutism, hair texture, sparse eyebrows
D. Skin texture, acne, intertriginous dermatitis, xanthoma
E. Eyes, visual fields, optic fundi, evidence of hypertensive or diabetic retinopathy or raised intracranial pressure
F. Thyroid size
G. Pulmonary function, dyspnea, plethora, cyanosis, somnolence
H. Cardiac function, blood pressure with a large cuff, evidence of congestive heart failure
I. Abdomen: confirm that size is due to fat and not to a mass or fluid
J. Extremities: evidence of arthritis, varicose veins, elbows with increased carrying angle, tapering extremities.

Biochemical Assessment
A. Blood count
B. Urinalysis
C. Electrolytes, uric acid
D. Liver and renal function tests
E. Cholesterol and fasting triglyceride
F. Morning plasma cortisol and, if elevated, dexamethasone suppression test
G. T_3, T_4, TSH
H. Fasting and 2-hr postprandial blood glucose
I. Lung function studies and blood gases if respiratory function severely impaired
J. Chest radiogram and EKG if cardiac function severely impaired
K. Skull radiogram and other CNS studies if evidence of neurologic disease
L. Gallbladder ultrasonogram if findings suggest cholelithiasis

of obese patients and incorporates tests to separate exogenous obesity from obesity syndromes. The work-up also includes tests to screen for hypertension, diabetes, hyperlipidemia, gallstones, and other recognized complications of severe obesity.

Pathophysiology of Exogenous Obesity

Since the laws of thermodynamics apply to man as well as to steam engines, obesity of all types implies a positive caloric balance which means a greater intake than expenditure. However, the term exogenous obesity is problematic because it infers that excessive eating is the primary etiology, whereas growing evidence suggests decreased energy expenditure as the major defect in most obese subjects. This is an important issue to the bariatric surgeon because it implies that obese people run at a lower energy cost than the rest of the population, which may explain the somewhat limited success of operations designed to restrict food intake.[19]

Table 1-5 summarizes the recent studies which have examined energy balance in obese subjects. It should be noted that most studies examining caloric intake find little difference between calories consumed by lean subjects and those consumed by weight-stable obese subjects. Hirsch (personal communication) found that weight-stable obese adults ate approximately the same number of calories as weight-stable lean subjects. It is possible that obese subjects have periods of overeating, especially during phases of accelerated growth; however, studies of caloric intake do not support this concept either in infants[52,53] or adults.[23-25]

If there are important intersubject differences in energy expenditure (Table 1-6) the question arises, what precisely are these differences and how are they controlled? Obesity commonly clusters in families. Whereas offspring of two normal-weight parents have only a 10% chance of becoming obese, the probability of obesity in the offspring when one or both parents are obese is increased to 50 and 80%, respectively.[54] The question is whether this family's tendency is an expression of shared genes or a shared environment? Griffiths and Payne[53] studied 4-year-old children of obese and normal-weight parents. At the time these children were studied, both groups were of similar height and weight; however, statistically the chil-

TABLE 1-5 Pathophysiologic Mechanisms in Obesity

Increased body fat can occur by increasing the triglyceride content of adipose cells (hypertrophy), by increasing the total number of adipose cells (hyperplasia), or by both mechanisms (hypertrophic-hyperplastic).[20,21] An enlarged fat cell exhibits increased glucose oxidation and synthesis of triglyceride, and increased lipolysis and release of free fatty acids. The hypertrophic cell has a decreased sensitivity to insulin.[22] Net lipid accumulation can result from increased lipid deposition or decreased lipid utilization.

Mechanisms Favoring Increased Lipid Deposition
A. Increased energy intake. Seen in genetically obese animal models.[23] Not an obvious component of most human types of obesity.[23-25] Obese people appear to respond more to external than internal cues.[26-28]
B. Hypothalamic lesions.[29] Ablative lesions of ventromedial nucleus (satiety center) cause hyperphagia and obesity, possibly secondary to vagally mediated increased basal insulin secretion and preabsorptive insulin release.[18,30] Stimulation of lateral hypothalamic nucleus (feeding center) induces hyperphagia, hyperdipsia, and other arousal reactions.[31]
C. Meal pattern. Frequency of eating inversely related to obesity, perhaps because large infrequent meals are a strong stimulus to insulin and lipogenesis,[32,33] or because metabolic cost of shunting substrate in and out of stores is greater with more fluctuations in fed–fasted state.[34]
D. Increased insulin levels (genetic, acquired, iatrogenic). Promote lipogenesis, inhibit lipolysis, and stimulate lipoprotein lipase activity.[35]
E. Cellular metabolic differences. Hepatocytes from genetically obese rats are more lipogenic.[36] Adipocytes from morbidly obese persons show exaggerated in vitro replication rates.[37]

Mechanisms Favoring Decreased Lipid Mobilization or Utilization
A. Depressed lipolysis. Lipolysis is normal in obese subjects;[38] however, after prolonged fasting adipocytes demonstrate reduced lipolysis due to an increase in alpha-2-receptor activity.[39] Decreased fatty acid oxidation and ketogenesis have been demonstrated in obese rats.[40]
B. Depressed thermogenesis. Reduced diet-induced thermogenesis in genetically obese animals is possibly secondary to abnormal hypothalamic control or a reduced insulin effect.[41-45] Reduced nonshivering thermogenesis due to cold stress is also seen in genetically obese animals.[46] Reduced futile cycles are suggested but not confirmed.[47,48] Reduced Na^+/K^+ ATPase activity is seen in some animal models,[47,48] but is probably not of major significance in humans.[50]
C. Depressed physical activity. Less activity in obese compared to lean subjects[51,52] may be a result rather than a cause.

TABLE 1-6 The Various Components of Energy Expenditure

Type of Energy Expenditure	Average kcal/day
Resting metabolic rate (RMR)	1500
Thermogenic effect of exercise (TEE)	750
Thermogenic effect of food (TEF)	250
Adaptive thermogenesis (AT)	±250

dren from the obese families were "preobese" subjects. The preobese children behaved very differently from the children with normal-weight parents. The preobese children ate 24% fewer calories per kilogram per day and expended 25% fewer calories per kilogram per day. As Griffiths and Payne correctly point out, their study could not distinguish between a learned or inherited trait which caused reduced energy expenditure.

The classic experimental model for separating "seed" from "soil" involves studies of adopted children. Currently such adoption studies provide conflicting results. Garn et al[55] found that adopted children seemed to gain weight in exactly the same manner as their genetically unrelated siblings, suggesting that peer and parent role models may be just as important as hereditary factors. Conversely Biron et al,[56] in a study of 374 families with adopted children, found a strong weight and weight/height correlation of adopted children with their natural parents, but only a weak correlation with their adopted parents.

Genetic control of obesity is clearly established in several animal models, where it appears to be regulated from at least four independent gene loci.[57-59] Genetic control implies some identifiable biochemical abnormality and genetically obese animal models have provided investigators with an important tool to test various biochemical hypotheses.[60]

Table 1-6 lists the various components of energy expenditure. Although reduced physical activity does occur in severe obesity it is not clear that this is a primary defect, since in modern Western society most obese and lean subjects are equally sedentary. Motion studies have shown decreased physical activity in obese adolescent girls,[61] but probably in the majority of obese persons physical inactivity is a consequence of obesity[62] and a factor which perpetuates the obese state.

In recent years the component of energy expenditure which has attracted a great deal of attention is cellular or nonshivering thermogenesis. Thermogenesis is a major component of energy expenditure, and is an inherent by-product of most biochemical reactions. In warm-blooded animals such heat production is partly essential for maintenance of body temperature and partly represents metabolic "inefficiency," a phenomenon which may be a key to regulation of energy balance. There are several mechanisms by which thermogenesis could be modulated to enable a person to stay in energy equilibrium despite some fairly wide swings in energy intake.[63] Defective modulation could then result in obesity. Newsholme[48] has hypothesized that various enzymes governing metabolic control points—e.g., those that control glycolysis and gluconeogenesis, such as phosphofructokinase and fructose diphosphatase (Fig. 1-1)—may be constantly cycling substrate up and down the glycolytic pathway. He postulates that alterations in substrate and hormone concentrations enhance this cycling and temporarily shift the equilibrium in one direction or another. Since the cycling generates heat, small intersubject differences in the rate of cycling could explain critical differences in metabolic efficiency. This hypothesis is so far unproven; however, like brown adipose tissue, which will be mentioned later, catecholamines do influence such metabolic cycling. Hence lean and obese differences in stress and diet-induced thermogenesis could be a reflection of altered "futile" cycles.

Although obese subjects have a slightly higher absolute resting metabolic rate (RMR) than their lean counterparts,[64] when this is expressed per kilogram of muscle mass, obese and lean subjects have the same RMR.[65] In other words, most obese subjects have a greater muscle mass, or a bigger engine. Eating induces a thermic response which continues for several hours afterward. Welle et al[66] have shown that the thermic response to the carbohydrate component of the diet is mediated by stimulation of the sympathetic nervous system (SNS). Protein and fat-induced thermogenesis apparently do not reflect sympathetic stimulation. It has been postulated that the thermogenic effect of food (TEF) might differ in lean and obese subjects, both in response to a single meal and in response to prolonged overfeeding (adaptive thermogenesis—AT.) Such a difference has been elegantly demonstrated in experimental animals,[42-46,67,68] where diet-induced norepinephrine

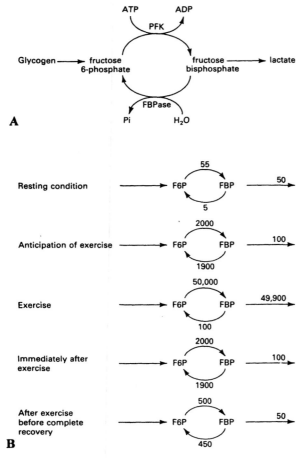

FIG. 1-1. Futile cycles: a possible metabolic basis for the control of body weight. **A** The fructose 6-phosphate–fructose bisphosphate cycle in the glycolytic pathway from glycogen to lactate. PFK, phosphofructokinase; FBPase, fructose 1,6 bisphosphatase; Pi, inorganic phosphate. **B** Hypothetical fluxes in the fructose 6-phosphate–fructose bisphosphate cycle and in glycolysis before, during, and after exercise. The numbers refer to the rates of the reactions shown, and those on the right represent glycolytic flux in nmole $\times$ min^{-1} $\times$ g^{-1}. F6P, fructose 6-phosphate, FBP, fructose bisphosphate. The ratios of cycling rate to flux can be readily calculated from the numbers given; the highest ratio is present during anticipation of exercise,[19] and the lowest during exercise. The rate of cycling is 90 times higher before complete recovery from exercise than it is at rest. From Newsholme EA: A possible metabolic basis for the control of body weight. N Engl J Med 302:401, 1980. Reprinted by permission of the New England Journal of Medicine.

secretion apparently stimulates uncoupled respiration in brown adipose tissue[69] by altering the binding of guanidine diphosphate to mitochondrial protein.[70] As lean animals overeat their heat production increases and this enhanced heat produc-

tion (AT) continues after overfeeding stops, until the genetically lean animal returns to its normal weight. The obese animal exhibits less heat production both during and after overfeeding and hence, on an increased energy intake, experiences a significant and sustained gain in weight.

Although it is far more difficult to study subtle changes in thermogenesis in humans, lean men who overeat demonstrate increasing inefficiency (AT) as judged by the excess caloric intake required to gain weight.[71] Recent studies in lean and obese subjects have shown that obese subjects (per kilogram of fat free mass) expend less energy after a single meal[65] and after prolonged overfeeding.[72] It remains to be demonstrated that these differences are present in preobese persons to confirm that this greater efficiency is a factor in developing obesity and not just secondary to the obese state, as are so many other metabolic changes.[71] In addition to the thermic effect of food (TEF), nonshivering thermogenesis may also occur in response to exercise (TEE) and acclimation to cold (AT). Although obese mice show an impaired thermogenic response to cold,[47] such a defect has not yet been demonstrated in obese humans or in exercising humans.[65]

Another thermogenic mechanism shown to be defective in the obese mouse is the reduced sodium–potassium pump activity of their muscle[73] and liver[74] cells. Na$^+$/K$^+$ ATPase maintains normal intracellular–extracellular sodium and potassium gradients in all cells and has a key role in many cellular transport mechanisms. Since the sodium pump accounts for 20–50% of total cellular thermogenesis,[75] alterations in the activity of this enzyme could readily explain lean and obese differences of energy efficiency. In 1980 DeLuise et al[49] reported similar reduced Na$^+$/K$^+$ ATPase activity in the red cells of obese human subjects both before and after weight reduction. Such a defect, if it occurred generally in obese tissues, could account for a lower energy expenditure in obese subjects. Since this defect was not confirmed in hepatocytes of obese subjects,[50] the relevance of the red cell defect to overall energy balance is probably not significant. The fact that obese and lean subjects have similar RMR/kg of lean body tissue supports the fact that there are no major lean/obese differences in sodium pump activity in the resting state.

Catecholamines and thyroid hormone have an important role in modulating cellular thermogenesis. They in turn are controlled by the anterior and posterior nuclei of the hypothalamus[76] and thus ultimately the defect in obesity may reflect hypothalamic dysfunction or afferent mechanisms which adjust hypothalamic signals. Since the ventral and lateral nuclei of the hypothalamus[77] control eating behavior, it seems highly probable that the hypothalamus is the ultimate integrator of energy balance.

There are a number of different functions which have been shown to be abnormal in obese subjects which may reflect the putative hypothalamic dysfunction. Obese subjects may be more responsive to food-related external cues and less sensitive to internal cues of satiety.[28] Food intake in obese subjects may alter central neurotransmitters, such as serotonin and norepinephrine, differently than in lean subjects.[78] Recent studies have implicated cholecystokinin as a satiety factor and brain levels of cholecystokinin have been shown to be reduced in ob/ob mice.[79] Obese mice and rats have elevated concentrations of pituitary and plasma β-endorphin[80] and this may be related to eating, since the opiate antagonist naloxone depresses their feeding behavior.

It is well recognized that people with established obesity who lose a lot of weight, by dieting or from jaw wiring or a surgical bypass procedure, tend to regain all this weight if their diet lapses, their jaws are unwired, or their bypass procedure is reversed. Such persons return to a weight very close to their preintervention weight level, which strongly suggests a hypothalamic "set point" and some mechanism which informs the brain about the level of adipose stores.[81] Present evidence suggests this is a circulating factor: in experiments on parabiotic animals when one member of the pair is made obese, the other undereats and loses weight, suggesting that it is responding to a circulating signal indicating overweight.[82] The nature of this satiety factor is presently unknown. This message is probably not transmitted from adipocytes directly, because large fat cells transplanted into lean mice and normal fat cells transplanted into obese mice take on the characteristics of the recipient animal and not vice versa.[83]

In addition to these physiologic factors which seemingly control energy balance via their influence on the hypothalamus, supratentorial factors such as emotional stress and behavioral patterns may also affect hypothalamic function. Obese people frequently comment that they can exhibit effective weight control when they are emotionally sta-

ble but experience rapid weight gain when they are psychologically depressed. While this might reflect changes in food intake and physical activity, it could also reflect a supratentorial influence on the hypothalamic regulating system.

Physical Consequences of Obesity

Bray[84] collected data on 16 cases of very severe obesity (average maximum weight, 811 lb) and found their average age at death was 35 years. Thus obesity of this magnitude markedly affects longevity. VanItallie[1] analyzed statistics from the three largest studies linking excess mortality to weight (Fig. 1-2) and showed that mortality accelerates steeply once the subject is 40–50% overweight.[85-87] Obviously if morbid obesity is characterized as 100% overweight, the risk of premature death is substantial. It is likely that insurance statistics understate the true mortality of extremely overweight persons, because relatively

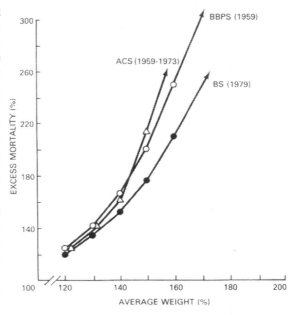

FIG. 1-2. The relationship between excess mortality and overweight. The segments of the lines beyond 140% of average weight in the case of the ACS study[86] and beyond 160% in the Build and Blood Pressure Study (BBPS)[87] and the Build Study (BS)[88] are extrapolations. From VanItallie TB: Morbid obesity: a hazardous disorder that resists conservative treatment. Am J Clin Nutr (Suppl) 33:359, 1980.

strict underwriting probably selects only the better risk cases. Drenick et al[88] studied mortality and morbidity in 200 morbidly obese men and showed the probability of dying is greatly affected by age. Thus morbidly obese men aged 25–34 have a 12-fold mortality excess, whereas morbidly obese men aged 65–74 have only a twofold increase over normal-weight men of the same age.

The principal causes of death in morbidly obese subjects are cardiovascular diseases, particularly strokes, and diabetes mellitus. As pointed out by Drenick et al,[88] very few morbidly obese subjects die as a direct consequence of their obesity—more commonly they die from degenerative diseases associated with being overweight (Table 1-7). In addition, treatment may be started late because obese patients appear reluctant to seek medical attention as a consequence of prior patient–physician frustration, and diagnosis may be delayed because of the clinical difficulty of examining the patient.

Hypertension is the commonest cardiovascular disease associated with obesity.[89] Indirect measurements with an inflatable cuff only reflect intraarterial blood pressure if a long cuff (42 cm) is used with a bladder that totally surrounds the arm. In a large study of 67,000 adults,[90] for every 10 kg increase in body weight, systolic pressure increased 3 mmHg and diastolic pressure increased 2 mmHg. Heyden et al,[91] in a prospective study of 3102 men, found that men who weighed more than 150 lb at age 20 and subsequently gained more than 30 lb had a stroke incidence of 90 per 1000, whereas those who weighed less than 150 lb at age 20 and subsequently gained less than 30 lb, there was a stroke incidence of 38 per 1000. In the Framingham study[92] obesity, independent of hypertension, was associated with angina pectoris and sudden death in young white males and with congestive heart failure in women. Apart from these situations obesity did not correlate strongly with coronary artery disease in the absence of hypertension and diabetes.

Increasing body weight and age are both associated with a rising frequency of diabetes mellitus. Only 1% of normal-weight women aged 25–44 have diabetes mellitus, but this increases to 7% in women of the same age who are 100% overweight.[93] Mortality from diabetes is highest in those populations that experience the greatest weight increase after age 25.[94] Obesity causes decreased binding of insulin to its receptors on target tissues which leads to hyperglycemia and greater insulin secretion. Administration of insulin to obese diabetics may further down regulate the number of insulin receptors exacerbating insulin resistance.

The main effect of obesity on pulmonary function is to reduce the expiratory reserve volume. In the Pickwickian syndrome, dyspnea, severe hypoventilation, and somnolence develop and patients appear to be insensitive to hypercarbia. Although the full-blown syndrome is quite rare, it is always unwise to prescribe sedatives for morbidly obese subjects, since this can precipitate respiratory failure. The Pickwickian syndrome has a mortality rate of about 30%.[95]

Gallbladder disease is three times commoner in obese men compared to lean men.[96] This probably reflects the increase in cholesterol synthesis in obese subjects, raising the lithogenic index.[97]

TABLE 1-7 Physical Consequences of Obesity

A. Cardiovascular
   Hypertension[90,92]
   Atherosclerotic heart disease in presence of ↑BP,
      ↑LDL, DM
   Cardiomegaly and congestive heart failure[93]
   Sudden death[93]
   Varicose veins and thromboembolism
B. Endocrine
   Diabetes mellitus,[94,95] adult onset, ↓insulin receptors, ↓postreceptor glucose metabolism, ↑glucose, hyperinsulinemia, ↑uric acid, cholesterol and triglycerides, ↑plasma amino acids (arg, leu, tyr, phe, val), ↑fasting glucagon, ↓growth hormone
   Virilization, hyperandrogenism probably reflect ↑ACTH, ↑cortisol and androgenic steroids from adrenals, ↑urinary 17-OHCS and 17-KS[99]
   Menstrual irregularities, amenorrhea and metrorrhagia
   Endometrial and breast cancer
   Complications of pregnancy: diabetes, hypertension, toxemia, thromboembolism
C. Respiratory
   Dyspnea
   Pickwickian syndrome,[96] alveolar hypoventilation
D. Gastrointestinal
   Cholelithiasis,[97,98] Fatty liver
   Colon cancer
E. Musculoskeletal
   Osteoarthritis
   Gout
F. Dermatologic
   Intertriginous dermatitis
   Venous stasis ulceration

The effect of obesity on endocrine function is well outlined in a recent review by Glass et al[98] and will be briefly summarized here. There is no evidence for any clinically significant abnormality of thyroid function in most obese subjects. Since T3 production is decreased by low carbohydrate diets, measuring thyroid hormone levels in an obese subject who is undergoing weight reduction can lead to a false diagnosis of hypothyroidism. Such individuals have a normal TSH, whereas true end-organ failure causes an elevated TSH.

Obese subjects have a slight increase in plasma ACTH, causing enhanced production of cortisol and an elevated urinary 17-OHCS, and also enhanced production of adrenal androgens and elevated urinary 17-KS. Plasma cortisol is readily suppressed by exogenous dexamethasone, which distinguishes obese patients from patients with Cushing's syndrome. Massively obese men have subnormal serum testosterone levels. This reflects a reduction in the binding protein; the free testosterone levels are usually normal. Some investigators have reported elevated estrogen production in obese males. This may reflect enhanced conversion of androgens to estrogens by adipose tissue. It has not been shown that increased estrogens cause feminization; however, studies of semen analysis in obese men are not available.

Obese women have an increased incidence of amenorrhea, but this is not due to primary ovarian failure and it is reversed by weight loss. This may reflect the hyperandrogenism seen in obese women from increased adrenal stimulation. The enhanced peripheral conversion of androgens to estrogens by adipose tissue may account for the greater incidence of endometrial carcinoma in obese women.

Growth hormone response to a variety of stimuli is blunted in obesity and these abnormalities are reversed by weight loss. Despite the low growth hormone levels, somatomedin levels are normal in obesity, perhaps as a result of the hyperinsulinemia. There is evidence for impaired release of prolactin in obese subjects and Kopelman et al[99] have shown that in some obese subjects this prolactin abnormality persists after weight reduction, confirming a possible primary hypothalamic defect in some forms of obesity.

Basal plasma parathyroid hormone levels are elevated in obese subjects and fall after weight reduction. Baseline plasma vasopressin levels are normal but water excretion after water loading is impaired. Plasma norepinephrine levels are elevated in obesity and the aldosterone increase after furosemide is exaggerated. These factors may contribute to the hypertension associated with obesity.

The Social Consequences of Obesity

The social and psychological consequences of obesity are often more important than the physical consequences, especially in young subjects. Richardson[100] and Goodman[101] showed that both lean and obese adults and children rate obese children as less likable than children with other physical deformities such as paraplegia, a missing hand, or a disfigured face. The explanation offered was usually that obese children are "responsible" for their plight.

Although there is no association between obesity and intelligence rating (IQ), Canning and Mayer[102] showed that obesity greatly affects educational opportunities, especially for women students. Of all female applicants to college, 92% of nonobese women are accepted whereas only 58% of obese women are accepted. The prejudice against obese male students is less severe. Interestingly, men who go to college tend to become fatter, whereas women who go to college tend to become thinner. Thin women move up the economic scale and fat women move down.[103] Obesity is six times more common in women of low socioeconomic status compared with high economic status.[104]

Employers are reluctant to hire fat people and overweight people are disproportionately represented in lower income brackets. Unemployment is very high among obese subjects. Although some of this discrimination may reflect the greater health hazards of employing obese subjects, probably the major factor is a deep societal prejudice against obesity. Drenick's[88] studies of mortality in morbidly obese subjects showed an increased risk of fatal accidents, indicating that morbid obesity can render people less alert and less mobile and therefore more vulnerable to unforeseen physical hazards.

Nonsurgical Treatment for Morbid Obesity

There are few reports on the long-term treatment of morbidly obese subjects by medical therapy and those studies which are available show discouraging results. This lack of medical success and the life-threatening consequences of morbid obesity are obviously the primary justifications for surgical treatment.

Drenick and Johnson[105] reported 7-year follow-up data on 121 morbidly obese men who underwent weight reduction by prolonged in-hospital fasting and subsequent semistarvation. Seventy-five percent of the men fasted for a month or longer and 25% continued for more than 2 months, achieving an average weight loss of 41.4 kg. Most of the weight-reduced men kept their weight off for 12–18 months and then gradually started to regain. After 7 years only seven of the 121 subjects remained at their reduced weight. The men who had been morbidly obese since childhood (hypercellularity) tolerated fasting the poorest and tended to regain lost weight most rapidly.

Blackburn[106] and Bistrian,[107] using a protein-sparing supplemented fast (1.5 g protein/kg of desirable weight), behavior modification techniques, and an exercise program, achieved an 18-kg (40-lb) weight reduction in 75% of their morbidly obese subjects. Two years later 30% of these reduced subjects (25% of the starting group) were maintaining their reduced weight. This study has not yet provided 5-year follow-up; however, it is worth noting that most of the successful patients retained physician contact, suggesting that this may be critical for any sustained medical success with morbidly obese subjects.

Kark reported on jaw wiring in 14 morbidly obese subjects.[108] After 4–20 months of maxillomandibular fixation, the average weight lost was 29.8 kg. Two years later 13 of the 14 subjects had regained all their lost weight. Because of these disappointing long-term results, Kark advised jaw wiring only for preoperative weight reduction of patients scheduled for more definitive bariatric surgery.

There may be a number of factors which account for the poor long-term results of medical management. The area which is currently receiving the greatest attention is the metabolic adaptive response of the hypothalamus; this adaptation apparently develops in any person who starves and reduces weight below the established "set point." The concept is that in every individual the hypothalamus has a set point for energy balance, above which energy conservation becomes increasingly *less* efficient and below which energy conservation becomes increasingly *more* efficient. This homeo-static mechanism accounts for the fact that most adults keep their weight remarkably constant, despite large swings in energy input and expenditure and an average intake, between 20 and 60 years, of some 40 tons of food!

Positive energy balance can increase fat cell number at any point in life,[109] although particularly, as mentioned earlier, during phases of maximal somatic growth in infancy and adolescence and to a lesser extent in pregnancy. Once formed, fat cells are apparently not lost even after years of sustained weight reduction,[110] and depleted fat cells or some circulating messenger which reflects their reduced energy stores appear to inform the hypothalamic control mechanism of their ongoing energy depletion. Thus while weight reduction may produce many medical benefits such as correction of high blood pressure and improved glucose tolerance, the weight-reduced subject, in regard to hypothalamic energy conservation, remains persistently abnormal. Hirsch (personal communication) has found that a reduced obese subject requires 30% fewer calories to maintain his weight, than the amount required for weight maintenance by normal subjects of similar weight. For subjects with hypercellular obesity this factor of conservation may be even greater than for subjects with hypertrophic obesity; this may explain the poorer medical results in early onset obese subjects.[111] These same adaptations are present in surgically weight-reduced subjects which may explain why few patients ever achieve their ideal weight, even after stringent food-curtailing surgical operations. It also explains weight regain if surgical procedures have to be reversed.

The most pertinent question for the future is to determine a possible means of resetting the hypothalamus and of inhibiting energy conservation mechanisms expressed by altered thyroid and catecholamine function. There is great interest in determining whether sustained physical training alters this biologic set point or whether pharmaceutical agents may be used for long-term manipulation of metabolic efficiency. It is intriguing that patients with cancer cachexia often fail to demonstrate the normal energy-conserving metabolic responses to starvation; thus a circulating substance may be discovered which can alter the hypothalamic set point. Until such a fundamental breakthrough is achieved, the best treatment for obesity is prevention. For established morbid obesity, surgery is currently the best guarantee of

TABLE 1-8   The Potential Benefits of Sustained Weight Reduction[112]

Improved glucose tolerance
Amelioration of hypertension
Amelioration of hyperlipidemia
Improved pulmonary function
Less stress on diseased weight-bearing joints
Improved self-esteem and social functioning
Possible prolongation of life

---

long-term weight reduction. The potential benefits of sustained weight reduction are listed in Table 1-8.

References

1. VanItallie TB: Morbid obesity: a hazardous disorder that resists conservative treatment. Am J Clin Nutr (Suppl) 33:358–363, 1980.
2. Howard LJ, Mendeloff AI: For whom is surgical treatment desirable and undesirable? Am J Clin Nutr (Suppl) 33:525–526, 1980.
3. Salans LB: The obesities. In Felig P, et al (eds): Endocrinology and Metabolism. New York: McGraw Hill, 1981, p. 891.
4. Strakova M, Markova J: Ultrasound used for measuring subcutaneous fat. Rev Czech Med 17:66–73, 1971.
5. Behnke AR: Anthropometric evaluation of body composition throughout life. Ann NY Acad Sci 110:45–464, 1963.
6. Lesser GT, Dentsch S, Markofsky J: Use of independent measurement of body fat to evaluate overweight and underweight. Metabolism 20: 792–804, 1971.
7. Cheek DB, Schultz RB, Pava A, Reba RC: Overgrowth of lean and adipose tissues in adolescent obesity. Pediatr Res 4:268–279, 1970.
8. Forbes GB, Lewis AM: Total sodium, potassium, and chloride in adult man. J Clin Invest 35:596–600, 1956.
9. Durnin JGVA, Womersley J: Body fat assessed from total body density and its estimation from skin fold thickness. Measurements on 481 men and women aged 16–72 years. Br J Nutr 32:77–97, 1974.
10. Parizkova J, Buzkova P: Relationship between skin fold thickness measured by Harpenden caliper and densitometric analysis of total body fat in men. Hum Biol 43:16–21, 1971.
11. Abraham S, Johnson CL: Prevalence of severe obesity in adults in the United States. Am J Clin Nutr (Suppl) 33:364–369, 1980.
12. Kissebah AH, Vydelingum N, Murray R, Evans D, Hartz A, Kalkhoff R, Adams P: Relation of body fat distribution to metabolic complications of obesity. J Clin Endocrinol Metab 54(2):254–260, 1982.
13. Keys A, Fidanza F, Karvonen MJ, Kimura N, Taylor HL: Indices of relative weight and obesity. J Chronic Dis 25:329–343, 1972.
14. Obesity in America. U.S. Department of Health, Education and Welfare. NIH Publication No. 79, 1979, p 359.
15. Roncari DAK, Lau DCW, Kindler S: Exaggerated replication in culture of adipocyte precursors from massively obese persons. Metabolism 30:425–427, 1981.
16. Charney E, Goodman HC, McBride M, Lyon B, Pratt R: Childhood antecedents of adult obesity. N Engl J Med 295:6–9, 1976.
17. Paulsen CA, Gordon DL, Carpenter RW, Ganoly HM, Drucker WD: Kleinfelter's syndrome and its variants: A hormonal and chromosomal study. Recent Prog Horm Res 24:321, 1968.
18. Inoue S, Bray GA, Mullen YS: Transplantation of pancreatic beta cells prevents development of hypothalamic obesity in rats. Am J Physiol 235:E266–E271, 1978.
19. Editorial: Metabolic obesity. Br Med J 282:172–173, 1981.
20. Sjostrom L: Fat cells and body weight. In Stunkard A (ed): Obesity. Philadelphia, Saunders, 1980, pp 72–100.
21. Hirsch J, Batchelor B: Adipose tissue cellularity in human obesity. Clin Endocrinol Metab 5:299–311, 1976.
22. Björntorp P: The fat cell: A clinical view. In Bray GA (ed): Recent Advances in Obesity Research: II. Westport, Ct., Technomic, 1979, pp. 153–168.
23. Levitsky A, Strupp B: Behavioral control of energy expenditure. In Gibbs L, James WPT, VanItallie T (eds): The Body Weight Regulatory System: Normal and Disturbed Mechanisms. New York, Raven Press, 1981, pp 125–135.
24. Forget P, Fernandes J, Begemann P: Plasma triglycerides clearing in obese children. Am J Clin Nutr 28:858–865, 1975.
25. James WPT, Trayhurn P, et al: Interactions of food intake and energy expenditure: An overview. In Gibbs L, James WPT, VanItallie T (eds): The Body Weight Regulatory System. Normal and Disturbed Mechanisms, New York, Raven Press, 1981, pp 147–152.
26. Schackter S: Obesity and eating: Internal and external cues differentially affect the eating behavior of obese and normal subjects. Science 161:751–756, 1968.
27. Herman CP, Polivy J: Anxiety, restraint, and eating behavior. J Abnorm Psychol 84(6):66–72, 1975.

28. Grinker J, et al: Taste sensitivity and susceptibility to external influence in obese and normal weight subjects. J Pers Soc Psychol 22:320, 1972.

29. Grossman SP: The biology of motivation. Ann Rev Psychol 30:209–242, 1979.

30. Bray GA, York DA: Hypothalamic and genetic obesity in experimental animals: An autonomic and endocrine hypothesis. Physiol Rev 59:719–809, 1979.

31. Grossman SP: Hypothalamic regulation: A re-evaluation. In Gibbs L, James WPT, VanItallie T (eds): The Body Weight Regulatory System. Normal and Disturbed Mechanisms, New York, Raven Press, 1981, pp 11–17.

32. Fabry, P, Tepperman J: Meal frequency—a possible factor in human pathology. Am J Clin Nutr 23:1059–1068, 1970.

33. Metzer HL, Lamphiear DE, Wheeler NC, Larkin IA: The relationships between frequency of eating and adiposity in adult men and women. The Tecumach Community Health Study. Am J Clin Nutr 30:712–715, 1977.

34. Flatt JP: Biochemistry of energy expenditure. In Bray GA (ed): Recent Advances in Obesity Research II. Westport, Ct., Technomic, 1979, p 211–229.

35. Pykalisto OJ, Smith PN, Brunzell JD: Determinants of human adipose tissue lipoprotein lipase: Effect of diabetes and obesity on basal and diet induced activity. J Clin Invest 56:1108–1117, 1975.

36. McCune SA, Durant PJ, et al: Comparative studies on fatty acid synthesis, glycogen metabolism, and gluconeogenesis by hepatocytes isolated from lean and obese Zucker rats. Metabolism 30:1170–1178, 1981.

37. Roncari DAK, Lan DCW, Kindler S: Exaggerated replication in culture of adipocyte precursors from massively obese persons. Metabolism 30:425–427, 1981.

38. Bogdade JD, Porte D, Bierman EL: The interaction of diabetes and obesity on the regulation of fat mobilization in man. Diabetes 18:759–772, 1969.

39. Arner P, Ostman J: Changes in the adrenergic control and the rate of lipolysis of isolated human adipose tissue during fasting and after re-feeding. Acta Med Scand 200:273–279, 1976.

40. Triscari J, Greenwood MRC, Sullivan AC: Oxidation and ketogenesis in hepatocytes of lean and obese Zucker Rats. Metabolism 31:223–228, 1982.

41. Jung RR, Shetty PS, James WPT, Barrand MA, Callingham BA: Reduced thermogenesis in obesity. Nature 279:322–323, 1979.

42. Rothwell NJ, Stock MJ: A role of brown adipose tissue in diet induced thermogenesis. Nature 281:31–35, 1979.

43. Trayburn P, Jones PM, McGucklin MM, Goodbody AE: Effects of overfeeding on energy balance and brown fat thermogenesis in (ob/ob) mice. Nature 295:323–325, 1982.

44. Perkins MN, Rothwell NJ, Stock MJ, Stone TW: Activation of brown adipose tissue thermogenesis by the ventromedial hypothalmus. Nature 289:401–402, 1981.

45. Rothwell NJ, Stock MJ: A role for insulin in the diet induced thermogenesis of cafeteria fed rats. Metabolism 30:673–678, 1981.

46. Thurlby PL, Trayhurn P: The role of thermoregulatory thermogenesis in the development of obesity in genetically obese (cb/cb) mice pair fed with lean siblings. Br J Nutr 42:377–385, 1979.

47. Stirling JL, Stock MJ: Non-conservative mechanisms of energy metabolism in thermogenesis. In Apfelbaum M (ed): Energy Balance in Man. Paris, Masson, 1972, p 219.

48. Newsholme EA: A possible metabolic basis for the control of body weight. N Engl J Med 302:400–405, 1980.

49. DeLuise M, Blackburn G, Flier JS: Reduced activity of the red cell sodium–potassium pump in human obesity. N Engl J Med 303:1017–1022, 1980.

50. Bray GA, Kral JG, Bjorntorp P: Hepatic sodium–potassium dependent ATPase in obesity. N Engl J Med 304:1580–1582, 1981.

51. Durnin JVGA: Body weight, body fat, and the activity factor in energy balance. In Apfelbaum M (ed): Energy Balance in Man. Paris, Masson, 1972, p 141.

52. Huenemann RL, Hampton MC, Shapiro LR, Behnke AR: Adolescent food practices associated with obesity. Fed Proc 25:4–10, 1966.

53. Griffiths M, Payne PR: Energy expenditure in small children of obese and nonobese parents. Nature 260:698–700, 1976.

54. Bowkin H: Obesity in children. J Pediatr 54:392–400, 1952.

55. Garn SH, Bailey SM, Cole PE: Similarities between parents and their adopted children. Am J Phys Anthropol 45:539, 1969.

56. Biron P, Mongeau I, Bertrand D: Familial resemblance of body weight and weight/height in 374 homes with adopted children. J Pediatr 91:555–558, 1977.

57. Ingalls AM, Dickie MM, Snell GD: Obese, new mutation in house mouse. J Heredity 41:317–318, 1950.

58. Assimacopoulos-Jeannet F, Jeanrenaud B: The hormonal and metabolic basis of experimental obesity. Clin Endocrinol Metab 5:474, 1976.

59. Bray GA, York DA: Genetically transmitted obesity in rodents. Physiol Rev 51:598, 1971.

60. Bray GA: Is corpulence catching? In Bjorntrop P, Cairella M, Howard AN (eds): Recent Advances in Obesity Research II. London, Libbey, 1981, pp 374–387.

61. Bullen BA, Reed RB, Mayer J: Physical activity of obese and nonobese adolescent girls appraised by motion picture sampling. Am J Clin Nutr 14:211–223, 1964.

62. Bray GA, Whipp BJ, Kayal SN, Wasserman K: Some respiratory and metabolic effects of exercise in moderately obese men. Metabolism 26:403–412, 1977.

63. Edholm OG, Adam JM, Healy MJR, Wolff HS, Goldsmith R, Best TW: Food intake and energy expenditure of army recruits. Br J Nutr 24:1091–1107, 1970.

64. James WPJ, Davies HL, Bailes J, Dauncey MJ: Elevated metabolic rates in obesity. Lancet 1:1122–1125, 1978.

65. Katzeff H, Danforth E: Norepinephrine sensitivity and energy expenditure in response to overnutrition in lean and obese men. Clin Res 30:245A, 1982.

66. Welle S, Lilavivat V, Campbell KG: Thermic effect of feeding in man: Increased plasma norepinephrine levels following glucose but not protein or fat consumption. Metabolism 30:953–958, 1981.

67. Himms-Hagen J: Cellular thermogenesis. Ann Rev Physiol 38:315–351, 1976.

68. Rappaport E, Young J, Landsberg L: Initiation, duration, and dissipation of diet induced changes in sympathetic nervous system activity in the rat. Metabolism 31:143–146, 1982.

69. Brooks SL, Rothwell NJ, Stock MJ, Goodbody AE, Trayburn P: Increased protein conductance pathway in brown adipose tissue mitochondria of rats exhibiting diet induced thermogenesis. Nature 286:274–276, 1980.

70. Lin CS, Klingenberg M: Isolation of the uncoupling protein from brown adipose tissue mitochondria. FEBS Lett 113:299–303, 1980.

71. Sims EAH, Danforth E, Horton ES, Bray GA, Glennon JA, Salans LB: Endocrine and metabolic effects of experimental obesity in man. Rec Prog Hormone Res 29:457–495, 1973.

72. Daniels RJ, Katzeff HL, Ravussin E, Garrow JS, Danforth E: Obesity in the Pima Indians: Is there a thrifty gene? Clin Res 30:244A, 1982.

73. Lin MH, Romsos DR, Akera T, Leveille GA: Na⁺-K⁺ ATPase enzyme units in skeletal muscle from lean and obese mice. Biochem Biophys Res Commun 80:398–404, 1978.

74. York DA, Bray GA, Yukimura Y: An enzymatic defect in the obese (ob/ob) mouse: loss of thyroid induced sodium- and potassium-dependent adenosine triphosphatase. Proc Natl Acad Sci 75:477–481, 1978.

75. Whittam R, Blond DM: Respiratory control by an adenosine triphosphatase involved in active transport in brain cortex. Biochem 92:147–158, 1965.

76. Reuler JB: Hypothermia: Pathophysiology, clinical setting, and management. Ann Intern Med 89:519–527, 1978.

77. Pauskepp J: Hypothalamic regulation of energy balance and feeding behavior. Fed Proc 33:1150–1165, 1974.

78. Wurtman J, Wurtman RJ, Growdon JH, Henry P, Lipscomb A, Zeisel SH: Carbohydrate craving in obese people: Suppression by treatments affecting serotoninergic transmission. T Int J Eating Disorders 1:2–15, 1981.

79. Straus E, Yalow RS: Cholecystokinin in the brains of obese and nonobese mice. Science 203:68–69, 1979.

80. Margules DL, Moisset B, Lewis MJ, Shibuya H, Pert C: β-Endorphin is associated with overeating in genetically obese mice (ob/ob) and rats (fa/fa). Science 202:988–991, 1978.

81. Woods SC, Smith PH, Porte D: The role of the nervous system in metabolic regulation and its effects on diabetes and obesity. In Brownlee M (ed): Handbook of Diabetes Mellitus, Vol. 3. New York, Garland STPM Press, 1982, Chap 5.

82. Fleming DG: Food intake studies in parabiotic rats. Ann NY Acad Sci 157:985–1002, 1969.

83. Meade CJ, Shwell MA, Sawter C: Is genetically transmitted obesity due to an adipose tissue defect? Proc R Soc Lond 205:395–410, 1979.

84. Bray GA: The Obese Patient. Philadelphia, Saunders, 1976, pp 1,219.

85. Society of Actuaries Build and Blood Pressure Study, Vol. 1, Chicago, 1959, p 1957.

86. Lew EA, Garfinkel L: Variations in mortality by weight among 750,000 men and women. J Chronic Dis 32:563–576, 1979.

87. Society of Actuaries and Association of Life Insurance Medical Directors Build Study. Chicago, 1979.

88. Drenick EJ, Bale GS, Seltzer F, Johnson DG: Excessive mortality and causes of death in morbidly obese men. JAMA 243:443–445, 1980.

89. Chiang BN, Perlman LV, Epstein FH: Overweight and hypertension, a review. Circulation 39:403–421, 1969.

90. Bjerkedal T: Overweight and hypertension. Acta Med Scand 159:13–26, 1957.

91. Heyden S, Hames CG, Bartel A, Cassel JC, Tyroler HA, Cornoni JC: Weight and weight history

in relation to cerebrovascular and ischemic heart disease. Arch Intern Med 128:956–960, 1971.

92. Kannel WB, Gordon T: Obesity and cardiovascular disease: In Burland W, et al (eds): The Framingham Study in "Obesity." London, Churchill Livingstone, 1974.

93. Rimui AA, Werner LH, Bernstein R, vanYserloo B: Disease and obesity in 73,532 women. Obesity Bariatric Med 1:77–84, 1972.

94. Hundley JM: Diabetes, overweight: U.S. problems. J Am Dietetic Assoc 32:417–422, 1956.

95. McGregor MI, Block AJ, Ball WC Jr: Topics in clinical medicine. Serious complications and sudden death in the pickwickian syndrome. Bull Johns Hopkins Hosp 126:279–295, 1970.

96. Sturdevant RAL, Pearce ML, Dayton S: Increased prevalance of cholelithiasis in men ingesting a serum cholesterol lowering diet. N Engl J Med 288:24–27, 1973.

97. Grundy SM: Effects of unsaturated fats in hypertriglyceridemia (type IV). Clin Res 22:469A, 1974.

98. Glass AR, Burman KD, Dahms WT, Boehm TM: Endocrine function in human obesity. Metabolism 30:89–104, 1981.

99. Kopelman PG, White N, Pilkington TRE: Impaired hypothalamic control of prolactin secretion in massive obesity. Lancet 1:747–750, 1974.

100. Richardson SA, Hastorf AH, Goodman N, Dornbusch SM: Cultural uniformity in reaction to physical disabilities. Ann Sociol Rev 26:241–247, 1961.

101. Goodman N, Richardson SA, Dornbusch SM, Hastorf AH: Variant reactions to physical disabilities. Am Sociol Rev 28:429–435, 1963.

102. Canning H, Mayer J: Obesity—its possible effect on college acceptance. N Engl J Med 275:1172–1174, 1966.

103. Elder GH Jr: Appearance and education in marriage mobility. Ann Sociol Rev 34:519–533, 1969.

104. Stunkard A, D'Aquili E, Fox S, Filion RDL: Influence of social class on obesity and thinness in children. JAMA 221:579–584, 1972.

105. Drenick EJ, Johnson D: Weight reduction by fasting and semistarvation in morbid obesity longterm follow-up. In Bray GA (ed): Obesity: Comparative Methods of Weight Control. Westport, Ct., Technomic, 1980, Chap 3.

106. Blackburn GL, Greenberg I: Multidisciplinary approach to adult obesity therapy. In Bray GA (ed): Obesity: Comparative Methods of Weight Control. Technomic, 1980, Chap 4.

107. Bristrian BR, Sherman M: Results of the treatment of obesity with a protein-sparing modified fast. In Bray GA (ed): Obesity: Comparative Methods of Weight Control. Technomic, 1980, Chap 5.

108. Kark AE: Jaw wiring. Am J Clin Nutr (Suppl) 33:420–424, 1980.

109. Faust I, Johnson P, Stern J, Hirsch J: Diet-induced adipocyte number increase in adult rats: A new model of obesity. Am J Physiol 235(3):E279–E286, 1978.

110. Bjorntorp P, Carlgren G, Isaksson B, et al: Effect of an energy-reduced dietary regimen in relation to adipose tissue cellularity in obese women. Am J Clin Nutr 28:445–452, 1975.

111. Krotkiewski M, Larsson B, Sjostrom L, Bjorntorp P: Adipose tissue cellularity in relation to prognosis for weight reduction. Int J Obesity 1:395–416, 1977.

112. Mancini M, Contaldo F, Mattoli P, Caprio S, Postiglione A, Rivellese A: Metabolic abnormalities associated with obesity: Effect of weight loss. In Enzi G, Crepaldi G, Pozza G (eds): Obesity: Pathogenesis and Treatment, New York, Academic Press, 1981.

CHAPTER 2

Psychiatric Considerations

DEANE C. MANOLIS

This chapter will describe the rationale for including the psychiatrist in the multidisciplinary team involved in the surgical treatment of obesity and define the role of the psychiatrist as a member of that team.

The prevalence of significant psychopathology in the morbidly obese will be reviewed, and post-surgical psychological adaptation and psychiatric morbidity will be discussed. Methods of assessment will also be reviewed, as will psychiatric contraindications to surgical treatment. Finally, the role of the psychiatrist in preoperative assessment and perioperative management of patients who have incipient or frank psychiatric disorders will be discussed.

Psychopathology in the Morbidly Obese

The association between obesity and psychological disturbance has long been assumed. The early psychoanalysts developed elaborate explanations for obesity, using startling labels such as "oral-aggressive character." Weight changes are commonly seen in depressive disorders, and it has been assumed by many that depression is common among the obese. Numerous early studies in the literature attempted to link obesity and psychological disorder, but the more careful the study, the less evidence for such an association was apparent.[1]

Over the past 10 years, a number of reports of careful preoperative psychological screening of morbidly obese patients have appeared in the literature.[2-8] It is impossible to make direct comparisons between these studies due to differences in assessment techniques and definition of psychopathology, and also to the fact that no control groups were utilized. The overall impression was that the prevalence of major psychopathology was low. Halmi et al[7] utilized the strictly defined diagnostic criteria of the new *Diagnostic and Statistical Manual III* (*DSM-III*) for psychiatric diagnosis. They found a 50% prevalence of *lifetime* psychiatric diagnosis in this retrospective study of 80 morbidly obese patients. There was no clustering except in the diagnosis of depressive disorder, which occurred in 29%. The investigators compared this to a standard control population from a study with similar diagnostic criteria, in which there was a 25% prevalence of lifetime depressive disorder. The difference in the two populations was thought not to be statistically significant.

Literature studies have shown milder personality trait and pattern disturbances to occur commonly, however. Passive-dependent and passive-aggressive personality styles are frequent,[11] along with disturbance of body image[2] and ideas of reference,[13] both of which are *realistic* in the morbidly obese.

Despite the above comments, there are some morbidly obese individuals to whom the surgeon must be alert, as for example, several small populations in whom emotional disorder and obesity are clearly related. These deserve careful psychiatric evaluation. Stunkard[1] points out that in young women of upper or middle socioeconomic status who are both obese and neurotic, there is a high likelihood that the disorders are related. (Both occur with much less frequency in upper compared to lower socioeconomic groups; thus when seen together, a relationship is likely.) Stunkard goes on to describe two examples of this phenomenon. The first includes "neurotic overeating" consisting of either nocturnal hyperphagia with insomnia or bulimia—sudden, episodic binge eating. The second includes those with *severe* neurotic distortion of body image—which goes much beyond the realistic negative perception of obesity.

It appears that the prevalence of major psychopathology in the morbidly obese is not much different from that in the general population. There does appear to be considerable minor distress in the so-called "obese personality"—anxiety, depression, disturbed body image, and low self-esteem—which may well be a result rather than a cause of obesity.[2,5]

Postsurgical Psychological Adaptation

In the early years of surgery for the morbidly obese there was considerable concern that rapid weight loss would deprive these individuals of a psychological defense, and that significant psychological disturbance would ensue. This concern was drawn from the observation of considerable psychological morbidity associated with dieting and weight loss.[9] Surgical experience and research studies have shown on the contrary that there is generally a low incidence of psychological complications following both jejunoileal bypass (JIB) and gastric bypass (GBP) procedures.[5-8,10-14]

Although differences in assessment techniques again make direct comparisons difficult, several salient findings are noteworthy. Several groups reported that patients with psychological impairment prior to surgery have no higher incidence of postoperative psychological complications than those viewed as well adjusted or "normal."[2,6,8] Halmi et al[7] who noted 23 of 80 patients with a lifetime diagnosis of depressive disorder, found none experienced the *onset* of their depression after GBP surgery. The question of whether postoperative physical complications or effects of surgery such as chronic diarrhea add to the incidence of psychological complications is unclear. There is a general sense that the struggle with physical complications can be emotionally draining,[11] but Kuldau and Rand found no direct correlation between physical and psychological complications, suggesting that most psychopathology in the postoperative period is environmentally determined.[13] Re-

searchers are cautioned about the "dropouts" who are unavailable and thus not counted in follow-up studies, with the suggestion that this group may represent treatment failures.[15] However, Leon et al[5] made a concentrated effort to contact dropouts, and even with these additions, found that only 12.5% of their study group reported severe psychological problems.

Despite the overall positive response during the weight loss period, most patients reported emotional lability with rapid mood fluctuation and irritability.[11] This was nowhere near the intensity seen with rigorous dieting, however.[12] Additionally, many patients noted much diminished eating behavior formerly associated with strong pleasant or unpleasant emotion.[1]

Reports suggesting an adverse effect on marital and sexual adjustment in the JIB postoperative period are exemplified by Neill et al in a small retrospective study.[16] However, a larger prospective controlled study[14] suggested a higher prevalence of dysfunctional marriage in the morbidly obese *before* surgery. There was a higher incidence of divorce postoperatively, but these were in marriages previously identified as dysfunctional.

There has been some speculation[6] that the GBP procedures may have a lower incidence of postoperative psychological disorder than the JIB procedures, but most of the reports in the literature are follow-ups of the JIB. There have been only two groups[6,12] reporting on the GBP procedures, both of which show that the incidence of psychological disturbance is similar to that of the JIB.

Psychological Assessment

Although the incidence of psychiatric disorder following obesity surgery is low, some surgeons believe that psychological evaluation is indicated prior to surgery.[8] The purpose for this screening is not only to rule out the rare individual for whom surgery is contraindicated, but also to identify those individuals who may need psychiatric attention in the perioperative and follow-up periods.

The literature describes multiple assessment techniques, from simple semistructured interviews, to a complex series of psychological tests and clinical interviews. Detailed assessment is necessary for research purposes, but impractical and expensive in clinical practice. Kuldau and Rand[13] note that a structured psychiatric interview using strict definitions (their "present state examination") is much more accurate in determining the significance of psychological symptoms, than self-rating paper and pencil scales which tend to overreport. On the other hand, the MMPI (described below), a true-false self-administered psychological test instrument, has been widely used and accepted as a screening device in this, as well as other medical settings.

In our institution, a screening technique has evolved that relies heavily on the MMPI (Minnesota Multiphasic Personality Inventory). This psychological test has been in use for over 40 years and has been validated repeatedly. The test has three scales that measure test-taking attitude as well as ten clinical scales measuring various personality characteristics. When interpreted by a competent psychologist, the test is a valid measure of an individual's psychological functioning. (A word of caution—various short forms of the MMPI are available which are not satisfactory substitutes for the standard forms; these short forms tend to overreport psychopathology.[17])

After initial evaluation by the surgeon, every bypass candidate with a history that suggests significant psychopathology is referred for administration of an MMPI. If this is normal, no further psychological assessment is done. If the MMPI is abnormal, further psychiatric evaluation is conducted. Psychiatric consultants utilized for this purpose are thoroughly familiar with the surgical procedure anticipated and its potential complications. (The expected results of the consultation will be outlined below.) Thus it is vital for the psychiatric consultant to have a firm medical orientation and to maintain close communication with the surgeon. If the patient has had previous psychological or psychiatric treatment, or is receiving current treatment, information is requested from the treatment source. Usually, the surgeon's psychiatric consultant will also see the patient as he knows more specifically what is needed in the assessment and subsequent therapy.

Certain patients in Minnesota require a prescribed structured assessment. These are individuals receiving medical care paid under several governmental programs. Because of some complications with early JIB procedures, the Minnesota Department of Public Welfare has required that all welfare patients have a careful medical/psychiatric evaluation, the results to be reviewed by a statewide screening committee. Based on these data, approval for surgery is determined. Thus each welfare patient must have an MMPI and a psychiatric consultation as minimum psychological data. This State Welfare Department requirement has not been accepted favorably by all surgeons, and the implication that the incidence of psychopathology is higher in the lower socioeconomic population is resented by some welfare recipients.

Psychiatric Contraindications

Experience has shown that there are few psychiatric contraindications for obesity surgery. In a long University of Minnesota series, only five of 850 surgical candidates were excluded for psychiatric reasons.[5] Other studies previously cited in this chapter have little to say about contraindications.

Rigden and Hagen[10] attempted to rank their series of 20 patients into "ideal," "intermediate," and "suboptimal" groups. The eight suboptimal criteria consisted of demographic and personality characteristics that tended to be vague and nonspecific. Kuldau and Rand[8] identified "active psychosis, alcoholism, and an obvious inability to comply with therapy" as the only psychiatric contraindications to surgery.

The authors would like to propose a three-level division as a way of conceptualizing psychiatric contraindications. These levels—(1) absolute contraindications, (2) relative contraindications, and (3) "red flags"—are not rigid; i.e., a patient may move from one level to another at different intervals, with appropriate psychiatric treatment. Thus a patient at the "absolute contraindication" level with an active psychosis or severe alcoholism might eventually drop to the "red flag" level with appropriate psychiatric or alcoholism treatment. With this concept in mind, we will now review the various contraindications gleaned from our experience.

Absolute Contraindications

1. *Active psychosis.* Psychosis is an obvious contraindication for any type of elective surgery. Both schizophrenia and bipolar-affective disorder (manic-depressive psychosis) are treatable with psychotropic medication and appropriate psychiatric management. When compensated and with continuing psychiatric

care, some of these patients can tolerate a bypass procedure.

2. *Alcoholism.* A patient actively drinking is incapable of cooperating with postsurgical follow-up. However, a medically cleared "arrested" alcoholic who has participated in an alcohol treatment program and/or is active in Alcoholics Anonymous could likely handle the stress of bypass surgery. Of importance here, however, is the need to assess for alcoholism *carefully* because of the high level of denial typical of this disorder.

3. *Severe paranoid disorder.* Paranoia is included at this level because this mental disorder can often be fixed and relatively untreatable. There may be a history of poor compliance with medical treatment, with hostility and paranoid ideas about physicians, whose actions in medical treatment may be misinterpreted as assaultive. There may be delusional expectations of surgical procedures. Additionally, these people are frequently litigious.

4. *Mental retardation.* Extreme retardation prevents surgical consent from being a truly informed consent. Retardation of this degree should be obvious.

5. *Personality or behavior disorder.* Here are included people with markedly impulsive behavior, sociopathic behavior, or with severe drug and/or alcohol abuse. Such disorders usually prevent compliance with the postoperative treatment plan.

Relative Contraindications

1. *Active depression or recent significant life stress.* These conditions require adequate psychiatric evaluation and treatment with delay of surgery until the mood disorder is stabilized or the life stress resolved. We have treated a number of these people with no significant psychiatric sequelae.

2. *Ambivalence.* Candidates for surgery who are uncertain or who appear to have made an impulsive decision about surgery (impulsive decisions are often a "solution" to ambivalence) should be given the benefit of time in the evaluation process. This is one of the advantages of a multidisciplinary evaluation, as some people will self-select out before they complete the evaluation process.

3. *Unrealistic expectations.* Such expectations may be mildly inappropriate to bordering on delusional. This type of patient would benefit from a temporizing approach in the evaluation process until the misconceptions can be corrected, or psychiatric treatment can be instituted. In this group may also be those who expect no change in their postoperative eating pattern, and who thus may potentially be able to "defeat" the gastric bypass procedure.

4. *"Neurotic obesity."* This group includes those people described earlier with neurotic eating disorders—nocturnal hyperphagia and bulimia. Also included are patients with adult-onset obesity related to a specific life stress. Surgery should not be contemplated in these groups unless vigorous attempts at treatment with psychotherapy or behavioral therapy have failed.

5. *Hysterical personality with hostility toward men.* We have retrospectively identified a small group of women with the above personality characteristics. These women had a history of marked ambivalence and fear in their relationships with men. They developed an ambivalent relationship with their surgeon and had a stormy postoperative course, marked by various psychosomatic and depressive symptoms. We speculate that surgery may have represented a psychological and bodily assault to these women. Close psychiatric evaluation is indicated with psychotherapy the treatment of choice.

6. *History of severe functional gastrointestinal disorder.* Persons who report multiple evaluations for gastrointestinal symptoms, especially nausea and vomiting, or who report gastrointestinal symptoms under stress, are prone to difficult management in the postoperative period. Careful assessment, by both a psychiatrist and a gastroenterologist, is in order before proceeding with surgery.

7. *Borderline intelligence.* Occasionally a surgical candidate may appear to have adequate intellectual functioning, but on close evaluation may have difficulty understanding the nature and expectations of the procedure. Intelligence testing may be necessary, with careful explanations to ensure informed consent. Signed consent by a relative may also be appropriate.

"Red Flags"

These criteria serve to raise the index of suspicion about more serious psychological disturbance.

1. *Abnormal MMPI with negative psychiatric history.* Psychiatric consultation is suggested.
2. *Denial of psychiatric history.* We have seen a few individuals who have flatly denied significant psychiatric history, apparently in order to obtain approval for surgery. A true history was elicited from other sources or not discovered until the postoperative period. One such patient had a stormy (months long) postoperative hospital course.
3. *Upper class women with concurrent neurotic disorder.* As described earlier, these patients may well have a "neurotic obesity" disorder and may need psychotherapy rather than surgery.
4. *History of complicated postoperative course with previous surgery.* Several of these patients have been found to have significant psychosomatic disorders with a need for combined medical–psychiatric management.
5. *History of chronic psychosis or recurrent depression.* These patients may be able to do quite well with surgery, but psychiatric management will be necessary.

As can be seen, the number of truly absolute contraindications for bypass surgery is small. We have included these numerous criteria as an aid to the surgeon, hoping to minimize psychiatric morbidity and thus helping to ensure a better postoperative course.

Role of the Psychiatrist

The foregoing has established the rationale for the psychiatrist's involvement in the surgical treatment of obesity. It is apparent that psychiatric evaluation is unnecessary in most cases, but there are some situations in which the psychiatrist's input can be extremely valuable to the surgeon. The nature of the psychiatrist's role has been given little attention in the literature; only Kuldau and Rand[8] attempt to define it, and they focus primarily on the consultation–assessment process. In our experience, the psychiatrist's role is twofold, with the second aspect being collaborative patient management with the surgeon at various stages of the surgical treatment.

In the assessment role, the psychiatrist acts as any other medical consultant, providing expert opinion after examination of the patient. The psychiatrist will be expected to perform a standard psychiatric interview with psychiatric history, psychosocial history, and mental status examination leading to a personality formulation and an estimate of current state of personality functioning. The surgeon must expect more of this particular type of assessment, however. The psychiatrist will need to differentiate the expected distress associated with marked obesity from more specific psychiatric disorders,[8] and must be alert to the potential contraindications for surgery discussed earlier. The psychiatrist also should assess the patient's motivation and level of ambivalence, and determine whether he has unrealistic or magical expectations of surgery. It is also vital for the psychiatrist to check the patient's understanding of the procedure and to clarify any misconceptions. From the interview, the psychiatrist should be able to document the patient's understanding of risks and benefits of the procedure and state whether the patient is capable of informed consent. If there is any question regarding the patient's suitability for surgery the psychiatrist is in a position to slow down the preoperative evaluation process to obtain more detailed psychological testing, to see the patient again, or to discuss the assessment in detail with the surgeon.

The second aspect of the psychiatrist's role—collaborative case management—may begin with the consultation or at any other point in the pre- or postoperative period. At times several preoperative psychiatric contacts will suffice, whereas on other occasions treatment over a number of months may be necessary. If a treating relationship has been established preoperatively, we have found it quite useful for psychiatric contact to continue in the hospital setting. The psychiatrist may also be needed for postoperative consultation or management for patients not seen in the assessment phase. Psychiatric management in the hospital may be helpful in minimizing or preventing psychiatric morbidity. An experienced "liaison psychiatrist" may work with the patient, the patient's family, the nursing staff, and other physicians in the hospital context. The psychiatrist should be able to continue collaborative management of these patients for as long as necessary.

With the above expectations of the psychiatric consultant, the surgeon will need to choose a consultant with some thought. Many psychiatrists do no hospital work and thus may not be experienced in, nor comfortable with, the concept of liaison psychiatry. The trend toward a more medically oriented psychiatry suggests that an appropriate consultant should be available in most locales, however. The surgeon must be explicit regarding expectations of the psychiatrist and the latter must become familiar with the medical, surgical, and psychiatric aspects of obesity surgery. Surgeons and psychiatrists must maintain good communication in both the consultative and collaborative phases of patient care.

Summary

Review of the prevalence of psychopathology in the morbidly obese shows little difference from the general population. Surgery for morbid obesity does not elicit a high incidence of psychological complications. Some do occur, however, and a few can be potentially serious, emphasizing the need for preoperative screening criteria to exclude a small number of poor risk surgical candidates, and to utilize psychiatric treatment, both pre- and postoperatively, when indicated. The medically oriented psychiatrist, familiar with morbid obesity and its surgical treatment, has an important role in presurgical assessment and collaborative medical management of this disorder.

References

1. Stunkard A: Obesity. In Kaplan H, Freedman A, Sadock B (eds): Comprehensive Textbook of Psychiatry III. Baltimore, Williams & Wilkins, 1980, pp 1872–1882.
2. Solow C, Silberfarb P, Swift K: Psychosocial effects of intestinal bypass surgery for severe obesity. N Engl J Med 290:300–304, 1974.
3. Castelnuovo-Tedesco P, Schiebel D: Studies of superobesity. I. Psychological characteristics of superobese patients. Int J Psychiat Med 6:465–480, 1975.
4. Castelnuovo-Tedesco P, Schiebel D: Studies of superobesity. II. Psychiatric appraisal of jejuno-ileal bypass surgery. Am J Psychiat 133:26–31, 1976.
5. Leon G, Eckert E, Teed D, Buchwald H: Changes in body image and other psychological factors after intestinal bypass surgery for massive obesity. J Behav Med 2:39–55, 1979.
6. Saltzstein E, Gutmann M: Gastric bypass for morbid obesity. Arch Surg 115:21–28, 1980.
7. Halmi K, Long M, Stunkard A, Mason E: Psychiatric diagnosis of morbidly obese gastric bypass patients. Am J Psychiat 137:470–472, 1980.
8. Kuldau J, Rand C: Jejuno-ileal bypass: General and psychiatric outcome after one year. Psychosomatics 21:534–539, 1980.
9. Gluckman M, Hirsch J: The response of obese patients to weight reduction: Clinical evaluation of behavior. Psychosom Med 30:1–11, 1968.
10. Rigden S, Hagen D: Psychiatric aspects of intestinal bypass surgery for obesity. Am Fam Physician 13:68–71, 1976.
11. Castelnuovo-Tedesco P: Jejuno-ileal bypass for superobesity. Adv Psychosom Med 10:196–206, 1980.
12. Halmi K, Stunkard A, Mason E: Emotional responses to weight reduction by three methods: gastric bypass, jejuno-ileal bypass, diet. Am J Clin Nutr 33:446–451, 1980.
13. Kuldau J, Rand C: Negative psychiatric sequelae to jejuno-ileal bypass are often not correlated with operative results. Am J Clin Nutr 33:502–503, 1980.
14. Rand C, Kuldau J, Robbins L: Surgery for obesity and marriage quality. JAMA 247:1419–1422, 1982.
15. Reed M: Medical news. JAMA 248:277–278, 1982.
16. Neill J, Marshall J, Yale C: Marital changes after intestinal bypass surgery. JAMA 240:447–450, 1978.
17. Newmark C: Brief synopsis of the utility of MMPI short forms. J Clin Psychol 37:136–137, 1981.

CHAPTER 3

Malabsorption Techniques

JOHN H. LINNER

Jejunoileal Bypass

In our first jejunoileal bypass (JIB) of 1954 (described in the preface) we were uncertain what the optimal lengths of the functioning bowel should be. We erred on the conservative side, making them longer than lengths which subsequently proved to be effective. Ninety cm of jejunum were anastomosed to 45 cm of ileum, and the distal end of the bypassed small intestine was anastomosed to the transverse colon.[1,2] In 1971, the patient's JIB was revised by shortening the functioning jejunum to 40 cm, and the ileum to 15 cm. Her weight then decreased from 240 lb to 171 lb, and leveled off in a few years at 190 lb. Although she was happy about her weight loss and increased mobility, she required intermittent supplementation with magnesium, calcium, and potassium. In addition, during the last year of her life she developed angina pectoris and electrocardiographic evidence of coronary insufficiency despite a low serum cholesterol (60 to 120 mg%) and a normal serum triglyceride. She died in 1981 of a myocardial infarction at the age of 61 years.

Payne et al[3] coined the term "malnutritional morbid obesity" to apply to the grossly obese patient, and provided the first extensive clinical studies in this field. From 1956 to 1966 they performed 13 jejunocolic bypass operations designed to be taken down when optimal weight loss had been achieved. The jejunocolic shunt resulted in "metabolic disasters," and when intestinal continuity was restored these patients regained all their weight. This method was then discontinued. From 1962 to 1966 these investigators performed a variety of end-to-side jejunoileostomies until they arrived at what they considered to be the ideal proportionate lengths of jejunum and ileum—35 cm (14 in) of proximal jejunum anastomosed to the side of the terminal ileum, 10 cm (4 in) from the cecum. Measurements were made along the stretched mesenteric border. Payne and DeWind added a minor modification in 1977, suturing the functional jejunum to the defunctional ileum for a distance of 15 cm, thus forming an acute angulation designed to inhibit reflux into the defunctional ileum (Figs. 3-1 and 3-2).[4]

Scott[5,6] attributed the poor weight loss in 11 of his patients with the Payne end-to-side procedure to reflux and therefore adopted the end-to-end JIB, anastomosing the distal end of the defunctional bowel to either the sigmoid or the transverse colon. He used three variations of the end-to-end operation: 30 cm of jejunum to 30 cm of ileum, 30 cm of ileum to 15 cm of ileum, and 30 cm of jejunum to 20 cm of ileum. In general the best and most sustained weight loss occurred with the short (45 cm) end-to-end functional lengths. This length was recommended for patients over 350 lb in weight and the 50-cm length for patients less than 350 lb (Fig. 3-3).

Buchwald[7] in a large series of obesity operations used one configuration that proved effective—40 cm of jejunum to 4 cm of ileum, end-to-end—with the distal defunctional limb anastomosed to the cecum.

Baddeley[8] in a randomized 5-year study of JIB compared the end-to-end with the end-to-side type, using the same lengths in both: 35 cm of jejunum and 10 cm of ileum. He reported that there was no statistical difference in weight loss or morbidity between the two groups. Following another study

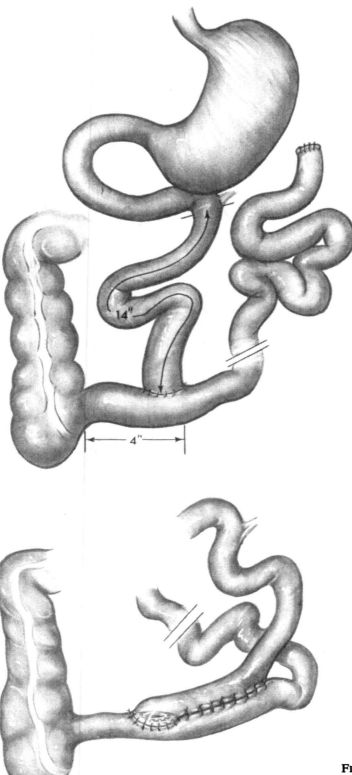

FIG. 3-1. Payne–DeWind end-to-side jejunoileal bypass (35 cm jejunum to 10 cm ileum).

14"

4"

FIG. 3-2. Payne–DeWind end-to-side JIB with an acute angulation, 15 cm in length, to inhibit reflux.

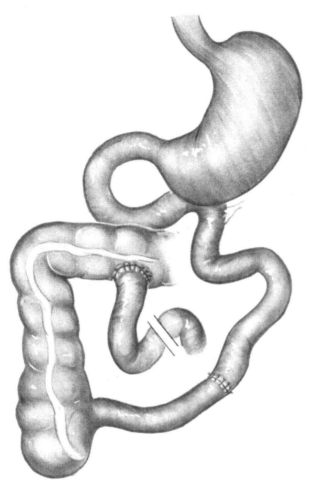

FIG. 3-3. Scott end-to-end JIB with defunctional bowel anastomosed to transverse colon. Sigmoid colon also used.

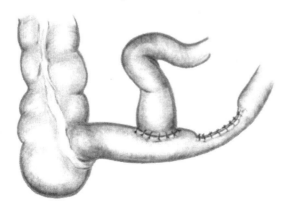

FIG. 3-4. End-to-side JIB with antireflux enteroplasty, 6 cm in length. The defunctional lumen is narrowed by approximately 50% to inhibit reflux.

in which the relative lengths of jejunum and ileum were varied, he found no difference in effectiveness or morbidity until the combined lengths either exceeded 50 cm or were less than 45 cm. With lengths greater than 50 cm, weight loss proved to be unsatisfactory, and with those shorter than 45 cm the incidence of protein malnutrition rose sharply. Based on this evidence, he recommended the use of 30 cm of jejunum anastomosed end-to-side to the ileum 20 cm from the cecum.

There have been many other contributors to this field, but space does not permit presenting their findings.[9-14]

From 1968 to 1976, 173 JIB operations were done by the author (Table 3-1). There were 14 patients who had an end-to-side (35 cm to 10 cm) operation (Fig. 3-1), 35 patients with the same operation plus an antireflux enteroplasty modification (Fig. 3-4), and the balance, end-to-end operations with varied lengths of jejunum and ileum. The defunctional limb was anastomosed to the cecum, ascending colon, or transverse colon. The sigmoid colon was used for the defunctional anastomosis in one patient, but she developed such severe diarrhea and distension of the bypassed small intestine that a revisional procedure was necessary. The functional ileum was moved from the sigmoid to the transverse colon with marked improvement in her symptoms.

Because we discontinued using the JIB in 1976 in favor of the gastric bypass operation (GBP), and currently do not recommend its use, the details of technique and of pre- and postoperative care will not be presented. A few general observations that have arisen out of our experience will be mentioned, and chronic complications will be addressed in some detail.

We found that unless an antireflux modification was added to the end-to-side JIB, weight losses were disappointing. The critical length of function-

TABLE 3-1   Patient Data: Jejunoileal Bypass

Age range (years)	17–64
Sex ratio (F:M)	7:1
Preoperative average weight (kg)	129.9 (87.3–252.7)
Ideal body weight (kg)	66.8 (47.3–95.4)
Preoperative excess weight (kg)	63.1 (35.4–171.8)
Preoperative excess weight (%)	98.5 (49.7–212.3)

Study includes 174 patients seen in the period 1954–1976.

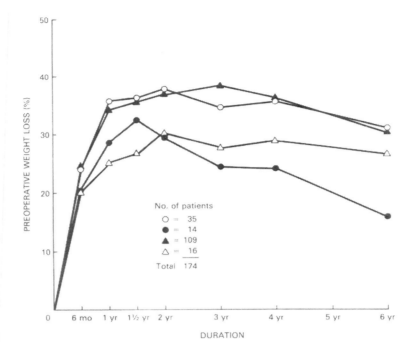

FIG. 3-5. Mean percentage *preoperative* weight loss over a 6-year period for 174 JIB patients of four different types: end-to-side, 35 cm jejunum to 10 cm ileum with antireflux modification (○); end-to-side, 35 to 10 cm without modification (●); end-to-end with total functioning length from 45 to 50 cm (▲); end-to-end with total length greater than 50 cm (△).

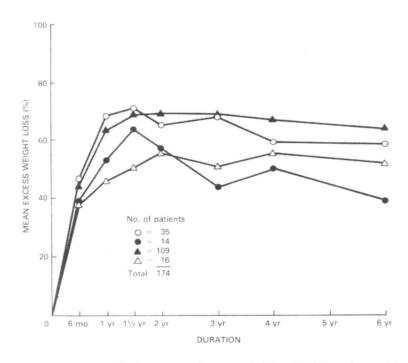

FIG. 3-6. Mean percentage *excess* weight loss over a 6-year period for 174 JIB patients of four different types: end-to-side, 35 cm jejunum to 10 cm ileum with antireflux modification (○); end-to-side, 35 to 10 cm without modification (●); end-to-end with total functioning length from 45 to 50 cm (▲); end-to-end with total length greater than 50 cm (△).

ing small bowel was found to be between 40 and 50 cm. We found, as had Baddeley, that shorter lengths resulted in an increased incidence of complications due to malabsorption, and lengths longer than 50 cm did not produce adequate weight losses. The mean percentage of preoperative weight loss at the end of 6 years for the operations that fell within the optimal length (45–50 cm) category was 30%, and the percentage of excess weight loss for the same period was 64%. In other groups with longer functioning small bowel lengths (> 50 cm), the average percentage of preoperative weight lost at 6 years was 28% and excess weight, 54% (Figs. 3-5 and 3-6). At the time we discontinued the JIB in 1976 we discovered that the most effective anatomic arrangement in our hands was the following: 10 in (25 cm) of jejunum anastomosed end-to-end to 9 in (22.5 cm) of ileum with the defunctional limb anastomosed to the ascending colon at an acute angle designed to inhibit reflux (Fig. 3-7). The end-to-side jejunoileal bypass with an antireflux modification was equally effective and had the advantage of not requiring a defunctional ileocolostomy (Figs. 3-2 and 3-4).

Maximum weight loss following a JIB occurred between 1 and 2 years and leveled off between 3 and 4 years. After 4 years there was a gradual gain in weight for some patients, with weight stabilizing at 20–40% above their ideal weight. A few reached their preoperative weight. The weight regained by any patient was dependent upon energy balance, which in turn was related to eating and exercise habits. Bray[15] has shown that weight loss following JIB is primarily due to a reduction in food intake rather than to calorie loss through malabsorption.

Although hyperplasia and hypertrophy of the functional small intestine a year or more after JIB have been routinely demonstrated, Fairclough[16] concluded that the principal reason for stabilization of weight loss and late weight gain was adaptation of the patient's feeding pattern rather than improved intestinal absorption, although both played a part. The excessive use of alcohol by several of our patients has been an important contributing factor in regain of weight.

It was not failure to obtain a satisfactory and sustained weight loss that caused us to discontinue use of the JIB, but rather the high late complication rate (Table 3-3). It was difficult to follow patients, particularly those from out of town, closely

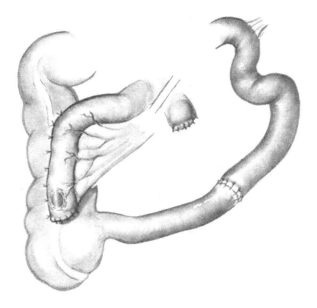

FIG. 3-7. End-to-end JIB with acute angle of defunctional ileum to ascending colon to inhibit reflux. Jejunal length, 25 cm; ileum length, 22.5 cm.

enough to insure that they would not develop a serious and irreversible complication. Although patients were exhorted to return to our office at least annually throughout their lifetimes, many have failed to do so for a variety of reasons. Telephone and mail contact is essential to maintain a reasonably good follow-up.

The other important factor causing us to abandon the JIB was the option we now had of offering the gastric reduction procedure as an alternative. After 1978, the complications and side effects of the JIB became so widely publicized in the lay press and the medical literature that patients seeking surgical treatment for their obesity insisted on having the "stomach stapling operation" instead of the "intestinal operation." For most of them, the choice had already been made by the time they arrived at our office.

Complications and Side Effects

Because 100,000 patients in the United States have had the JIB operation,[17] and any one of them may present with a wide variety of symptom complexes involving almost any organ system, both surgeons and primary physicians should familiarize themselves with the possible long-term complications and side effects of this procedure.

The attending physician or surgeon must be aware of the possible metabolic derangements, the best approach to their diagnosis, and the most appropriate treatment. A surgeon experienced in bariatric surgery should be consulted if the patient has a potentially life-threatening complication requiring restoration of small bowel continuity, because most reconstitutions today involve the addition of a synchronous gastric reduction operation. The indications and technique for this procedure are discussed in Chapter 7.

Early Complications

These will be briefly presented and are further documented in Table 3-2. Generally, except for thromboembolism, wound infections, and small bowel obstruction, the incidence of early complications is lower following JIB than after gastric reduction (GR) procedures. We have attributed the decrease in thromboembolism in our GR cases to the use of minidose heparin, which was not used during the earlier JIB period. There was one perioperative death following a JIB (5th day) due to a massive pulmonary embolism.

The incidence of wound infection is higher in JIB than in GR operations, probably because of increased contamination from the distal small bowel and colon anastomoses, and the less effective use of prophylactic antibiotics prior to 1976. There were two patients with wound dehiscence in the JIB group and none in the GR group, despite the fact that in the former, two-layer transverse incisions were used, and in the latter, single-layer horizontal midline incisions were performed.

Respiratory complications—atelectasis and pneumonitis—are more common after GR than after JIB. This is most likely related to the high midline incision in the gastric procedure, with increased splinting of the diaphragm and lower chest.

Late Complications

The principal disadvantage of JIB, and the reason this operation has been discontinued by most surgeons, is the serious long-term complications and sometimes intolerable side-effects (Table 3-3).[18,19] A complete presentation of the pathophysiology underlying the metabolic derangements, deficiency states, and immunologic manifestations found in these patients is beyond the scope of this book. However, most of the complications likely to be

TABLE 3-2 Perioperative Complications: Jejunoileal Bypass

	No. of Cases	%
Wound infection	10	5.8
Thrombophlebitis	8	4.6
Anastomotic leak and fistula formation	4	2.3
Pulmonary embolism (1 death)	3	1.7
Obstruction: functional limb	3	1.7
Wound dehiscence	2	1.2
Intraabdominal abscess	1	0.6
Postoperative intraabdominal hematoma	1	0.6
Deaths	1	0.6

Study includes 174 patients seen in the period 1954–1976.

TABLE 3-3 Late Complications of Jejunoileal Bypass

	No. of Cases	%
Kidney stones	22	12.8
Arthritis	17	9.9
Severe persistent diarrhea	13	7.6
Malnutrition and dehydration	11	6.4
Hernia (incisional)	10	5.8
Cholecystitis and cholelithiasis	8	4.6
Hypomagnesemia (requiring intramuscular MgSO$_4$)	3	1.7
Acidosis (symptomatic)	2	1.2
Intussusception (reoperated)	2	1.2
Pancreatitis	2	1.2
Hypocalcemia	2	1.2
Temporary hepatic dysfunction	2	1.2
Hepatic failure with death	2	1.2
Dermatitis	2	1.2
Duodenal ulcer with massive hemorrhage (2 episodes)	1	.6
Gastric ulcer	1	.6
Erythema nodosum	1	.6
Persistent vomiting	1	.6
Perforated sigmoid diverticulitis	1	.6
Carcinoma, sigmoid colon	1	.6
Encephalopathy	1	.6
Deaths	3	1.7

Study includes 174 patients seen in the period 1954–1976.

encountered will be described briefly, with an emphasis on diagnosis and treatment. Renal complications will be discussed in more detail in the appendix to this chapter.

Hepatic Complications

Liver failure is the most feared complication of JIB, and the most common cause of late postoperative death.[20] The incidence of clinically significant liver dysfunction following JIB has been estimated to vary between 3 and 10%. Twenty-five to 75% of all post-JIB deaths are attributed to liver failure.[21] Unless acute liver failure can be diagnosed early, and treatment started promptly, the mortality rate is excessive.

In one reported series, 50% of post-JIB patients who required reanastomosis of their small bowel due to liver failure died from progressive liver necrosis.[22] In a report from the University of Minnesota, 5% of 351 patients with JIB developed clinical and biochemical liver failure, but with vigorous therapy, only approximately 0.5% of the entire series died. Of 604 patients with JIB from seven different centers, Marubbio et al[23] reported 31 (5.2%) deaths. Ten (1.7%) of the total number of patients, or approximately 30% of the deaths, were due to liver failure.

Liver failure occurs most often during the first postoperative year, frequently associated with a period of rapid weight loss, and is infrequent after the second year. Nevertheless, it can occur at any time.

There were two deaths from liver failure in our series of 174 JIB patients, and a third death in a patient with cirrhosis and advanced liver failure from another medical center upon whom we performed a small bowel reconstitution procedure. This death will be discussed in Chapter 7. The first two deaths may have been prevented by earlier diagnosis and treatment. They will be presented in brief.

Death Due to Liver Failure: First Case Report The patient was a 31 year old caucasian female who was 67 in (157.5 cm) tall and weighed 267 lb (121 kg). In October 1974 she had an end-to-end JIB with 11 in (27.5 cm) of jejunum anastomosed to 8 in (20 cm) of ileum. The distal end of the defunctional small bowel was connected to the transverse colon. Liver biopsy showed 2+ fatty metamorphosis. Her postoperative course was complicated by a fecal fistula and an infected subhepatic hematoma, the latter thought to be related to the liver biopsy. She was discharged to her home after 5 weeks, and returned again to the hospital in January 1975 for a fistula excision

and colostomy closure. She recovered well from this operation and was discharged to her home in February 1975. At the time of this discharge her SMA-12 profile was normal except for an elevated alkaline phosphatase, 300 mU/liter ($N = 80$); SGOT, 80 mU/liter ($N = 45$); and serum bilirubin, 1.6 ($N = 1$). Her total protein was 5.5 g% and albumin 2.6 gm%. She did well at home, her weight loss averaging 10 lb per month.

In June she developed an upper respiratory infection which was followed 2 weeks later by weakness, anorexia, nausea, and vomiting. She refused hospitalization, but when she became semistuporous was readmitted at her husband's insistence. On examination at the hospital her skin and sclerae appeared jaundiced and a firm liver edge was palpable 10 cm below the costal margin. She responded only to painful stimuli. Her laboratory findings were grossly abnormal as follows: serum calcium, 6.8 mg%; total protein, 4.5 mg%; albumin, 1.6 mg%; alkaline phosphatase, 250 mU/ml; LDH, 700 mU/ml ($N = 200$); SGOT, 140 mU/ml; BUN, normal; serum creatinine, 3.1 mg%. The prothrombin time was 17.9 s (control, 11); partial thromboplastin time, 59.1 s (control, 30.9). Her serum sodium was 132; chloride, 87; potassium, 3.3; and CO_2 content, 29.2 mEq/liter. Arterial blood gases were as follows: Po_2, 58.4 mmHg, with 87% oxygen saturation; Pco_2, 35 mmHg; pH, 7.225; hemoglobin, 10.8 g; hematocrit, 33%; WBC, 11,100.

Her condition rapidly deteriorated with progressive jaundice and renal shutdown. She died 2 days after admission of hepatorenal failure. Autopsy examination revealed a large (3850 g) yellow fatty liver which showed on microscopic examination severe fatty change with mixed inflammatory infiltrate within the portal triads. There was no evidence of cirrhosis, and almost no identifiable normal hepatic tissue. Microscopic sections of the kidneys revealed tubular nephrosis. There was bilateral pulmonary edema and bronchopneumonia.

If this patient could have been convinced to enter the hospital 2 weeks—or even a week—earlier and resuscitative measures (parenteral hyperalimentation plus broad spectrum antibiotics) had been initiated at that time, death might have been averted.

Second Case Report The second patient was a 31-year-old black female who was 60 in (150 cm) tall and weighed 304 lb (138 kg). In September 1976, she had an end-to-end JIB with the functioning component made up of 10 in (25 cm) of jejunum and 9 in (22.5 cm) of terminal ileum. The distal end of the defunctional ileum was anastomosed to the ascending colon. An intraoperative liver biopsy revealed minimal fatty change, and no other abnormalities. She made an uneventful postoperative recovery and was discharged from the hospital on the 7th postoperative day. She was then examined in the office at 2-month intervals and seemed to be doing quite well. She was losing weight at approximately 12 lb (5.4 kg) per month. She was instructed to eat a high protein, low fat, low oxalate diet, and was taking the following medications: a liquid potassium supplement (Kaon), calcium carbonate (Titralac, t.i.d.), multivitamins, and Cantil for diarrhea. At 7 months postoperatively she complained of being tired and was somewhat anorexic, but otherwise seemed normal.

Laboratory examinations were as follows: SGOT, 81 mU/liter; LDH, 319 mU/liter; serum calcium, 7.1 mg%; ionic calcium, 3.7 mg% ($N =$ 4.0–4.8 mg%); total protein, 5.8 g%; albumin, 2.5 g%; A/G ratio, 0.8/1 ($N =$ 1.1–2.2); cholesterol, 86 mg%; potassium, 3.0 mEq/liter; magnesium, 1.3 mg% ($N =$ 1.8–2.9 mg%); BUN, 4 mg% ($N =$ 8–25 mg%). The hemoglobin was low at 11.7 g%, and the indices showed a normochromic normocytic anemia. The WBC was 5700 with 28% PMNs and 64% lymphocytes. Serum bilirubin and alkaline phosphatase were normal.

Examination in the office 2 months later (9 months postoperatively) revealed the patient to be feeling stronger. She had complained of arthralgia a week or so earlier which had responded to doxycycline hyclate (Vibramycin). At her last visit to the office, 10 months postoperatively, her strength was only fair and she was having six to seven stools daily. She had lost 105 lb (47 kg) since her operation.

Approximately 2 weeks after this visit she was found unresponsive by her mother, and was admitted to the hospital. Resuscitative measures were started, but the patient's condition deteriorated rapidly, and she died 10 h after admission.

At postmortem examination, the liver was found to weigh 1280 g, and was finely nodular. The parenchyma was medium brown with small yellowish nodules throughout. It had a normal lobular architecture. On microscopic examination,

there was evidence of severe fatty metamorphosis with portal cirrhosis and fibrous bridging between portal areas. The parenchyma was organized in a micronodular pattern, and there was a significant amount of bile duct proliferation. The kidneys were pale with normal glomeruli, but marked tubular necrosis. There was some dependent congestion of both lungs.

This patient's postoperative course did not seem particularly unusual to us, even though her laboratory tests were abnormal in April. In retrospect, a technetium sulfa colloid scan or a percutaneous liver biopsy would have revealed the extent of her liver disease, and would have prompted earlier treatment in the hospital. Reconstitution of her JIB would probably have been necessary to prevent death.

Diagnosis of Liver Failure These case reports illustrate how quickly a patient who seems to be recovering satisfactorily may progress rapidly to hepatic failure and death. Liver failure should be suspected on the basis of clinical findings because liver function tests often do not reflect the true status of the liver.[24] Patients with severe hepatic dysfunction present with weakness, lethargy, anorexia, nausea, vomiting, and in late stages, ascites, jaundice, and peripheral edema. They may have a tender enlarged liver.[25] The earliest most accurate diagnostic examination is a technetium sulfa colloid scan. A large, poorly opacified liver shadow with a more intense splenic image is diagnostic of severe liver dysfunction. Sulfobromophthalein retention is usually elevated early, as are the liver enzymes SGOT, SGPT, and alkaline phosphatase.[26] Hypoalbuminemia, hypokalemia, and hyperbilirubinemia are later manifestations. Hepatitis-associated antigens are not present in this type of involvement. An elevated serum ammonia level with encephalopathy occurs in late stages of acute liver failure, but is more commonly found in patients with advanced cirrhosis and esophageal varices. A liver biopsy is the most reliable method of evaluating the status of the liver, particularly in chronic disease.[24,26] There is often a discrepancy between liver function tests and the liver biopsy, the biopsy usually indicating more extensive involvement than suggested by function tests alone.[27] A percutaneous liver biopsy must be done with caution if coagulation studies are abnormal.

Baker et al[28] presented two case reports of patients with extensive hepatitis, steatosis, cirrhosis, and liver failure who were first treated aggressively with parenteral hyperalimentation and antibiotic therapy, and after improvement in liver function underwent reanastomosis of their small bowel with recovery. Subsequent liver biopsies revealed definite regression of the histopathologic abnormalities.

Treatment of Liver Failure As soon as the diagnosis of impending liver failure is reasonably assured, the patient should be started on a high protein diet and a broad spectrum antibiotic such as metronidazole (Flagyl), or doxycycline hyclate (Vibramycin). Often the patient is too nauseated to eat, in which case parenteral hyperalimentation should be used. Heimburger et al[29] recommend a glucose-free amino acid solution when treating liver failure, which can be administered via a peripheral vein. If parenteral hyperalimentation is used, at least 1 liter daily of the hyperalimentation fluid should be glucose free.[30] If, after this intensive therapeutic regimen the patient does not improve, or relapses, restoration of the small bowel should be done. More specific indications for reconstitution are set forth in Chapter 7.

Chronic Liver Disease The diagnosis of chronic progressive cirrhosis and hepatitis is unreliable by any method except percutaneous liver biopsy. Ideally, this should be done semiannually or annually on every JIB patient but this is difficult to attain because many patients will not return for routine biopsy after the first year or two, especially if they feel well. A small amount of fatty metamorphosis (1+ to 2+) with triaditis (1+) is a common postoperative finding and may be permanent. Steatosis in moderate degree does not affect liver function adversely, nor does it cause progressive liver disease.[31-33] Steatosis and cirrhosis are not causally related, but both result from the same metabolic derangement.[33]

In an excellent study from the University of Minnesota, Marubbio et al[23] reported the following preoperative findings in 351 JIB patients: fatty metamorphosis in 81%, triaditis in 19.6%; portal fibrosis in 9.8%; and central lobular pericellular fibrosis in 8.5%. This was similar to the pericellular fibrosis seen in alcoholic hepatitis, but without the inflammation. They also pointed out that the presence of portal fibrosis, triaditis, or biliary proliferation did not necessarily portend progressive liver disease. These lesions were found to disappear

following JIB in some patients and to appear in others. We have found this to be true in our serial liver biopsies as well. The lesion that did predict invariable progression after JIB according to Marubbio et al was central pericellular fibrosis. This begins with the formation of collagen fibrils between the hepatic cells and the sinusoidal cells near the central vein in the spaces of Disse. As the collagen fibrils coalesce, they form basement membranes not normally present except within portal triads and in the central veins. The presence of basement membranes in this location interferes with nutrition and oxygenation of the hepatocytes. The central pericellular fibrosis is a precursor lesion to the scar that links portal and central areas, subdividing the liver into the pseudolobules of nodular cirrhosis.

Steatosis The cause of the high incidence of steatosis of the liver in obesity is unknown, but it is thought to represent either another area of fat storage or possibly a relative protein insufficiency in patients who tend to consume large quantities of carbohydrate and fat.[34]

Serial postoperative liver biopsies revealed the liver abnormalities found pre- or intraoperatively to increase up to 2 years after operation, when they usually returned to their preoperative state. Some remained the same, and a small percentage increased in severity.[23,34]

Liver function tests or the patient's clinical appearance often do not mirror the hepatic histopathology and should not be substituted for serial liver biopsies in the determination of liver status, as stressed earlier.[26,34]

Etiology of Progressive Liver Failure Although the cause of liver failure or chronic progressive hepatic pathology in patients who have been submitted to JIB is unknown, the most prominent hypotheses are the following.

1. *Circulating endotoxin or other toxic products from bacterial overgrowth in the excluded segment of small intestine.* At the time of JIB reanastomosis in our series of patients we obtained cultures from the defunctional bowel which yielded large numbers of colon-type bacteria, mostly anaerobic forms (unpublished data). This has been reported by others.[32] It has not been proved whether the bacteria within the excluded intestine produce a hepatotoxic endotoxin, secondary metabolites such as bile acids, or endogenous ethanol which could damage

the liver.[21] The endotoxin theory is considered the most plausible but the etiology could be multifactorial.

Drenick et al[32] in a clinical study of steatosis after JIB found that a broad-spectrum antibiotic, metronidazole, caused it to regress, and concluded that the etiology of post-JIB steatosis was related to bacterial endotoxins produced by anaerobic organisms in the excluded loop. Protein malnutrition was considered a permissive factor only. Direct bacterial colonization of the liver from the portal circulation is considered remote, but involvement of the liver by circulating immune complexes,[21] implicated in JIB arthritis,[42] dermatitis,[41] and glomerulonephritis,[35] is considered possible. The presence of granulomata in the postshunt liver would tend to suggest the immune complex theory, but liver granulomata can be drug-induced or from a number of other causes.[31,36,37] We have found granulomata in 10% of our post-JIB patients, and in several patients who have had a gastric bypass revision. The presence of granulomata has had no detectable clinical significance in our experience.

Buchwald et al[7] pointed out, on the other hand, that hepatic failure is extremely rare in patients who have had a partial ileal bypass for hyperlipidemia. They have a long (200 cm) bypassed segment of small intestine, which if the endotoxin theory is correct, should be expected to result in as high an incidence of liver failure as that following JIB for obesity. He advanced the belief that before liver dysfunction develops, a prolonged period of negative caloric balance must have occurred.

Yost et al[27] in a prospective randomized clinical trial in 45 JIB patients found that doxycycline hyclate was not of value in preventing hepatic dysfunction. They concluded that the antibacterial spectrum of doxycycline was not sufficiently broad to effectively reduce or eliminate the offending anaerobic organisms such as *Bacteroides fragilis*. They did not believe their study disproved the possible etiologic relationship between bacterial endotoxins and hepatic dysfunction.

2. *Nutritional (protein deficiency)*. The second hypothesis of liver dysfunction is based on the similarity between kwashiorkor, also called "protein energy malnutrition," characterized by a large fatty liver, and a deficiency of certain essential and nonessential amino acids. During the early catabolic phase following JIB, the same amino acid deficiency is noted, but returns to normal as protein energy balance is achieved. Steatosis and abnormal liver function tests are seen during this period of rapid weight loss, but protein deficiency alone has not been shown to cause hepatocellular necrosis, inflammation, or fibrosis.[21,32]

3. *Hepatic collagen proline hydroxylase activity*. This was found to be increased in patients with hepatocellular necrosis following JIB and was associated with severe liver damage. This enzyme was also found to be increased in experimental fibrosis caused by carbon tetrachloride and in alcoholic hepatitis. The enzyme was not increased in patients with fatty infiltration alone or in hepatic fibrosis.[38]

4. *Alcoholism*. Alcoholism is a well-recognized cause of hepatic necrosis and cirrhosis.[25] Its role in the etiology of liver failure following JIB in some patients is not appreciated because their abuse of alcohol has been so well concealed.

Prevention and Management of Liver Dysfunction The essential aspects of prevention and management have been discussed. The indications and techniques for reanastomosis are presented in Chapter 7. Careful clinical follow-up and serial liver biopsies are essential preventive measures. Treatment consists of a high protein, low fat diet, broad spectrum antibiotics, hyperalimentation when necessary, and in some patients, reanastomosis.[21,23,32]

Arthritis; Myositis; Tenosynovitis; Dermatitis
The joint and skin involvement following JIB resembles that associated with ulcerative colitis and Crohn's disease and probably has a similar origin.[39] Polyarthritis as a sequela of intestinal bypass (jejunocolic) was first reported by Shagrin et al in 1971, present in 23% of 31 patients.[40] The incidence of post-JIB arthritis, tenosynovitis, and myositis has been reported as high as 25%. Dermatitis is less common, and when present is usually associated with arthritis.[41]

The etiology of these inflammatory responses is unknown, but it is thought to be related to the absorption of noxious bacterial products from the excluded intestinal limb.[42,49] Circulating immune complexes have been demonstrated in patients with polyarthritis and dermatitis, usually in the developing phase of the disease.[43] Immunofluorescent studies of skin lesions have shown the presence of IgG and C3 in various locations within the lesions, but a specific antigen has never been demonstrated in any published report; therefore the significance of the immune complexes as primary etiologic agents has not been established.[41] Wands et al[43] showed that immune complexes in post-JIB arthritis contained IgG reactive with *Escherichia coli* and *Bacteroides fragilis* which suggests an etiologic relationship with these organisms.

The fact that both the arthritis and dermatitis can be ameliorated, at least temporarily, by broad spectrum antibiotics such as metronidazole or tetracycline, strongly suggests that bacteria play an important role in these complications.[42,49] The overgrowth of colonic bacteria in the excluded limb, also thought to be an etiologic factor in post-JIB hepatic failure,[32] bypass enteritis,[47] and glomerulonephritis,[35] is considered the underlying if not the immediate cause.[49] Polyarthritis or dermatitis can occur at any time after JIB, is usually evanescent, but can be constant and of long duration in some patients. Polyarthritis involves primarily the extremity joints—wrists, elbows, shoulders, fingers, knees, and ankles—and seldom the spine. There is often an associated tenosynovitis and myositis.[41] The joints are usually swollen, tender, occasionally red, and infrequently contain fluid; when present, fluid is usually found in the knee. Tests for rheumatoid factor and antinuclear antibodies are negative.[49] The sedimentation rate may be elevated, but most other laboratory findings are noncontributory. Symptoms are usually most severe during the early hours after rising, during periods of fatigue, and when there are weather changes.

Dermatitis

Bypass dermatitis is usually first manifested by small, red, macular lesions located on the extensor surface of the arms, thighs, buttocks, and lower abdomen. They do not involve the palms, plantar surface of the foot, face, genitalia, or mucous membranes.[41] The macules either disappear in a few days or gradually form vesicles and pustules, approximately 1 cm in diameter. These gradually disappear spontaneously over the course of 2 to 3 weeks or after antibiotic therapy, without a residual scar. They can recur as single lesions or in extensive crops, and are characterized by burning pain and itching. Often they are mistaken for insect bites.[44]

The most common histopathologic finding in the skin lesion is a high concentration of PMNs causing a sterile pustule. The dermal capillaries and venules show a mild degree of damage, but necrotizing vasculitis is not usually seen as in other immune complex vasculitides, and the pustules do not progress to pyoderma gangrenosum.[41]

Erythema nodosum–like skin involvement can also occur with large, dusky red, raised nodules on the anterior aspect of the legs, usually below the knees. These lesions are more chronic and painful than the superficial lesions, but also heal without a scar following treatment.[45,49]

Treatment The milder forms of arthritis can be adequately managed with analgesics and rest. More severe involvement will respond only to a course of broad spectrum antibiotics. Prednisone is effective in reducing the pain, but we have used it sparingly because of its long-term side-effects. Dermatitis usually is self-limited, but when severe, must be treated by oral antibiotic therapy. Local application of either antibiotic or hydrocortisone ointment is ineffective.

Occasionally neither condition responds adequately to any conservative treatment, and the JIB must be taken down. This is always followed by the prompt disappearance of symptoms.

Of 85 patients in our series who had a reconstitution of their JIB for unacceptable sequelae, 11 (12%) were done for recalcitrant arthritis, one for erythema nodosum, and one for recurrent dermatis with arthritis.

Gastrointestinal Tract Complications

Included in this category are the following conditions: megacolon, bypass enteritis, pneumatosis cystoides intestinalis, gas bloat syndrome, intussusception, ulceration and fibrosis of the excluded bowel, and severe diarrhea. Peptic ulceration has been an infrequent complication of JIB.[46]

Megacolon Megacolon is universally present in JIB patients after a year or two and is a normal adaptation of the colon to the increased undigested food load. Frequently the dilated colon results in abdominal distention with pain and flatulence. There may be intermittent colonic pseudoobstruction and copious foul-smelling flatus. Surgical management is seldom necessary, but unless the attending physician or the radiologist is aware of this condition, the diagnosis of distal colonic obstruction may be made. Toxic megacolon as seen with ulcerative colitis is rarely a complication of JIB.[49] A low fat diet and broad spectrum antibiotic therapy are often helpful. Milk should be eliminated from the diet on a trial basis.

Bypass Enteritis   Passaro et al[47] first described and named this "new complication" in 1975. It is characterized clinically by diffuse abdominal distension and tenderness, fever, and increased frequency of diarrhea. Plain radiographs of the abdomen reveal gaseous distension of the small bowel without fluid levels. In two of four patients described, pneumatosis cystoides intestinalis was seen, and in one, pneumoperitoneum. Two patients were explored for possible abscess formation or perforation, but the principal finding at surgery was an edematous, inflamed, and dilated segment of excluded small bowel. There was no evidence of obstruction at the ileosigmoid anastomosis.

Although the etiology of this complication could not be proved it was Passaro's belief that the overgrowth of anaerobic bacteria in the bypassed small bowel caused an ileus, and in a few patients, passage of gas through the bowel wall. The condition responded to a broad spectrum antibiotic (cephalothin) which was the recommended therapy. It was felt that surgical management should seldom be necessary for this entity even in the presence of pneumoperitoneum.

Leung et al[46] reported complications involving the defunctional small bowel in 119 intestinal bypass patients evaluated between 1972 and 1980. There was a 66% incidence of bypass enteropathy (bypass enteritis) with three patients in this group exhibiting pneumatosis cystoides intestinalis. The signs and symptoms were those noted above. In addition they reported severe blood loss in three patients presumably due to diffuse mucosal inflammation, although the exact cause was never established. The bleeding responded to reanastomosis. In one patient an ulceration was found in the defunctional ileum several centimeters proximal to the ileosigmoid anastomosis.

Intussusception and Obstruction   Ten patients in the series of Leung et al[46] developed signs and symptoms of intussusception, and three required surgical correction. In one patient obstruction developed in the previously excluded bowel after reanastomosis secondary to extensive fibrous adhesions and multiple areas of obstructive luminal narrowing. One segment of the formerly excluded bowel was totally atretic with a pinpoint lumen. Histologic examination of the stenotic segments showed atrophy of the mucosa, fibrous adhesions, and foreign body granuloma in the serosa. (We have never seen this degree of obstructive pathology in any of our 85 patients who have had a JIB reconstitution.)

Bacterial overgrowth in the bypassed small bowel was considered to be the primary cause for most of the lesions except intussusception.[46,49] A suitable broad spectrum antibiotic (metronidazole) was found to relieve the various inflammatory conditions, but surgical management was necessary for recurrent intussusception, continuing hemorrhage, or obstruction.

It should be noted that in the technique employed for the JIBs in the abovementioned series (Passaro–Leung), the defunctional bowel was anastomosed to the sigmoid colon. Except for one of our patients where the defunctional intestine was shunted into the sigmoid colon, we have used the ascending colon, cecum, or transverse colon for this purpose. As mentioned earlier, this patient developed symptoms similar to those described with bypass enteritis, and improved when the defunctional anastomosis was moved from the sigmoid to the transverse colon. Otherwise, bypass enteritis has not been a significant complication in our series of 174 patients. Buchwald,[7] who used the cecum to drain the defunctional bowel, did not mention this entity as a significant complication. Although bypass enteritis has apparently been reported following almost any type of JIB, it seems to be more prevalent in those series where the excluded bowel is connected to the sigmoid colon.[48]

Severe Diarrhea and Flatulence   Diarrhea is considered a side-effect rather than a complication of JIB unless it becomes incapacitating. It is usually severe the first 3 to 6 months but gradually improves, until after a year most patients have from 3 to 10 movements daily depending to a large extent upon their diet. Some patients find that diarrhea does not impair their life style significantly, and others consider it intolerable. The diet should be low in fat and roughage, and milk should be temporarily discontinued. Calcium carbonate in the form of powder or tablets (Titralac) taken three to four times daily together with diphenoxylate (Lomotil) is often helpful. Intractable, severe diarrhea is an occasional indication for reanastomosis.

Severe diarrhea is often accompanied by proctitis, symptomatic hemorrhoids, and anal fissure. These complications occasionally become the primary indication for JIB takedown.[50]

Gas Bloat Syndrome This entity, with copious foul flatulence, is a common side-effect of JIB and becomes intolerable in some situations to both patient and family. Avoiding fat and using broad spectrum antibiotics are frequently helpful, but only on a temporary basis.

Dehydration, Electrolyte Imbalance, Acidosis Complications related to malabsorption are most severe during the first 3 to 6 months following JIB, and tend to improve after a year as adaptation of the functioning small bowel occurs.[52] It is therefore essential to rehospitalize the depleted patient as often as necessary during the first postoperative year for parenteral fluid and electrolyte replacement, because early deficiencies are reversible. Recurrent dehydration, electrolyte deficiency, or acidosis after the first year that does not respond to oral management at home will usually require takedown of the JIB. These patients must be followed closely.

A detailed description of the diagnosis and management of fluid and electrolyte imbalance following JIB is not within the scope of this book. A few general observations however, may prove helpful.

Of the many causes of post-JIB weakness and lassitude, *hypokalemia* is perhaps the most common.[51] Unfortunately, most forms of oral potassium are unpalatable in the liquid form and not absorbed in tablet form. Patients should be encouraged to eat foods high in potassium, such as bananas and tomatoes, and try different brands of liquid potassium until they find the one least objectionable. Hypokalemia is most common during the first postoperative year.

Hyperchloremic Acidosis This is an occasional cause of weakness, dizziness, and lethargy. Most patients with acidosis respond to oral or parenteral sodium bicarbonate.[52]

Metabolic Acidosis Metabolic acidosis caused by D-lactic acid, a product of enteric bacterial metabolism, can cause an intermittent encephalopathy that does not respond to administration of either oral or parenteral sodium bicarbonate. This syndrome is characterized by episodes of confu-sion, slurred speech, marked lethargy, and impaired coordination closely mimicking alcoholic intoxication, but without detectable ethanol in the blood or respired air.[53,54] These patients do not have any consistent fluid or electrolyte abnormalities, nor evidence of hepatic failure, and the serum ammonia levels are normal. The most effective conservative treatment is to fast the patient and administer broad spectrum antibiotics. The only permanent resolution for the problem is takedown of the bypass.

We encountered one such patient from outside our series who had had a JIB 3 years earlier. He was accused by his family and friends of being inebriated despite his vigorous denial of alcohol usage. His "inebriation" was eliminated only after reconstitution of his small bowel. This condition can occur at any time postoperatively and is undoubtedly more common, at least in its milder forms, than heretofore realized.

Hypocalcemia This is relatively common and manifested in a few patients by tetany. Often the only symptom is muscle cramps, especially involving the legs, noted most frequently after the patient has gone to bed. Oral calcium and vitamin D will provide adequate treatment for most patients. Calcium serves the dual purpose of minimizing oxylate reabsorption, which aids in preventing kidney stones, and allaying diarrhea, by complexing with fatty acids. Intravenous calcium is required for the initial treatment of tetany. Often other serious deficiencies accompany tetany and comprehensive parenteral management is necessary.[50,51]

Hypomagnesemia This is often undiagnosed and overlooked because magnesium is not included in the routine SMA laboratory analysis. Symptoms of deficiency of this cation include muscle cramps, arthralgia, tetanic contractures of hands and feet, dizziness, blurring of vision, and muscle incoordination.[51] These symptoms are reversible following magnesium ion repletion, but the oral route of administration has not proved satisfactory in our experience. We have had several patients who have required intramuscular magnesium on a continuing basis, usually 2–4 ml of 50% magnesium sulfate administered daily in moderately severe cases, for a week or so or three times weekly in those less severe for a 2- to 3-month period. Rarely it is necessary to hospitalize the patient for intravenous replacement. A 24-h urine excretion study of magnesium is helpful in assessing magnesium deficiency. The normal 24-h excretion is from 3 to 15 mEq/day, and if magnesium deficiency is present, 0 to 1 mEq/day.[55]

Skeletal Disease   A number of investigators [56-58] have reported the presence of hypovitaminosis D, secondary hyperparathyroidism, and osteomalacia in patients 1 to 7 years after JIB. Clinical symptoms, biochemical findings, and radiologic evaluations did not correlate well with bone histology. Bone biopsy was the only reliable method of establishing a diagnosis of bone disease.

Compston et al[59] reported that of 12 patients with proved osteomalacia, eight responded with return to normal or almost normal bone histology after 4–9 months of oral 1-hydroxyvitamin D_3 therapy. Of the four that did not respond to 1-OHD$_3$, two were given additional broad spectrum antibiotics—metronidazole and cotrimoxazole (Trimethoprim 80 mg + sulphamethoxazole 400 mg)—which resulted in clinical and biochemical improvement in both, and documented histologic improvement in one.

Jejunoileal bypass frequently results in vitamin D deficiency, and all patients should be given a vitamin D supplement. Serum determinations of 25-hydroxyvitamin D and parathormone should be obtained occasionally to identify patients who may require a larger dose. The use of 1-OHD$_3$ rather than the parent vitamin D has the advantage of a narrower therapeutic dose range and a shorter half-life. There were no serious side-effects or hypercalcemia encountered by Compston even when the supplement was used for over 6 months after the bone disease had healed. Patients who do not respond to treatment with vitamin D or one of its derivatives should be given an additional trial with a broad spectrum antibiotic. Compston advanced the intriguing theory that variability in the degree of bacterial colonization of the excluded small bowel after JIB might explain the rapid development of bone disease in some patients, and its absence even after many years in others. It might also explain the so-called "resistance" to vitamin D therapy in some patients.[59]

Protein Malnutrition   This is most severe during the first 3 to 6 months following JIB, and occasionally necessitates establishing tube feeding via a small nasogastric tube, a tube gastrostomy, or a tube jejunostomy brought out from the defunc-

tional bowel. Parenteral hyperalimentation is another alternative. A few patients will require several hospitalizations during the first postoperative year to ensure adequate protein intake. Protein malnutrition delays healing, blunts the immune response, serves as a cofactor in the etiology of liver failure, and causes loss of lean body mass with attendant muscle weakness.[60]

Vitamin Deficiency   Fat-soluble vitamins A and D are lost in the stool, and should be provided as daily replacement therapy, usually as a multivitamin tablet. A chewable or liquid form may be necessary to enhance absorption.[51] Parenteral vitamin B_{12} is required for life in patients whose functioning terminal ileum is less than 10 cm.[7]

Tuberculosis and Fungus Infections
An increased incidence over that of the general population of tuberculosis, blastomycosis, and histoplasmosis has been reported by several investigators presumably due to a defective immune response, although the exact etiology was not established.[61-63] These infections were most common in males who had sustained a greater-than-usual weight loss. Reconstitution of the bowel may be necessary to effect a cure in some patients.

Although this discussion of complications has been lengthy, it is of interest to note that 50% of our JIB patients have done well with good long-term weight losses and no serious complications. There is obviously a wide variation in tolerance among patients to the physiologic impact of jejunoileal bypass. Unfortunately there is no available method of selecting the "tolerant" patient.

Biliary Intestinal Bypass

Hallberg[64,65] reported a modification of the JIB in ten patients in which the proximal end of the defunctional small bowel was anastomosed to the gallbladder (Fig. 3-8). The advantage of this method was said to be preservation of the enterohepatic circulation of bile acids and much less diarrhea than following the standard JIB.

An end-to-side JIB was constructed with 40–45 cm of jejunum connected to the side of the terminal ileum 15–20 cm proximal to the cecum. The proximal end of the defunctional jejunum was

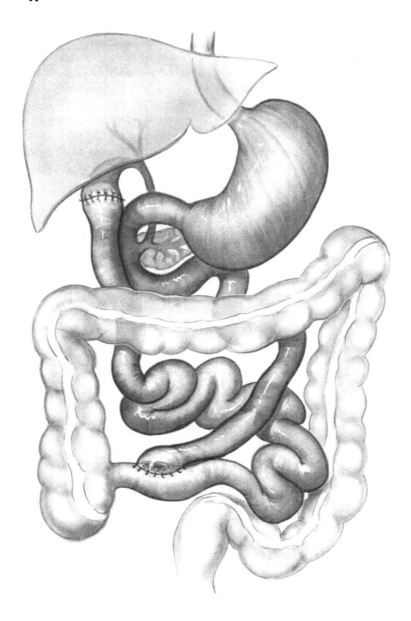

FIG. 3-8. Biliointestinal bypass. This permits normal enterohepatic bile salt circulation and less diarrhea than with JIB.

anastomosed to the gallbladder with as large an anastomosis as possible. If the gallbladder contained stones they were removed. A previous cholecystectomy, of course, precludes the use of this procedure.

An existing JIB can be converted to the biliary intestinal bypass in patients with severe intractable diarrhea with apparently some benefit.

Biliopancreatic Bypass

Scopinaro et al[66] developed an operation for obesity based on "selective" malabsorption, as opposed to the "indiscriminate" malabsorption of JIB. Several variations of the operation were evaluated in humans by Scopinaro, but only the most effective will be described here.

Biliopancreatic bypass (BPB) is the most extensive and complex surgical approach yet developed for the treatment of morbid obesity, but in the series presented by Scopinaro et al the morbidity was low (one wound dehiscence) with no deaths in 18 patients operated. As can be seen from Fig. 3-9, the operation consists of a two-thirds gastrectomy and a very long Roux-en-Y enteroenterostomy. The gastrectomy is necessary to prevent sto-

mal ulceration, which would otherwise be a frequent complication. The addition of a vagotomy to further protect against stomal ulceration was found by Holian[67] to cause diarrhea and was not recommended. The currently recommended length of intestine from the gastrojejunostomy to the ileocecal valve is 250 cm measured along the mesenteric border, with the end-to-side enteroenterostomy 50 cm proximal to the cecum.

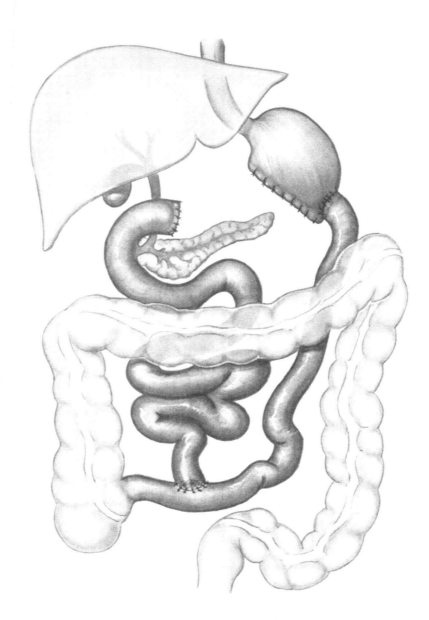

FIG. 3-9. Biliopancreatic bypass of Scopinaro which causes selective malabsorption, principally of fat. Enterohepatic bile salt circulation is normal and there is less diarrhea than with JIB. This is the most extensive bariatric operation.

The purported superiority of BPB over the standard JIB is related to the selective malabsorption of fat and starch while maintaining the enterohepatic circulation of bile salts intact. In addition, the flow of bile and pancreatic juice through the excluded small intestine allegedly reduces bacterial growth in this segment, minimizing the pathogenic effect of coliform bacterial metabolism that frequently occurs with the standard JIB.

Weight loss following BPB was reported to be comparable to that of JIB. There was an average of 60% of excess weight lost in 11 patients reported at the end of 1 year.[67] The diarrhea was reported to be less severe with only two to three fatty-type stools daily, and seldom any liquid movements. The principal disadvantage of the operation was the large amount of foul flatus resulting from starch digestion in the colon.

Kidney stones were not seen in this series even though oxalate excretion was elevated. This is apparently due to the absence of dehydration and the increased urine output with this operation. Compared to JIB the effect of the steatorrhea on fat-soluble vitamin absorption or bone metabolism is not known because follow-up has been short.

Summary

Although jejunoileal bypass is an effective weight-reducing operation, the long-term complications are so frequent and occasionally so severe that it should not be used, except possibly in the management of the few hyperphagic patients who have successfully outeaten their gastric bypass plus several revisions, or by a few surgeons who are devoted to the JIB and have the facilities and personnel to conduct an adequate follow-up.

The primary involvement a surgeon or attending physician will have with JIB today is the management of long-term complications and the selection of patients who need to have their intestinal tract restored. This aspect is discussed more extensively in Chapter 7.

Most of the long-term complications of JIB are related directly or indirectly to malabsorption from the short functioning intestine or to the toxic effects from overgrowth of coliform bacteria in the excluded bowel, or combinations of these factors. The most serious and difficult complication is hepatic failure, either acute or chronic. Serial liver biopsy is the most accurate method to evaluate liver status.

References

1. Kremen AJ, Linner JH, Nelson CH: An experimental evaluation of the nutritional importance of proximal and distal small intestine. Ann Surg 140:439–1954.
2. Linner JH: A summary of 24 years experience with surgery for morbid obesity. Am J Clin Nutr 33:504, 1980.
3. Payne JH, DeWind LT, Commons RR: Metabolic observations in patients with jejunocolic shunts. Am J Surg 106:273, 1963.
4. Payne JH, DeWind L, Schwab CE, Kern WH: Surgical treatment of morbid obesity, 16 years of experience. Arch Surg 106:432, 1973.
5. Scott HW Jr, Dean R, Shull HJ, Abram HS, Webb W, Younger RK, Brill AB: New considerations in use of jejunoileal bypass in patients with morbid obesity. Ann Surg 177:723, 1973.
6. Scott HW Jr: Surgical modifications of jejunoileal bypass. In: Surgical Management of Obesity. New York, Academic Press, 1980, pp 17–27.
7. Buchwald H, Varco RL, Moore RB, Schwartz MZ: Intestinal bypass procedures. Curr Prob Surg 12:1–51, Ap.1975.
8. Baddeley RM: The management of gross refractory obesity by jejuno-ileal bypass. Br J Surg 66:525, 1979.
9. Salmon PA: The results of small intestine bypass operations for the treatment of obesity. Surg Gynecol Obstet 132:965, 1971.
10. Benfield JR, Greeway FL, Bray GA, Barry RE, Lechago J, Mena I, Schedewie H: Experience with jejunoileal bypass for obesity. Surg Gynecol Obstet 143:401, 1976.
11. Hallberg D, Backman L, Espmark S: Surgical treatment of obesity. Prog Surg 14:46–83, 1975.
12. Nachlas MM, Crawford DT, Pearl JM: Current status of jejunoileal bypass in the treatment of morbid obesity. Surg Gynecol Obstet 150:250, 1980.
13. Wills CE Jr: Small bowel bypass for obesity. A discussion of four different procedures. J Med Assoc Ga 61:322, 1972.
14. Starkloff GB, Donovan JF, Ramach R, Wolfe BM: Metabolic intestinal surgery: its complications and management. Arch Surg 110:652, 1975.
15. Bray GA, Barry RE, Benfield JR, Castelnuovo-Tedesco P, Rodin J: Intestinal bypass surgery for obesity decreases food intake and taste preferences. Am J Clin Nutr 29:779, 1976.
16. Fairclough PD, Kumar PJ, Clark ML, Aggis A, Rimmer D, Pilkington TRE, Gazet JC: Intestinal adaptation. In: Surgical Management of Obesity.

New York, Academic Press, 1980, pp 103–114.

17. Mason EE: Development of gastric bypass and gastroplasty. In: Surgical Management of Obesity. New York, Academic Press, 1980, p 29.

18. Van Itallie TB, Kral JG: The dilemma of morbid obesity. JAMA 246:999, 1981.

19. Clayman CB, O'Reilly DJ: Jejunoileal bypass: Pass it by. JAMA 246:988, 1981.

20. Andersen T, Juhl E, Quaade F: Fatal outcome after jejunoileal bypass for obesity. Am J Surg 142:619, 1981.

21. Maxwell JD: Intestinal bypass and the liver. In: Surgical Management of Obesity. New York, Academic Press, 1980, pp 235–255.

22. Iber FL, Cooper M: Jejunoileal bypass for the treatment of massive obesity. Prevalence, morbidity, and short- and long-term consequences. Am J Clin Nutr 30:4, 1977.

23. Marubbio HT, Rucker RD Jr, Schneider PP, Horstmann JP, Varco RL, Buchwald H: The liver in morbid obesity and following bypass surgery for obesity. Surg Clin North Am 59:1079–1093, 1979.

24. Hocking MP, Duerson MC, Alexander RW, Woodward ER: Late hepatic histopathology after jejunoileal bypass for morbid obesity. Relation of abnormalities to clinical course. Am J Surg 141:159, 1981.

25. Peters RL, Gay T, Reynolds TB: Post-jejunoileal-bypass hepatic disease. Its similarity to alcoholic hepatic disease. Am J Coll Phys 63:318, 1975.

26. Brown RG, O'Leary JP, Woodward ER: Hepatic effects of jejunoileal bypass for morbid obesity. Am J Surg 127:53, 1974.

27. Yost RL, Duerson MC, Russell WL, O'Leary JP: Doxycycline in the prevention of hepatic dysfunction. An evaluation of its use following JIB in humans. Arch Surg 114:931, 1979.

28. Baker AL, Elson CO, Jaspan J, Boyer JL: Liver failure with steatonecrosis after jejunoileal bypass. Recovery with parenteral nutrition and reanastomosis. Arch Intern Med 139:289, 1979.

29. Heimburger SL, Steiger E, LoGerfo P, Biehl AG, Williams MJ: Reversal of severe fatty hepatic infiltration after intestinal bypass for morbid obesity by calorie-free amino acid infusion. Am J Surg 129:229, 1975.

30. Mason EE: Surgical treatment of morbid obesity. Major Probl Clin Surg. Philadelphia, Saunders, 1981, p 422.

31. Peters RL: Hepatic morphologic changes after jejunoileal bypass. In: Progress in Liver Diseases, Vol. 6. New York, Grune & Stratton, 1979, pp 581–594.

32. Drenick RJ, Fisler D, Johnson D: Hepatic steatosis after intestinal bypass. Prevention and reversal by metronidazole, irrespective of protein calorie malnutrition. Gastroenterology 82:535, 1981.

33. Thaler H: Relation of steatosis to cirrhosis. Clin Gastroenterol 4:273, 1975.

34. Salmon PA: Fatty metamorphosis in patients with jejunoileal bypass. Surg Gynecol Obstet 141:75, 1975.

35. Drenick EJ, Stanley TM, Border WA, Zawada ET, Dornfield LP, Upham T, Llach F: Renal damage with intestinal bypass. Ann Intern Med 89:594, 1978.

36. Wieland RG, Geraci K, Jones JC, Elkhaivi S: Intestinal bypass for obesity. JAMA 247:2098, 1982.

37. O'Reilly DJ, Clayman CB: Reply. Intestinal bypass for obesity. JAMA 247:2098, 1982.

38. Mezey E, Imbembo AL: Hepatic collagen proline hydroxylase activity in hepatic disease following jejunoileal bypass for morbid obesity. Surgery 83:345, 1978.

39. Buchanan RF, Willkens RF: Arthritis after jejunoileostomy. Arthritis Rheum 15:644, 1972.

40. Shagrin JW, Frame B, Duncan H: Polyarthritis in obese patients with intestinal bypass. Ann Intern Med 75:377, 1971.

41. Kennedy C: Inflammatory skin and joint disease after intestinal bypass. In: Surgical Management Of Obesity. New York, Academic Press, 1980, pp 273–286.

42. Drenick EJ, Ament ME, Finegold SM, Corrode P, Passaro E: Bypass enteropathy. Intestinal and systemic manifestations following small bowel bypass. JAMA 236:269, 1976.

43. Wands JR, LaMont JT, Mann E, Isselbacher KJ: Arthritis associated with intestinal bypass procedure for morbid obesity. Complement activation and characterization of circulating cryoproteins. N Engl J Med 294:122, 1976.

44. Troy JL: The bowel bypass syndrome. Am J Dermatol Pathol 3:361, 1981.

45. Kennedy C: Inflammatory skin and joint disease after intestinal bypass. In: Surgical Management Of Obesity. New York, Academic Press, 1980, p 276.

46. Leung FW, Drenick EJ, Stanley TM: Intestinal bypass complications involving the excluded small bowel segment. Am J Gastroenterol 77:67, 1982.

47. Passaro E, Drenick EJ, Wilson SE: Bypass enteritis: a new complication of jejunoileal bypass for obesity. Am J Surg 131:169, 1976.

48. Martyak SN: Pneumotosis intestinalis. A complication of jejunoileal bypass. JAMA 235:1038, 1976.

49. Thayer WR, Kirsner JB: Enteric and extra-enteric complications of intestinal bypass and inflammatory bowel disease. Are there some clues? Gastroenterology 78:1097, 1980.

50. Joffe SN: Surgical management of morbid obesity. Progress report. Gut 22:242, 1981.

51. Phillips RB: Small intestinal bypass for the treatment of morbid obesity (collective reviews). Surg Gynecol Obstet 146:455, 1978.

52. Baddeley RM: Indications for reversal of jejuno-ileal bypass. In: Surgical Management Of Obesity. New York, Academic Press, 1980, pp 293–303.

53. Ayub A, Faloon WW, Heinig RE: Encephalopathy following jejunoileostomy. JAMA 246:970, 1981.

54. Carr DB, Shih VE, Richter JM, Martin JB: Encephalopathy following jejunoileostomy. JAMA 247:1127, 1982.

55. Mason EE: Surgical treatment of morbid obesity. Major Probl Clin Surg. Philadelphia, Saunders, 1981, pp 94–95.

56. Mosekilde L, Melsen F, Hessov I, Christensen MS, Lund BJ, Sorensen OH: Low serum levels of 1,25-dehydroxyvitamin D and histomorphometric evidence of osteomalacia after jejunoileal bypass for obesity. Gut 21:624, 1980.

57. Hey H, Lund B, Sorensen OH, Lind BJ, Christenson MS: Impairment of vitamin D and bone metabolism in patients with bypass operation for obesity. Acta Med Scand (Suppl) 624:73, 1979.

58. Teitelbaum SL, Halverson JD, Bates M, Wise L, Haddad JG: Abnormalities of circulating 25-OH-vitamin D after jejunoileal bypass for obesity. Ann Intern Med 86:289, 1977.

59. Compston JE, Horton LWL, Laker MF, Merrett AL, Woodhead JS, Gazet JC, Pilkington TRE: Treatment of bone disease after jejunoileal bypass for obesity with oral L-hydroxy-vitamin D3. Gut 21:669, 1980.

60. MacLean LD: Host resistance in surgical patients. Trauma 19:297, 1979.

61. Pickleman JR, Evans LS, Kane JM, Freeark RJ: Tuberculosis after jejunoileal bypass for obesity. JAMA 234:744, 1975.

62. Yu VL: Onset of tuberculosis after intestinal bypass surgery for obesity. Guidelines for evaluation, drug prophylaxis, and treatment. Arch Surg 112:1235, 1977.

63. Tustin AW, Kaiser AB, Bradsher RW, Herrington JL: Unusual fungal infections following jejunoileal bypass surgery. Arch Intern Med 140:643, 1980.

64. Hallberg D, Holmgren U: Bilio-intestinal shunt for treatment of obesity. Acta Chir Scand 145:405, 1979.

65. Hallberg DA: Survey of surgical techniques for treatment of obesity and a remark on the bilio-intestinal bypass method. Am J Clin Nutr (Suppl) 33:499, 1980.

66. Scopinaro N, Gianetta E, Civalleri D, Bonalumi U, Bachi V: Biliopancreatic bypass for obesity. II, Initial experience in man. Br J Surg 66:618, 1979.

67. Holian DK: Biliopancreatic bypass for morbid obesity. Contemp Surg 21:55, 1982.

Renal Complications Following Jejunoileal Bypass Surgery

CHARLES L. SMITH

Renal complications following jejunoileal bypass contribute 0.1% to the mortality rate of bypass surgery[1] and are the indication for reanastomosis in 4–13% of patients.[2,3] Although numerous renal complications have been reported (Table 3A-1), most of this appendix will deal with calcium oxalate urolithiasis since this is the most frequent renal problem.

Calcium Oxalate Urolithiasis

The incidence of calcium oxalate urolithiasis after intestinal bypass has been reported to be 2–32%.[4,5] The lower number is an underestimate since it includes only clinically evident stone disease. The higher value represents a more accurate estimate since it includes both symptomatic stones and clinically silent but radiologically present calculi.

An important component of this form of calcium oxalate stone disease is enteric hyperoxaluria. Modigliani et al[6] found hyperoxaluria in 91% of a group of patients with ileal resection. Hyperoxaluria has been reported to occur in 60–77% of bypass patients.[7,8] An incidence of 88% in stone formers and 60% in non–stone formers has been reported,[9] and in a group of 32 patients studied in this laboratory, 84% were hyperoxaluric by 12 months postbypass.

Mechanism of Hyperoxaluria

The mechanism of hyperoxaluria has been studied extensively. Hodgkinson[10] states that the average daily oxalate intake in the English diet is 130 mg (American diet, 80–100 mg/day[11]) of which only

TABLE 3A-1   Renal Complications of Jejunoileal Bypass

Calcium oxalate urolithiasis
Uric acid urolithiasis
Postoperative acute renal failure
Tubular proteinuria
Renal tubular acidosis
Uric acid nephropathy
Renal granulomas
Glomerulonephritis
Interstitial nephritis
Chronic renal failure

4–6 mg/day is absorbed. Between 10 and 50 mg/day is lost in the feces and 70 to 100 mg/day destroyed in the bowel by bacteria. Endogenous production amounts to 15–45 mg/day. Urinary oxalate is a product of endogenous production and gastrointestinal absorption and hyperoxaluria can occur if there is an increase in either of these sources.

The original hypothesis for hyperoxaluria in the short bowel syndrome implicated increased endogenous production. It was proposed that malabsorption led to an increased production of glycine-conjugated bile acids. Glycine was liberated from the bile acids by colonic bacteria and served as a source of glyoxylate. Since glyoxylate is a precursor of oxalate, an increase in this material would result in an increased endogenous production of oxalate.[12-14] This hypothesis became untenable when it was demonstrated that oral glycine appeared in the urine as oxalate at the same level in both patients with ileal resection and in controls.[15,16]

Another potential cause of increased endogenous production of oxalate is pyridoxine deficiency, which has been reported to cause hyperoxaluria in animals[17] and man.[18] Pyridoxine deficiency was not found in a patient reported by Smith et al[19] nor in five patients tested in our laboratory.

Increased endogenously produced oxalate could occur as an acquired metabolic defect similar to the genetic defects seen in primary hyperoxaluria.[20] In type I primary hyperoxaluria urinary excretion of glycolate is increased, whereas in type II glyceric acid excretion is increased. Neither is increased in ileal resection.[12] Also against increased endogenous production is the fact that urinary excretion of oxalate has been shown to decrease to normal levels on total parenteral nutrition.[21]

Since increased endogenous production did not seem to be the cause of hyperoxaluria, attention was directed to alterations in intestinal absorption of oxalate. Normally 3–5% of ingested oxalate is absorbed[22] and absorption occurs throughout the intestine by passive diffusion.[23] Absorption of oxalate is therefore dependent on the concentration of unbound oxalate within the intestine and the permeability of the intestinal mucosa.

Chadwick et al[15,16] were the first to demonstrate that orally administered radioactive oxalate appeared in the urine in increased amounts in patients with ileal dysfunction. This finding has been substantiated by other investigators.[24,25]

There are two hypotheses, which are not mutually exclusive, to explain intestinal hyperabsorption of oxalate. The first is the "solubility" hypothesis first proposed by Chadwick et al[26] and supported by Anderson and Jagenburg.[27] Low levels of free calcium within the intestine lead to high concentrations of unbound oxalate which will promote oxalate absorption.[22] Fat malabsorption occurs following intestinal bypass. Lipids within the intestinal lumen bind calcium lowering intraluminal free calcium concentration and leading to an increase in the concentration of unbound oxalate and subsequent increased absorption of oxalate. In support of this hypothesis are the following observations: (1) there is a good correlation between the degree of steatorrhea and hyperoxaluria;[27,28,29,30] (2) a low fat diet decreases oxalate excretion;[27] (3) substitution of medium chain triglycerides for fat in the diet reduces oxalate excretion;[31] (4) sodium oleate increases the solubility of calcium oxalate;[31] and (5) oral calcium supplementation reduces oxalate excretion.[25,31]

The "permeability" hypothesis was proposed by Dobbins and Binder.[26] They demonstrated that bile salts and long chain fatty acids caused a nonspecific increase in colonic mucosal permeability resulting in increased oxalate absorption, and felt this change in permeability was responsible for enteric hyperoxaluria. In support of this hypothesis are the following observations: (1) the colon is the primary site of oxalate hyperabsorption in ileal dysfunction;[6,28] (2) perfusion of bile acids into the colon of rhesus monkeys increases oxalate absorption;[32] (3) administration of an agent which binds bile acids (cholestyramine) reduces oxalate excretion*;[33] and (4) substitution of medium chain triglycerides for 50% of dietary lipids decreases colonic exposure to long chain fatty acids, and a fall in oxalate excretion has been observed.[34]

Probably both of these hypotheses play a role in enteric hyperoxaluria following jejunoileal bypass. The level of dietary oxalate, fat, and calcium along with the degree of malabsorption of long chain fatty acids and bile salts determine the degree of hyperoxaluria present.

Other factors can potentially play a role in stone formation in these patients. These include low urine volumes and decreased excretion of citrate and magnesium. During the first few months postbypass the urine volume drops significantly.[35] A combination of decreased intake and loss of fluids with frequent watery stools contributes to the low urine volume. Low urine volumes lead to an increase in the state of saturation of the urine increasing the likelihood of stone formation.[36]

Urinary citrate excretion begins to fall 1 month postbypass[35] and is significantly depressed at 2 months and 6 months. Concentration of citrate also decreases. Citrate is an inhibitor of calcium oxalate stone formation. The fall in citrate concentration could increase the propensity of the urine to precipitate calcium oxalate.

Citrate is handled in the kidney by filtration and reabsorption. Decreased excretion could be accounted for by decreased filtered load or increased renal tubular reabsorption.

Filtered load of citrate is decreased if there is a fall in glomerular filtration rate or a decrease

---

* Cholestyramine has also been shown to bind oxalate.[25] This may be the mechanism by which it has lowered urinary oxalate excretion in some studies.

in the blood level. The glomerular filtration rate is increased in obesity and decreases after jejunoileal bypass. Stockholm et al[37] found a 19% decrease at 49 ± 8.7 (SEM) months after bypass and we found a 19% decrease as early as 1 month postbypass. A decreased blood citrate level has also been reported.[38] Both the fall in glomerular filtration rate and decrease in blood citrate contribute to hypocitraturia by decreasing filtered load, but do not account for the marked fall seen (63% at 2 months in patients studied in this institution).

Renal handling of citrate has been shown to be affected following bypass with increased renal tubular reabsorption.[38] Tubular reabsorption of citrate is increased by hypokalemia and acidosis.[39] Normal blood potassium levels and blood pH in our patients and those of others[38] would rule out these causes. Rudman et al[38] proposed that the low urinary magnesium excretion found postbypass plays a role in hypocitraturia. Magnesium binds citrate making it less available for tubular reabsorption. Low urinary magnesium would increase the level of free citrate in the urine available for reabsorption and thus decrease citrate excretion.

Magnesium excretion is decreased in patients with inflammatory bowel disease.[40] Following intestinal bypass it falls within 1 month[35] and remains low as long as the bypass is in place. Decreased urinary magnesium could contribute to stone formation by altering tubular citrate handling (see above). Magnesium is also an inhibitor of calcium oxalate stone formation[41] and increases the solubility of calcium oxalate.[42] Deficiency of urinary magnesium has been shown to increase precipitation of calcium oxalate[43] and magnesium in pharmacologic doses has been used to treat idiopathic calcium oxalate stone disease.[44]

Several changes take place in the renal excretion of other substances which protect against the occurence of calcium phosphate and uric acid stone disease. Urinary calcium and phosphorus excretion fall following bypass, a reflection of decreased intake and malabsorption.[45] When saturation studies were done in our laboratory, the urines were undersaturated for calcium phosphate but supersaturated for calcium oxalate, reflecting the predominance of calcium oxalate stone disease.[46]

Uric acid stones are unusual after bypass but do occur.[9,47] Uric acid excretion was decreased postbypass at 1, 2, and 6 months in our patients. Other researchers have shown either no change[40]

or an increased uric acid excretion[48] when patients were studied after a longer period of time. Uric acid stones can form when urine volumes are low and the urine pH is acidic,[49] and these may be the major contributing factors when such stones have formed.

In summary, calcium oxalate urolithiasis can occur in up to 32% of patients following intestinal bypass surgery[5] and accounted for 13% of the patients requiring dismantling of their intestinal bypass in one recent study.[3] This stone disease is due to the development of enteric hyperoxaluria and a low urine volume. There is also a decrease in the excretion of citrate and magnesium which may lower the capacity of the urine to inhibit calcium oxalate stone disease.

Management of Urolithiasis

Management of stone disease following intestinal bypass surgery has been primarily directed to decreasing the hyperoxaluria. Taurine was initially reported to decrease oxalate excretion.[12,13] The proposed mechanism was a decrease in glycine-conjugated bile acids due to increased taurine-conjugated bile acids. Taurine was not found to lower oxalate excretion in later studies.[33,48]

Cholestyramine was used to lower oxalate excretion[25,33] and has been shown to bind oxalate within the intestine making it unavailable for absorption.[25] It may have an added effect of binding bile salts, decreasing the effects of bile salts on colonic mucosal permeability. Others have not been able to demonstrate a decrease in oxalate excretion with cholestyramine[50,51] and the expense and lack of patient acceptance make this an unsatisfactory long-term therapy.

High dose pyridoxine therapy aimed at decreasing endogenous production of oxalate has not altered hyperoxaluria in this group of patients in the absence of pyridoxine deficiency.[12,33]

Based on the accepted mechanism for enteric hyperoxaluria, low fat diets are recommended to patients following intestinal bypass and have been shown to lower urinary oxalate excretion.[27,31] Substituting medium chain triglycerides for 50% of the dietary fat also decreases hyperoxaluria.[31] Added benefits of the low fat diet are less diarrhea and an increase in urine output.

Low oxalate diets are obviously a rational form of therapy since hyperoxaluria is due to increased absorption of dietary oxalate. Oxalate is common in many foods and adherence to restriction of these foods is difficult to obtain. One of the criteria for acceptance for bypass surgery is failure of dietary therapy to control obesity.[50] This previous failure of dietary therapy usually continues postbypass when attempting a low fat, low oxalate diet to control enteric hyperoxaluria.

Supplemental oral calcium has been shown to decrease oxalate excretion.[30,31] The mechanism is presumably one of oxalate binding in the intestine to make oxalate insoluble and therefore nonabsorbable. The dose must be titrated to the maximum benefit of lowering urinary oxalate without significantly increasing urinary calcium excretion. This usually does not result in decreasing oxalate excretion to normal levels.

Other agents will bind oxalate within the intestine and aluminum antacids have been shown to lower oxalate excretion.[52] This therapy should be approached cautiously. Hypophosphatemia can be induced by antacid use.[53,54] The malabsorption following intestinal bypass also leads to hypophosphatemia.[55] The combined effects of malabsorption and antacids can lead to an increased incidence of hypophosphatemia with a number of severe metabolic abnormalities[56] including hypercalciuria[57] thus promoting stone formation.[53]

Gregory[58] has used alkali therapy. He feels this leads to increased formation of soluble calcium complexes in the urine making calcium unavailable to combine with oxalate. Further studies of this therapy are warranted.

Attention should also be directed to the other factors promoting stone formation, i.e., low urine volume, hypomagnesiuria, and hypocitraturia. Increasing urine volume has been shown to decrease states of saturation.[36] Maintaining a urine volume of 2–3 liter/day is the goal but difficult to achieve since increased fluid intake frequently stimulates diarrhea.[55,59]

Oral supplements of magnesium should be tried to increase magnesium excretion. Severe cases of hypomagnesemia require parenteral magnesium therapy.

Oral supplements of sodium bicarbonate or citrate solutions alone have not been effective in increasing urinary citrate excretion to normal. One study suggests that citrate excretion can be brought to normal levels by the use of parenteral magnesium and oral citrate.[38]

Short-term success in preventing recurrent stone disease has been reported with each of these treatments. However, in our experience none of these therapies has been successful in those who recurrently form stones and restoring bowel continuity is usually required.

Following reanastomosis stone formation should cease. Because of the calcium malabsorption that occurs when the bypass is in place, urinary calcium remains low after reanastomosis. Combined with a fall in oxalate excretion to normal, the degree of supersaturation for calcium oxalate will decrease. A case of in situ dissolution of calcium oxalate stones has been reported following reanastomosis.[19] The urinary calcium and oxalate excretions should be measured after reconstitution surgery because if urinary calcium rises to normal levels, preexisting stones could grow.

Other Renal Complications

Although nephrolithiasis is the most common renal complication of jejunoileal bypass, a number of other disturbances have been reported.

The incidence of early postoperative renal failure has been reported to be from 0 to 9%.[60] Evidence of renal tubular dysfunction includes cases of tubular proteinuria[61] and renal tubular acidosis.[62,63,64]

One case of gouty nephropathy has been recorded.[59] Liver granulomas have occured in 7% of patients[65] and a case of renal granulomas associated with liver granulomas has been reported.[66] Glomerulonephritis associated with mixed cryoglobulinemia and immune deposits in the glomeruli[67,68,69] has been reported. These studies suggest that the antigen involved is bacterial in origin and from the bypassed segment of the intestine.

An early report showed normal renal biopsies in three patients[70] but a later study showed 17 of 18 patients to have interstitial nephritis.[67] In addition eight of 18 had tubular atrophy, 16 of 18 had glomerular hyalinosis, and eight of 18 had oxalate deposits. Only four of 18 had functional renal impairment, suggesting significant histologic disease can be present with normal renal function as assessed by endogenous creatinine clearance.

Renal failure has been reported late in the course.[47,71,72,73,74,75] Most often this has been associated with renal oxalosis but has also been associated with glomerulonephritis.[68]

Follow-up of patients after jejunoileal bypass

should include investigations for renal complications. We recommend yearly monitoring with a flat plate of the abdomen, urinalysis, and serum creatinine. Radiologic evaluation will detect those patients with clinically silent calcium oxalate stones. The urinalysis will detect hematuria, pyuria, or proteinuria and a rising serum creatinine will indicate impairment of renal function. If renal function is deteriorating in the absence of stone disease and especially if proteinuria or sterile pyuria is present, consideration should be given to a renal biopsy to define the cause. When impairment of renal function occurs, continuity of the bowel should be restored.

Renal complications following jejunoileal bypass are frequent and varied. Calcium oxalate urolithiasis is the most common problem and is difficult to manage in recurrent stone formers. Other complications, however, are also significant and not infrequently lead to impairment of renal function.

References to Appendix

1. Anderson T, Jukl E, Quaade F: Fatal outcome after jejunoileal bypass for obesity. Am J Surg 142:619–621, 1981.
2. Griffen WO, Hostetter JM, Bell RM, Birins BA, Bannon C: Experiences with conversion of jejunoileal bypass to gastric bypass: its use for maintenance of weight loss. Arch Surg 116:320–324, 1981.
3. Halverson JD, Gentry K, Wise L, Ballinger WF: Reanastomosis after jejunoileal bypass. Surgery 84:241–249, 1978.
4. Dickstein SS, Frame B: Urinary tract calculi after intestinal shunt operations for treatment of obesity. Surg Gynecol Obstet 136:257–260, 1973.
5. Gourlay RH, Reynolds C: Complications of surgery for morbid obesity. Am J Surg 136:54–57, 1978.
6. Modigliani R, Labayle D, Aymes C, Denvil R: Evidence for excessive absorption of oxalate by the colon in enteric hyperoxaluria. Scand J Gastroenterology 13:187–192, 1978.
7. Fikri E, Casella RR: Hyperoxaluria and urinary tract calculi after jejunoileal bypass. Am J Surg 129:334–336, 1975.
8. Starkloff GB, Wolfe BM, Ramach KR: Management of complications following intestinal bypass for morbid obesity. Missouri Med 71:119–121, 1974.
9. Gregory JG, Starkloff ZG, Miyai K, Schoenberg HW: Urologic complications of ileal bypass operation for morbid obesity. J Urol 113:521–524, 1975.
10. Hodgkinson A: Oxalate metabolism in animals and man. In: Oxalic Acid in Biology and Medicine. New York, Academic Press, 1977, p 159.
11. Ney DM, Hoffman AF, Fischer C, Stubblefield N: The Low Oxalate Diet Book for Prevention of Oxalate Kidney Stones. San Diego, California, University of California, 1981.
12. Admirand WH, Earnest DL, Williams HE: Hyperoxaluria and bowel disease. Trans Assoc Am Physicians 84:307–312, 1971.
13. Dowling RH, Rose GA, Sutor DJ: Hyperoxaluria and renal calculi in ileal disease. Lancet 1:1103–1106, 1971.
14. Hoffman AF, Thomas PI, Smith LH, McCall JT: Pathogenesis of secondary hyperoxaluria in patients with ileal resection and diarrhea. Gastroenterology 58A:960, 1970.
15. Chadwick VS, Modha K, Dowling RH: Pathogenesis of secondary hyperoxaluria in patients with ileal resection. Gut 13A:840, 1972.
16. Chadwick VS, Elias E, Modha K, Dowling RH: Pathogenesis and treatment of secondary hyperoxaluria in patients with ileal resection. Q J Med 42A:826, 1973.
17. Gershoff SN, Faragalla FF, Nelson DA, Andrus SB: Vitamin B_6 deficiency and oxalate nephrocalcinosis in the cat. Am J Med 27:72–80, 1959.
18. Ludwig GD: Renal calculi associated with hyperoxaluria. Ann NY Acad Sci 104:621–637, 1963.
19. Smith CL, Linner JH: Dissolution of calcium oxalate renal stones in patients with jejunoileal bypass and after reanastomosis. Urology 19:21–23, 1982.
20. Williams HE: Oxalic acid and the hyperoxaluric syndromes. Kidney Int 13:410–417, 1978.
21. Bachman L, Eliasson B, Larsson L: Studies on endogenous oxalate production after jejunoileostomy for treatment of obesity. In Brockis JG, Finlayson B (eds): Urinary Calculus: International Urinary Stone Conference. Little Town, Mass., PSG, 1979, p 169.
22. Zarembski PM, Hodgkinson A: Some factors influencing the urinary excretion of oxalic acid in man. Clin Chim Acta 25:1–10, 1969.
23. Binder HJ: Intestinal oxalate absorption. Gastroenterology 67:441–446, 1974.
24. Earnest DL, Williams HE, Admirand WH: Excessive absorption of oxalate contributes to hyperoxaluria in patients with ileal disease. Gastroenterology 64A:723, 1973.
25. Stauffer JQ, Humphreys MH, Weir GJ: Acquired hyperoxaluria with regional enteritis after ileal resection: role of dietary oxalate. Ann Intern Med 79:383–391, 1973.
26. Chadwick VS, Modha K, Dowling RH: Mecha-

nism for hyperoxaluria in patients with ileal dysfunction. N Engl J Med 289:172–176, 1973.

27. Anderson H, Jagenburg R: Fat-reduced diet in the treatment of hyperoxaluria in patients with ileopathy. Gut 15:360–366, 1974.

28. Earnest DL, Johnson G, Williams HE, Admirand WH: Hyperoxaluria in patients with ileal resection: An abnormality in dietary oxalate absorption. Gastroenterology 66:1114–1122, 1974.

29. McDonald GB, Earnest DL, Admirand WH: Hyperoxaluria correlates with steatorrhea in patients with celiac sprue. Gastroenterology 68A:949, 1975.

30. Stauffer JQ, Stewart JR, Bertand F: Acquired hyperoxaluria: relationship to dietary calcium content and severity of steatorrhea. Gastroenterology 66A:783, 1974.

31. Earnest DL, Williams HE, Admirand WH: A physiochemical basis for treatment of enteric hyperoxaluria. Trans Assoc Am Physicians 88:224–232, 1975.

32. Chadwick VS: Hyperoxaluria and ileal dysfunction. N Engl J Med 290:108, 1974.

33. Smith LH, Fromm H, Hoffman AF: Acquired hyperoxaluria, nephrolithiasis, and intestinal disease: description of a syndrome. N Engl J Med 286:1371–1375, 1972.

34. Dobbins JW, Binder HJ: Effects of bile salts and fatty acids on the colonic absorption of oxalate. Gastroenterology 70:1096–1100, 1976.

35. Smith CL, Linner JH, Wathen RL: Urinary oxalate excretion following ileo-jejunal bypass surgery for morbid obesity. Clin Res 24:370A, 1976.

36. Pak CYC, Sakhu K, Crowther C, Brinkley L: Evidence justifying a high fluid intake in treatment of nephrolithiasis. Ann Intern Med 93:36–39, 1980.

37. Stockholm KH, Hoilund-Carlson PF, Brochner-Mortenson J: Glomerular-filtration rate after jejunoilel bypass for obesity. Int J Obes 5:77–80, 1981.

38. Rudman D, Dedonis JL, Fountain MT, Chandler JB, Gerron GG, Fleming GA, Kutner MH: Hypocitraturia in patients with gastrointestinal malabsorption. N Engl J Med 303:657–661, 1980.

39. Cohn JJ, Barac-Nieto M: Renal metabolism of substrates in relation to renal function. IV. Renal metabolism of citrate. In Orlaff J, Berliner RW (eds): Handbook of Physiology. Section 8: Renal Physiology. Washington, D.C., American Physiological Society, 1973, pp 948–961.

40. Farmer RG, Mir-Madjlessi SH, Kiser WS: Urinary excretion of oxalate, calcium, magnesium, and uric acid in inflammatory bowel disease. Cleve Clin Q 41:109–117, 1974.

41. Fleisch H: Inhibitors and promoters of stone formation. Kidney Int 13:361–371, 1978.

42. Hammarstein G: On calcium oxalate and its solubility in the presence of inorganic salts with special reference to the occurrence of oxaluria. CR Travaux Lab Carlsberg 17:1–83, 1929.

43. Hallson PC, Rose GA, Sulaiman S: Magnesium reduces calcium oxalate crystal formation in human whole urine. Clin Sci 62:17–19, 1982.

44. Johansson G, Backman U, Danielson BG, Fellstrom B, Ljunghall S, Wikstrom B: Biochemical and clinical effects of the prophylactic treatment of renal calcium stones with magnesium hydroxide. J Urol 124:770–774, 1980.

45. Crisp AH, Kalucy RS, Pilington TRE, Gazet JC: Some psychosocial consequences of ileojejunal bypass surgery. Am J Clin Nutr 30:109–119, 1977.

46. Clayman RV, Williams RD: Oxalate urolithiasis following jejunoileal bypass: mechanism and management. Surg Clin North Am 59:1071–1077, 1979.

47. Gelbart DR, Brewer LL, Fajardo LF, Weinstein AB: Oxalosis and chronic renal failure after intestinal bypass. Arch Intern Med 137:239–243, 1977.

48. O'Leary JP, Thomas WC, Woodward ER: Urinary tract stone after small bowel bypass for morbid obesity. Am J Surg 127:142–147, 1974.

49. Pyrah LN: Uric acid calculi. In: Renal Calculus. New York, Springer-Verlag, 1979, pp 320–338.

50. Halverson JD: Obesity surgery in perspective. Surgery 87:119–127, 1980.

51 Starkloff GG, Donovan JF, Ramaeh R, Wolfe BM: Metabolic intestinal surgery: its complications and management. Arch Sug 110:652–657, 1975.

52. Earnest DL: Perspectives on incidence, etiology, and treatment of enteric hyperoxaluria. Am J Clin Nutr 30:72–75, 1977.

53. Cooke N, Teitlbaum S, Avioli LV: Antacid-induced osteomalacia and nephrolithiasis. Arch Intern Med 138:1007–1009, 1978.

54. Insogna KL, Bordley DR, Caro JF, Lockwood DH: Osteomalacia and weakness from excess antacid ingestion. JAMA 244:2544–2546, 1980.

55. Franck WA, Hoffman GS, Davis JS, Alpern HD, Olson JE: Osteomalacia and weakness complicating jejunoileal bypass. J Rheumatol 6:51–56, 1979.

56. Knochel JP: Hypophosphatemia. Clin Nephrol 7:131–137, 1977.

57. Coburn JW, Massry SG: Changes in serum and urinary calcium during phosphate depletion: studies on mechanisms. J Clin Invest 49:1073–1087, 1970.

58. Gregory JG: Hyperoxaluria and stone disease in the gastrointestinal bypass patient. Urol Clin North Am 8:331–351, 1981.

59. Dean RH, Scott W, Shull HJ, Gluck FW: Morbid obesity: problems associated with operative management. Am J Clin Nutr 30:90–97, 1977.

60. Bray GA, Benfield JR: Intestinal bypass for obe-

sity: a summary and perspective. Am J Clin Nutr 30:121–127, 1977.

61. Hey H, Skaarup P, Solling K, Christensen MS, Lund B, Sorensen OH, Lund B: Tubular proteinuria following jejunoileal bypass surgery. Int J Obes 5:155–161, 1981.

62. Jensen JB, Nielsen IL, Hensen HE, Nielsen B: Renal tubular acidosis as a complication of jejunoileostomy in obese patients. Ugeskr Lalger 138:2742–2745, 1977.

63. Payne JH, DeWind L, Schwab CE, Kern WH: Surgical treatment of morbid obesity: 16 years of experience. Arch Surg 106:432–436, 1973.

64. Vainder M, Kelly J: Renal tubular dysfunction secondary to jejunoileal bypass. JAMA 235:1257–1258, 1976.

65. Halverson JD, Wise L, Wazna MF, Ballinger WF: Jejunoileal bypass for morbid obesity: A critical appraisal. Am J Med 64:461–475, 1978.

66. Sweet RM, Smith CL, Berkseth RB, Crosson JT, Wathen RL: Jejunoileal bypass surgery and granulomatous disease of the kidney and liver. Arch Intern Med 138:626–627, 1978.

67. Drenick EJ, Stanley TM, Border WA, Zawada ET, Dornfield LP, Upham T, Llach F: Renal damage with intestinal bypass. Ann Intern Med 89:594–599, 1978.

68. Gamble CN, Kinichi A, Dynn TA, Christensen D: Immune complex glomerulonephritis and dermal vasculitis following intestinal bypass for morbid obesity. Am J Clin Pathol 77:347–352, 1982.

69. Utsinger PD: Systemic immune complex disease following intestinal bypass surgery. J Am Acad Dermatol 2:488–495, 1980.

70. Payne JH, DeWind LT, Commons RR: Metabolic observations in patients with jejunocolic shunts. Am J Surg 106:273–289, 1963.

71. Cryer PE, Garber AJ, Hoffstein P, Luca B, Wise L: Renal failure after small intestinal bypass for obesity. Arch Intern Med 135:1610–1612, 1975.

72. Das S, Joseph B, Dick AL: Renal failure owing to oxalate nephrosis after jejunoileal bypass. J Urol 121:506–509, 1979.

73. DeWind LT, Payne JH: Intestinal bypass surgery for morbid obesity: long-term results. JAMA 236:2298–2301, 1976.

74. Ehlers SM, Posalaky Z, Strate RG, Quattlebaum FW: Acute reversible renal failure following jejunoileal bypass for morbid obesity: a clinical and pathological (EM) study of a case. Surgery 82:628–633, 1977.

75. Scott, HW, Dean RH, Shull HJ, Gluck F: Results of jejunoileal bypass in 200 patients with morbid obesity. Surg Gynecol Obstet 145:661–673, 1977.

CHAPTER 4

Gastric Operations: General Principles

JOHN H. LINNER

Gastric reduction operations, with and without distal gastric exclusion, were developed by Mason and Ito[1,2] at the University of Iowa from 1965 to 1971. These procedures have undergone a host of modifications by their originators as well as by others.[3-6,46] The prototype was a Billroth II gastric bypass but without resection of the distal stomach (Figs. 4-1 and 4-2). The stomach was transected horizontally across the upper fundus, totally separating the distal stomach from the proximal gastric pouch, which was anastomosed to a loop of jejunum. Suture technique was used. In 1971 Mason altered the procedure by partially transecting the stomach from the lesser curvature, leaving a channel on the greater curvature—the first gastroplasty (Fig. 4-3).[3] Alden[7] introduced the use of the staple instrument to provide an in-continuity division between the upper pouch and distal stomach. This simplified the operation and made it safer (Fig. 4-4). Griffen[6] was among the first to use a Roux-en-Y gastrojejunostomy instead of a loop (Fig. 4-5). Gomez[8] is credited with improving the Mason gastroplasty, which led the way to a number of variations and continuing evaluation (Figs. 4-6–4-13).[9-14,39] The failure rate was high in the early generation of operations, and there is to date no clear consensus among surgeons as to which procedure is the best. All have advantages and disadvantages, and most have too short a follow-up to permit a conclusive judgment.

At the University of Iowa Bariatric Colloquium, June 2–3, 1983,[50] a questionnaire responded to by 149 surgeons revealed that 112 (75%) were doing some form of gastroplasty, and 37 (25%) either a Roux-en-Y or loop gastric by-pass. Although a large majority indicated a current preference for gastroplasty over gastric bypass, it does not necessarily follow that the former will prove to be the better operation over the long term. The current popularity of gastroplasty-type operations relates primarily to their simplicity, shorter operating time, and preservation of normal gastrointestinal tract continuity.[13-15] On the other hand, few if any long-term gastroplasty series have shown weight loss results equal to those with gastric bypass. Most comparative studies of 2 years or longer have revealed a much higher incidence of weight loss failure with gastroplasty than gastric bypass.[28,38,49] There are, of course, various types of gastroplasties, some more effective than others,[45] and these, together with gastric bypass operations, will be discussed in more detail later.

At least as important as the type of operative technique is patient selection, education, and follow-up. Any one of the many recommended operations can be defeated by a poorly motivated, uncooperative patient.

Selection Criteria

Intractable Morbid Obesity

The surgical treatment of obesity should be limited to morbidly obese patients who have failed to respond to conservative methods, as stressed in Chapter 1.

At the National Institutes of Health Consensus Development Conference on Surgical Treatment of Morbid Obesity,[15] this subset of obese patients

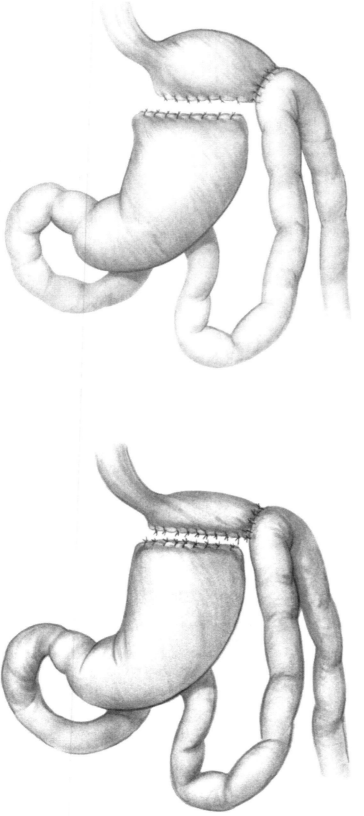

FIG. 4-1. Mason: gastric bypass (1966–70).

FIG. 4-2. Mason: gastric bypass—smaller pouch (1975).

FIG. 4-3. Mason: gastroplasty (1971).

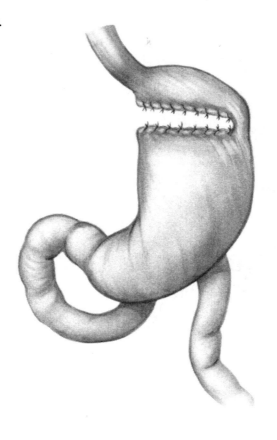

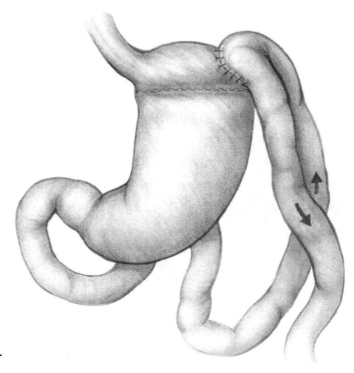

FIG. 4-4. Alden: loop-type incontinuity gastric bypass with staple partition (1977).

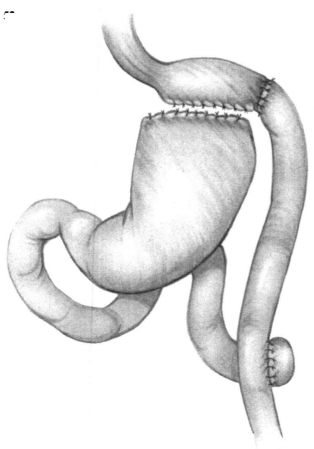

FIG. 4-5 Mason–Griffen: Roux-en-Y gastric bypass (1977). A. Transecton of upper stomach. B. Stomach stapled in continuity.

A

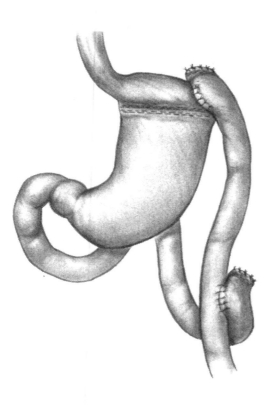

B

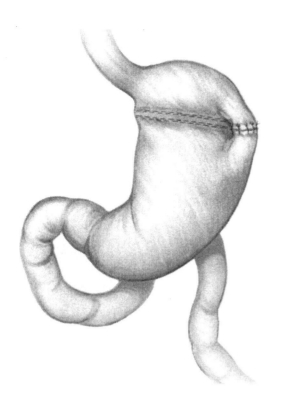

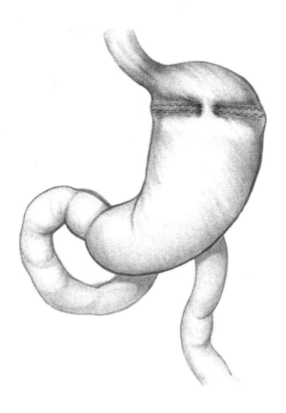

FIG. 4-6. Gomez: greater curvature gastroplasty (1978).

FIG. 4-7. Pace–Martin–Carey: gastric partition operation (1979).

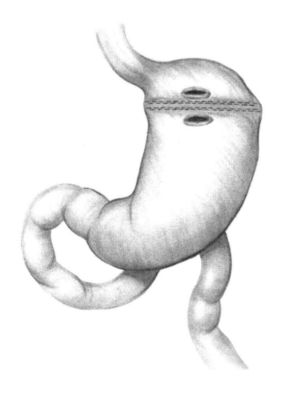

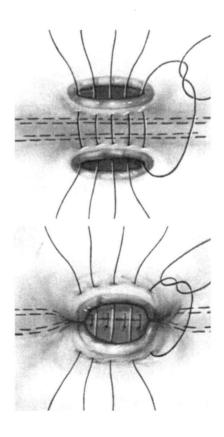

FIG. 4-8. LaFave–Alden: gastrogastrostomy: anterior type (1979).

53

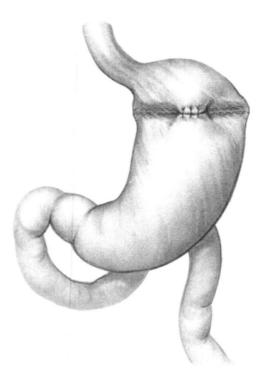

FIG. 4-9. Gastrostomy: anterior type complete.

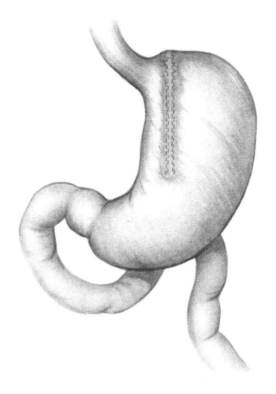

FIG. 4-10. Tretbar: tubular–vertical gastroplasty.

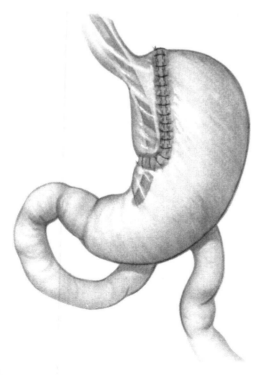

A

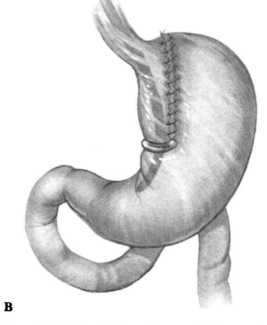

B

FIG. 4-11. Fabito–Eckhout–Laws: vertical gastroplasty (1979). **A** Purse string. **B** Silastic catheter–supported outlet.

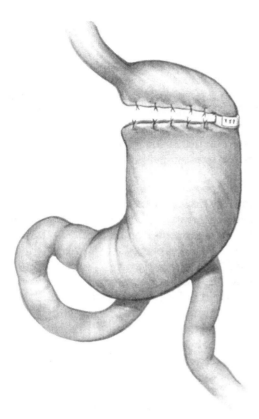 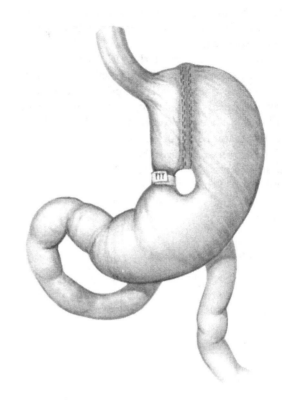

FIG. 4-12. Mason: horizontal-supported gastroplasty (1977–80).

FIG. 4-13. Mason: vertical-banded gastroplasty (1980–83).

was characterized as those who were 100 lb or 100% or more over ideal weight, with serious physical and psychosocial problems, who have failed to improve on adequate trials of nonsurgical treatment, or who have repeatedly relapsed after initial periods of weight loss. "Surgery may then be viewed as a final attempt at weight control in which the risks inherent to the procedure are accepted as an alternative to a life of incapacity, dysfunction, and accelerated mortality."[16]

Standards for Overweight

The two generally accepted standards used by most surgeons as well as third party payers in the United States as the minimal eligible overweight for surgical treatment are 45.2 kg (100 lb) over or double the ideal weight based on Metropolitan Life Insurance Company tables for normal height and weight.[17] The higher figure for the weight range at any particular height or body build

is used to determine excess weight; usually the "medium frame" category is chosen. If the patient's height is measured in stocking feet, 2 in are added to the height for females and 1 in for males. An approximation of the tables can be derived by assuming an ideal weight of 100 lb for a 5-ft female, and 110 lb for a 5-ft male, and adding 5 lb for each inch over 5 ft, plus 5 lb for a medium frame and 10 lb for a heavy frame.[18]

The use of the body-mass index (BMI = Weight in kg/Height in meters^2)[18] or the Broca index (BI = Weight in kg/Height in centimeters − 100) yields a numerical value that reflects both height and weight and is more meaningful than weight alone. The normal BMI would be from 20 to 25, and morbid obesity would be over 40. The normal BI would be 0.8 to 1.0, with morbid obesity over 1.7

Despite the theoretical advantage of these indices, however, most surgeons in the United States use the 100 lb or double ideal weight standards because they are simpler and accepted by most medical insurance companies as criteria for reimbursement.

Although at present the risk/benefit equation justifies selecting for surgery only the morbidly obese patient who fulfills the criteria noted above, sound clinical judgment must be applied, and occasionally an exception to this rule is justifiable, as for example, a patient who may not be quite 100 lb overweight but has painful degenerative arthritis involving one or more joints of the lower extremity. Prosthetic joint replacement would be an added indication for preliminary obesity surgery.

Associated Conditions

Other commonly associated medical conditions that are improved by this type of surgery and are a further indication for it are the following:

1. Hypertension
2. Pickwickian syndrome
3. Diabetes mellitus
4. Gout
5. Venous stasis with edema and ulcerations
6. Family history of arteriosclerotic heart disease with possible premature stroke or myocardial infarction

Contraindications

Contraindications to surgery are as follows:

1. Enteropathies (granulomatous enteritis, ulcerative colitis)
2. Malignancies
3. Certain systemic diseases (lupus erythematosus, cirrhosis of the liver, Cushing's disease, severe atherosclerotic heart disease with congestive failure)
4. Drug dependency or alcoholism, unless the patient has undergone treatment and is at least 1 year into an ongoing sobriety program such as Alcoholics Anonymous.
5. Almost all psychoses, and certain psychoneurotic conditions, particularly paranoia and conversion hysteria; patients who exhibit unrealistic expectations should not be operated upon until they completely understand what to expect from the operation and the role they must play in its successful outcome (see Chapter 2)

Relative Contraindications

Peptic Ulcer Disease
If the patient has a healed duodenal ulcer and there are no recent complications such as bleeding or perforation, gastric bypass can be combined with truncal vagotomy and pyloroplasty. We have done this successfully in six patients. More recently we have eliminated the pyloroplasty unless peptic ulceration is accompanied by pyloric obstruction.

Alveolar Hypoventilation Syndrome
Patients with pickwickian syndrome should not be operated upon until they have undergone careful respiratory function studies, and have achieved maximum benefit from a 2- to 4-week period of intensive respiratory therapy, preferably in the hospital. Sleep laboratory studies should be done to rule out the sleep apnea syndrome due to obstructive disease of the upper airway, which is best treated by a tracheostomy prior to surgery.[19]

Other patients with restrictive or obstructive lung disease, with or without hypercarbia, should be on a very low calorie (VLC) diet or a protein-sparing modified fast (PSMF),[16] respiratory physiotherapy, diuretics, and where indicated, digitalis. Smoking, of course, must be discontinued.

Lyons and Huang[20] found in eight morbidly obese patients that alveolar hyperventilation was improved by the administration of 100 mg progesterone intramuscularly daily. Although the mechanism of action is unknown, progesterone apparently acts as a respiratory stimulant, as it does in the last trimester of pregnancy, improving blood gas concentrations and restoring normal respiratory center sensitivity to hypercarbia with an increase in oxygen consumption. These patients should be informed that it may be necessary for them to remain on a respirator in the intensive care unit for several days following surgery.

Coronary Artery Disease with Congestive Heart Failure
The risk of surgery is too great for the possible benefit unless intensive medical therapy with a VLC or PSMF diet, diuretics, digitalis, and respiratory physiotherapy results in sufficient improvement.

Multiple Sclerosis
Obese patients with multiple sclerosis can benefit by surgery, although they often do not achieve an optimal result owing to lack of exercise.

Junk Food Consumers

Some patients consume an excessive number of soft drinks, usually in the form of nondiet caffeine-containing colas, up to eight bottles and more a day. The soda is usually accompanied by junk foods. These patients must understand that if they are unable to eliminate such items from their diet they should not have the operation because it will most likely fail. They should discontinue the use of these products for at least 1 month preoperatively to demonstrate to themselves as well as the surgeon that they can control this habit. This is particularly true for any gastric reduction operation without a gastrojejunal anastomosis (gastroplasty), because with these procedures there is no deterrent to sweets as there often is with the gastric bypass.

Age

Eighteen to 50 years is the optimal age span, but exceptions are made quite frequently. We have operated on patients from 14 to 63 years of age. Older patients usually do not lose as much weight as those in the optimal age group, and the risk of surgery is increased.

Education and Informed Consent

A technically perfect operation may end in failure unless the patient has been thoroughly indoctrinated preoperatively. Although important, it is not enough to have covered only the perioperative and remote complications of surgery. The ramifications peculiar to these procedures involve almost every aspect of the patient's life: marital, sexual, emotional, interpersonal, occupational, but most importantly, their capacity to eat, and they must be made aware of the possible consequences. If they have been properly informed these effects are usually positive, and the majority of patients accept surprisingly well the drastic restrictions imposed upon their eating habits. In fact, they are delighted with the prompt postprandial satiety resulting from small food portions, and the freedom they now experience from the usual bête noire of the obese: diet–depression–gluttony–guilt. The reduced gastric capacity serves as a regulator that protects most patients from the tyranny of compulsive overeating.

Patient education begins with the first visit. In our practice patients fill out a form (Appendix 1) that includes questions such as age at onset of obesity, family history, associated medical conditions, and the extent and type of weight-reduction methods already employed. They are also given a nine-page informed consent pamphlet (Appendix 2) that describes the indications and rationale for surgery, the risks and benefits, the impact surgery has on dietary habits, the necessity of energy expenditure to achieve optimal results, and the importance of lifetime follow-up. The most commonly used operations are diagramed in the pamphlet. The recommended procedure is then explained in detail during this visit. The pamphlet is primarily designed for the patient to study at home, and to raise any questions at a later date.

The process of patient education is time consuming and cannot be rushed or curtailed. Patients vary considerably in their ability to comprehend, and some are so excited during the first visit they remember little of what was said. A few are incapable of reading the pamphlet, and this situation must be ascertained early and appropriate verbal education substituted. Paramedical personnel are frequently involved as a part of the teaching process, but the surgeon must become involved on a one-to-one basis with the patient at some time preoperatively to establish the rapport which is absolutely vital for an optimal result. The surgeon must also be assured that the patient thoroughly comprehends all the significant consequences of the operation. In some of the larger clinics patient education becomes a multidisciplinary effort involving many health care personnel: a psychiatrist, dietitian, internist, patient representative, and others.[16] The initial education is often in the form of a group session, which is a time-saving technique, but at some point each patient must have the opportunity to discuss his or her particular situation with the surgeon on an individual basis.

The surgical candidate can often be reassured by talking to patients who have had the operation.

The Medical Work-up

The preoperative work-up varies in complexity depending on the patient's age, weight, and associated medical conditions. Obviously a patient who is three times ideal weight with chronic respiratory insufficiency is going to require a longer and more extensive work-up than a young, healthy patient who is twice ideal weight and has no other serious medical problems. In the interest of cost effectiveness some surgeons recommend an abbreviated work-up in otherwise healthy patients.[21] This usually includes a routine history and physical examination, chest x ray, complete blood count, partial thromboplastin time, prothrombin time, blood type and screen, and urinalysis. At the other extreme, some large centers prefer an elaborate series of examinations in every case.[16] We have adopted a middle course between these extremes, with a standard work-up for all patients and additional studies when indicated. We usually request the referring primary physician to carry out our standard preoperative protocol if he is interested and qualified to do so. Otherwise the patient is referred to a medical consultant with a known interest in this field. In either case the surgeon must be assured that the preoperative work-up has been satisfactory.

Patients with known or suspected psychoneurotic disease are referred to a psychiatrist for evaluation, who usually includes a Minnesota Multiphasic Personality Inventory as part of the examination. Those with schizophrenia, schizoid personalities, paranoid neuroses, conversion hysteria, or active drug dependency are rejected for surgery. Patients with endogenous depression or severe anxiety neurosis who undergo surgery must be followed by a psychiatrist for an indefinite period depending upon the severity of the condition (see Chapter 2).

The preoperative work-up for our patients includes the following studies and must be individualized, some patients requiring a more detailed evaluation than others.

* 1. History and physical examination, including dental evaluation (a dentist is involved only if dental care is required)
  2. Proctoscopic examination (patients with colorectal symptoms)
  3. Barium enema examination (patients with a change in bowel habits or other colon symptoms)
  4. IVP (in patients with hypertension, or with a history of renal calculi, gout, or hematuria)
*5. Upper GI tract examination
*6. Cholecystogram

---

* These tests are most important and are usually done on all patients.

*7. Chest x-ray examination
*8. EKG
 9. Pulmonary function studies (selected symptomatic patients)
*10. CBC
*11. SMA-12
*12. Electrolytes
 13. Serum lipids (triglycerides, total cholesterol, HDL, LDL, VLDL)
 14. Serum cortisol (when Cushing's disease is suspected; when indicated additional adrenocortical laboratory studies are conducted)
 15. Glucose tolerance test (selected patients)
*16. Urinalysis
 17. T3, T4 examination (usually has already been done)
 18. MMPI and psychiatric evaluation when indicated

Preoperative Management

Most patients are admitted shortly after noon on the day prior to surgery.

Immediate Preoperative Gastric Bypass–Gastroplasty Orders

1. Low residue diet entire preoperative day: clear liquid diet for JIB reconstitution; nothing by mouth after midnight
2. Hemoglobin, WBC, differential, urinalysis, type and screen, coagulation survey, serum electrolytes (recent outpatient tests do not need to be repeated if normal)
3. Magnesium citrate, 8 oz, or castor oil, 60 ml, 6–8 P.M.
4. Flurazepam hydrochloride (Dalmane) 30 mg or temazepam (Restoril) 30 mg. h.s. (after laxative action is over); repeat once p.r.n.
5. Shower bath the night before surgery
6. Dulcolax suppository early A.M.
7. Insert No. 16 Foley catheter (5-ml bag) early A.M. (if patient objects, it can be done in the operating room)
8. Elastic (TED) stockings or 6-in Ace bandage, foot to knee, early A.M.
9. Call anesthesiologist for preoperative medication or diazepam (Valium), 10-mg oral tablet, 1.5 h preoperatively with a sip of water
10. If arm veins are poor, hot pack arms before

laboratory draws blood and just before patient goes to the preoperative preparation room

11. Sign permit for gastric bypass or gastroplasty, needle biopsy of liver, and when appropriate, tubal ligation, appendectomy, cholecystectomy, or other concomitant procedures

12. If patient has been on any cortisone drug within the past 6 months give cortisone acetate, 50 mg intramuscularly, at 6 P.M. and repeat at 6 A.M.

13. 5000 U heparin, deep subcutaneous, 2 h preoperative, except in patients with a history of abnormal bleeding or abnormal coagulation, or when patient is also scheduled for reconstitution of small bowel—in the latter case 3000 U of heparin is given; heparin should never be given if the patient has cirrhosis of the liver or evidence of liver dysfunction

14. Start broad spectrum antibiotic (cephalosporin or doxycycline hyclate) intravenously in preoperative preparation room (patients with inadequate arm veins should have either an internal jugular or subclavian catheter inserted, usually the day before surgery)

Poor Risk Patients

Patients with symptomatic respiratory dysfunction, cardiac decompensation, or those weighing in excess of three times ideal weight are admitted 1 to 4 weeks before surgery for extensive cardiopulmonary evaluation and medical treatment depending upon the severity of the disease. Respiratory function studies include forced vital capacity, forced expiratory volume, maximum voluntary ventilation, peak flow rate, maximum midexpiratory flow rate, arterial blood gases, and in some cases, sleep apnea studies.[19] Mean pulmonary arterial pressures and pulmonary capillary wedge pressures are obtained on these severely involved patients. Respiratory response to ordinary exertion serves as a helpful clinical approximation of cardiorespiratory function: e.g., exertional dyspnea on walking down the hall, or inability to hold the breath for 30 s. Patients with pulmonary dysfunction whose PaO_2 is less than 50 mmHg or whose $PaCO_2$ is greater than 45 mmHg require a period of preoperative weight reduction, pulmonary physiotherapy, diuretics, and in some cases,

digitalis. Pickwickian patients should also be given a 1- or 2-week trial of progesterone, 100 mg intramuscularly daily.[20] Sleep apnea syndrome patients with obstructive airway involvement may require a tracheostomy. To date we have not found this necessary in our patients.

Family Cooperation

It is important whenever possible to solicit the cooperation of significant family members during this work-up period. If a spouse or family member is negatively oriented toward the intended surgery an effort should be made to obtain their understanding and acceptance. Unfortunately this is not always possible, and in this situation surgery is best postponed.

Patients must discontinue smoking at least 2 weeks prior to surgery, and the operation is delayed or cancelled until this requirement has been met.

All patients should be instructed in the use of the incentive spirometer and the intermittent positive pressure breathing (IPPB) machine before surgery.

It has been seldom necessary, in our experience, to start intravenous fluids the day prior to surgery in the average patient, although this has been recommended by Mason[22] and Bothe.[16]

Principles of Surgical Technique

Although details of technique vary considerably with different surgeons, several basic principles have emerged that are considered to be of vital importance in achieving long-term success.[23]

1. A small measured pouch size, less than 50 ml in volume (ours currently are made 12–15 ml in volume)

2. A calibrated outlet (channel or anastomosis) of between 10 and 12 mm (30–36 F).

3. A secure partition between the pouch and the distal stomach or transection

4. Some type of reinforcement around the outlet to prevent dilatation; this is particularly important in the gastroplasty operation

Also of importance is whether the channel or stoma empties into the distal stomach or a limb of jejunum, i.e., gastroplasty or gastric bypass.

Each of these factors has an important bearing on the success of the operation and will be considered in some detail.

The Pouch

A small pouch is of paramount importance for several reasons:

(1) better weight losses;
(2) lower incidence of stomal ulceration in gastric bypass procedures (less acid produced); and
(3) less tendency to dilate and fail later (Laplace's law—this states in effect that the smaller the diameter of a tube (or pouch), the greater the tensile strength of the wall)[24]

What constitutes a "small" or an "ideal" pouch is open to considerable debate. Many surgeons now refer to the pouch as a conduit or channel because its size has been reduced from "10% of stomach size" to a volume of less than 50 ml. Hornberger was one of the early proponents of the very small pouch, "about the size of a 1-oz shot glass, or about as small as possible and still usable for an anastomosis."[25] Mason[23] recommends a pouch size of 50 ml or less, and others mention sizes from 15 to 100 ml.[27,28]

Measuring Pouch Size

Alder and Terry emphasized the importance of standardizing gastric bypass surgery by calibrating pouch volume.[26]

For several years we depended upon linear (ruler) measurements for determining pouch size. Now, however, we depend upon volume measurements because "eyeballing" the pouch can be deceiving. Linear measurements do not indicate the anterior–posterior dimension, or the distensibility of the pouch. After measuring a large number of pouches, however, we have found that it is seldom necessary to alter the position of the TA90 staple instrument. Volume measurement requires only a few extra minutes, and establishes an accurate basis for later comparison. Recently we have not used the pressure manometer, but have accepted full distension of the pouch as the end point, with a volume measuring 12–15 ml at approximately 70 cm H_2O. A 50-ml pouch is too large in our opinion, and will frequently fail from late dilatation. Considering the difference in size between a 15-ml and a 50-ml syringe, it becomes immediately apparent that the former is much closer to what most experienced surgeons would consider the appropriate size.

Satiety

It might be argued that if a tiny pouch is more effective, why not eliminate the pouch entirely and simply make an esophagojejunal anastomosis bypassing the entire stomach, or place a constricting type ring of one sort or another around the lower esophagus to inhibit eating by causing dysphagia? The objection to this approach is that an obstructive ring around the distal esophagus would eventually produce esophageal dilatation and a situation similar to advanced achalasia with serious morbidity and potential mortality.

There may be an optimal pouch size somewhere between 10 and 30 ml, which when full, produces an afferent satiety reflex response that would be lost with no pouch. Meredith[29] reported an obese (275 lb) patient with achalasia and a huge esophagus who had never experienced satiety until after a Heller procedure plus a gastroplasty was performed. She lost 87 lb in 6 months and claimed that after this operation she experienced satiety for the first time. The esophagus remained dilated and apparently satiety resulted from fullness of the gastric pouch. Balloon studies on gastric bypass patients suggested that "fullness" seemed to be secondary to distension of the upper pouch rather than to an increase in upper pouch pressure.[30] These experiments, however, were not correlated with variations in pouch size so the conclusions were not entirely clear on this point. In clinical practice the degree and duration of satiety vary considerably in different patients and with different operative procedures. A few patients never experience a "full" sensation even when they have reached the point of vomiting.

To prevent dilatation of the pouch we recently performed a Nissen type gastric wrap around the pouch and anastomosis in one patient without complication, and plan to obtain annual upper gastrointestinal tract radiographs on this patient to evaluate its effectiveness. Our primary concern would be restoration of gastric anatomy should that become necessary in a patient with a Nissen wrap.

Vertical Pouch

A vertical tubular-shaped pouch formed by placing the staple lines parallel and quite close to the lesser curvature has become popular and the merits of this procedure will be discussed in detail later.

The Stoma

The size of the stoma (anastomosis, channel, outlet) is as important as pouch size. A small stoma and pouch are of more critical importance in gastric reduction type operations, i.e., gastroplasty, than in the gastric bypass. In the former, these are the only two technical factors that influence caloric intake, and ultimately weight loss. In the latter, other factors limit (although they do not eliminate) the importance of stomal size.

Stomal size reported in the literature for gastric partition and gastroplasty procedures varies from 12 mm[31] to as small as 3 mm.[32] Most of these very small stomas are accompanied by obstructive symptoms and the patients are limited to a liquid diet which in time becomes unpalatable, and if highly caloric, as is frequently the case, attended by a disappointing weight loss.

Because there is more likelihood of scarring and narrowing of a gastric bypass anastomosis than a gastroplasty channel where the mucosa is unbroken, an anastomosis should be slightly larger, varying between 10 and 12 mm. The most satisfactory size for a gastroplasty channel in our experience has been 32 F (10.6 mm), and 34 F (11.3 mm) for the gastric bypass anastomosis. Outlet enlargement is a common cause of failure, especially with the gastroplasty.[33]

Anastomosis Size

The importance of a small gastrojejunal anastomosis was not appreciated during the early development of the gastric bypass.[34] Even with these large, unmeasured, and unreinforced anastomoses, failure rates were not as high as might be expected, apparently owing to the deterrent effect of the dumping syndrome and other unknown factors related to the size of the adjacent jejunal limb as opposed to the distal stomach, as well as to the elimination of the digestive and absorptive capacity of the distal stomach, duodenum, and proximal 20 to 25 cm of jejunum. Kirkpatrick and Siegel[47] reported in a nonrandomized study of 44 Roux-en-Y patients, followed for an average of 22 months, that with a pouch size of 45 ml stomal size could be as large as the diameter of the jejunum (2.5–4 cm) and weight losses were still satisfactory. Our own experience,[33] however, as well

as that of Mason,[34] has demonstrated the importance of having a small gastrojejunal anastomosis of measured size, usually from 10 to 12 mm. Obstruction or functional stenosis has not been a significant problem in our patients.

Stoma Support

Some type of stomal reinforcement has proved to be essential in all gastric reduction type operations. Gastroplasties or gastric partitioning procedures without stomal support have had an excessively high failure rate. A variety of methods have been described to provide stomal support, and only a few will be mentioned here. Gomez[8] recommended the use of a purse-string suture of 3–0 or 2–0 Prolene around the gastroplasty channel to prevent dilatation. Mason[35] suggested that this be sutured around a previously placed circumferential chromic ligature with a 30-F Hurst dilator in place. The chromic tie would form a groove to guide the purse-string suture and was thought to cause fibrosis. An additional running Prolene suture was later added to form a seromuscular "pseudopylorus" to delay pouch emptying and prevent subsequent dilatation. O'Leary[14] used a 2–0 Dexon (polyglycolic acid) ligature around a 32-F dilator for the same purpose. To prevent obstruction it is essential, of course, that a dilator be in place when the channel is reinforced. Strips of Marlex, Merseline, Prolene, or Teflon have also been used with varying success to surround the channel. Gomez[8] discontinued using a Merseline band because it too frequently resulted in obstructive stenosis. Kroyer,[36] who used a Marlex band, pointed out that in his patients the obstruction was related to kinking of the outlet due to external adhesions rather than to any stricturing effect from the Marlex. He recommended that the greater curvature of the distal stomach be sutured to the anterior abdominal wall to prevent obstruction, a technique he called "gastric partitioning pexy." Obstructing adhesions to the Marlex band can also be prevented by covering it with adjacent fat or omentum. Silastic tubing of approximately 6-F to 12-F size with an inner suture that can be ligated around the channel has been recommended by Eckhout,[13] Fabito,[12] and Laws.[48]

Anastomosis Support

External reinforcement of the gastrojejunal anastomosis of the gastric bypass has not been commonly utilized because, as stated earlier, the size of the anastomosis has not been considered as critical a factor in achieving success as it has been in the gastroplasty. There are failures, however, due to dilatation of the gastric bypass anastomosis, and thus, for the past 2 years, we have used either a No. 1 Prolene suture ligated around the anastomosis, or more recently (past 12 months) a No. 12 radioopaque Silastic catheter with a 34-F dilator in place, which has improved our results. A few of the sutures migrated into the lumen, but most apparently remained within the scarred tissue around the anastomosis. There have been 2 erosions of the Silastic ring in our patients.

Mason[34] stated he was convinced that "the stoma cannot be made small enough to prevent an excessive diameter later, and that the specifications should include an adequate (12 mm) stoma, surrounded by a nonabsorbable suture that will prevent stretching of the diameter for as long as possible."

The Partition

The primary objective in the selection of a technique for incontinuity partitioning of the stomach is *durability*, i.e., preventing staple line disruption (SLD). The attainment of this objective has been approached from three directions.

1. The number, type, location, and reinforcement of the staple line(s)
2. Maintenance of decompression of the distal stomach by gastrostomy tube drainage[37]
3. The timing and type of postoperative diet allowed
   a. Nothing by mouth for a minimum of 4 weeks (tube feeding–gastrostomy or –jejunostomy)[38]
   b. Liquids only for 8 weeks[39,40]

Stapling Technique
One of the principal advantages of the staple instrument, i.e., that it does not crush mucosa, can become a disadvantage when it is used to separate, in continuity, one part of the stomach from another. Failure to crush the mucosa results in minimal fibrosis and lack of a firm scar.[41] Peristalsis, vomiting, and stretching of the pouch cause staples to pull out and migrate. If this happens before fibrosis or healing develops, a disruption will occur. Printen[42] reported migration of staples with

areas of disruption as early as 2 h after surgery in dogs. The staple line is particularly vulnerable at points where staples have been removed to form a channel as with the partitioned staple line. The only certain method to prevent SLD is to *divide* the stomach completely between staple lines, totally separating the upper pouch from the lower stomach (Fig. 4–5). The increased operating time and morbidity from leaks reported with this technique, however, have caused most surgeons to eschew dividing the stomach.[7,21] Some, however, have gained confidence through experience and prefer the transection technique.[43,49]

There are proponents of each of the many methods of creating a durable partition and most report a low incidence of SLD. Alden[37] uses a single application of the TA90 staple instrument, but states that postoperative gastrostomy drainage of the distal stomach is of key importance in preventing SLD. Most surgeons do not depend upon a single unreinforced staple line, especially with the gastroplasty. Gomez[8] reported a much higher incidence of SLD with the single than with double staple lines.

Suture Reinforcement

We have used both single and double staple lines but most of our primary procedures have been done with a single TA90 staple line reinforced with interrupted through-and-through 2–0 silk sutures placed at 1-cm intervals along the staple line. Since starting this technique 2 years ago, to our knowledge there have been two of 185 patients with staple line disruptions. One patient was reoperated and the disruption closed. In the other, the disruption was small and closed spontaneously. This patient has had an excellent weight loss at 1 year. Apparently the sutures fix the staple line in position and promote an inflammatory-fibrotic response which results in a firm scar. There have been no leaks or apparent abscess formation resulting from the through-and-through sutures. In patients who are having a revision of a gastric bypass or reconstitution of a jejunoileal bypass, we place two closely applied TA90 staple lines plus interrupted 2–0 silk sutures at 1.5 cm intervals because the incidence of SLD is higher in these patients.[11] Recently we have applied this technique to primary GBP operations as well.

Fischer[44] reported similar findings in dogs, i.e.

that a single staple line without suture reinforcement failed 100% of the time, and a double staple line 60% of the time. The only part of the staple line that remained intact was the segment reinforced with 2–0 silk or Prolene sutures. He recommended the use of transgastric suture support of the staple line in humans to prevent SLD.

Distance Between Staple Lines

There are many advocates of the double staple line and the primary controversy with this technique relates to the optimal distance between the lines, which varies from a maximum of 2 cm to immediately adjacent lines.

O'Leary[14] noted in a fluorescent microsphere study of blood flow in dogs that at the 2-cm distance, no ischemia could be noted in the intervening segment, but that at a distance of 1 cm there was considerable ischemia. He reported one patient who developed necrosis and leak with a 1-cm separation, and concluded that this distance was unsafe, but that a 2-cm interval was no stronger than a single staple line. In his opinion, immediately adjacent staple lines were the most satisfactory.

Printen[42] found some necrosis between staple lines in dogs at 1 cm but none at 2 cm, which suggested to him that 2 cm was perhaps the best distance. He also noted, however, that in humans the width of the intervening segment was not significant, because double applications had been reported at a variety of distances with no necrosis.

Eckhout[13] reported using a double application of the TA90 instrument with two vertical staple lines placed immediately adjacent and reinforced with running 2–0 Prolene suture. His SLD rate was slightly over 2% in 90 patients, but was 14.4% in gastric bypass patients with a single, unreinforced staple line. The latter group had a longer follow-up period.

In his new "vertically banded gastroplasty" technique, Mason[45,46] places two vertical staple lines less than 1 cm apart without suture reinforcement. No disruptions or leaks were reported, but follow-up has been short. Using the same technique Doherty[45] reported one early disruption in his series of patients.

Summary

A number of methods for creating a firm, durable, incontinuity partition have been reported in the literature, none of which are infallible. Division of the stomach between staple lines is the only certain way to avoid SLD, but at this time most surgeons believe the potential morbidity is too high to warrant its use.

Our current recommendation is either a single TA90 4.8-mm staple line reinforced with interrupted 2–0 silk sutures placed at 1-cm intervals, or closely applied double staple lines with the silk sutures placed 1.5 cm apart. Double application of the staple instrument plus reinforcing sutures is recommended in revision or reconstitution operations.

If double staple lines are used, they should be closely adjacent (less than 1 cm). Whether suture reinforcement of double staple lines will offer additional protection against SLD has not as yet been proved. The only apparent disadvantage is the additional time involved.

References

1. Mason EE, Ito C: Gastric bypass in obesity. Surg Clin North Am 47:1345, 1967.
2. Mason EE, Ito C: Gastric bypass. Ann Surg 170:329, 1969.
3. Mason EE, Printen KJ, Blommers TJ, Lewis JW, Scott DH: Gastric bypass for obesity. Am J Clin Nutr 33:395–405, 1980.
4. Mason EE, Printen KJ, Hartford CE, Boyd WC: Optimizing results of gastric bypass. Ann Surg 182:405, 1975.
5. Mason EE: Surgical treatment of morbid obesity. Major Probl Clin Surg 26:39–57, 1981.
6. Griffen WO Jr: Gastric bypass for morbid obesity. Surg Clin North Am 59:1103, 1979.
7. Alden JF: Gastric and jejunoileal bypass: a comparison in the treatment of morbid obesity. Arch Surg 112:799, 1977.
8. Gomez CA: Gastroplasty in the surgical treatment of morbid obesity. Am J Clin Nutr 33:406, 1980.
9. Pace WG, Martin EW Jr, Tetirick T, Fabri PJ, Carey LC: Gastric partitioning for morbid obesity. Ann Surg 190:392, 1979.
10. Tretbar LL, Taylor TL, Sifers EC: Weight reduction: Gastric plication for morbid obesity. J Kans Med Soc 77:488, 1976.
11. LaFave JW, Alden JF: Gastric bypass in the operative revision of the failed jejunoileal bypass. Arch Surg 114:438, 1979.
12. Fabito DC: Vertical stapling gastroplasty for obesity. Presented to Bariatric Surgery Workshop, Iowa City, May 29–30, 1980.
13. Eckhout GV: Surgery for morbid obesity. Compar-

ison of gastric bypass with vertically stapled gastro-plasty. Colo Med 78:117, 1981.

14. O'Leary JP: Partition of the lesser curvature of the stomach in morbid obesity. Surg Gynecol Obstet 134:85, 1982.

15. VanItallie TB, Burton BT: National Institutes of Health Consensus Development Conference on Surgical Treatment of Morbid Obesity. Am Surg 189:455, 1979.

16. Bothe A Jr, Bistrian BR, Greenberg I, Blackburn GL: Energy regulation in morbid obesity by multidisciplinary therapy. Surg Clin North Am 59:1017–1031, 1979.

17. Metropolitan Life Insurance Company: New weight standards for men and women. Stat Bull 40:1, 1959.

18. Drenick EJ: Definition and health consequences of morbid obesity. Surg Clin North Am 59:963–976, 1979.

19. Walsh RE, Michaelson ED, Harkleroad LE, Zeghelboim A, Sackner MA: Upper airway obstruction in obese patients with sleep disturbance and somnolence. Ann Intern Med 76:185, 1972.

20. Lyons HA, Huang CT: Therapeutic use of progesterone in alveolar hypoventilation associated with obesity. Am J Med 44:881, 1968.

21. Griffen WD, Bivins BA, Bell RM, Jackson KA: Gastric bypass for morbid obesity. World J Surg 5:817–822, 1981.

22. Mason EE: Surgical Treatment of Obesity. Major Probl Clin Surg 26:150, 1981.

23. Mason EE: Surgical Treatment of Obesity. Major Probl Clin Surg 26:449–500, 1981.

24. Guyton AC: Textbook of Medical Physiology, 5th ed. Philadelphia, Saunders, 1976, pp 231–232.

25. Hornberger HR: Personal communication. Gastric Bypass Workshop, Iowa City, April 28–29, 1977.

26. Alder RL, Terry BE: Measurement and standardization of the gastric pouch in gastric bypass. Surg Gynecol Obstet 144:762, 1977.

27. Freeman JB, Burchett HJ: A comparison of gastric bypass and gastroplasty for morbid obesity. Surgery 88:433, 1980.

28. Lechner GW, Callender AK: Subtotal gastric exclusion and gastric partitioning: a randomized prospective comparison of 100 patients. Surgery 90:637, 1981.

29. Meredith JH: Achalasia: case report. Presented to Bariatric Surgery Workshop, Iowa City, May 29–30, 1980.

30. Villar HV, Wangensteen SL, Burks TF, Patton DD: Mechanisms of satiety and gastric emptying after gastric partitioning and bypass. Surgery 90:229, 1981.

31. Gomez CA: Gastroplasty in morbid obesity: a progress report. World Surg 5:823–828, 1981.

32. MacLean LP, Rhode BM, Shizgal HM: Gastroplasty for obesity. Surg Gynecol Obstet 153:200, 1981.

33. Linner JH: Comparative effectiveness of gastric bypass and gastroplasty: a clinical study. Arch Surg 117:695, 1982.

34. Mason EE: Surgical treatment of obesity. Major Probl Clin Surg 26:156, 1981.

35. Mason EE: Surgical treatment of morbid obesity. Major Probl Clin Surg 26:391–393, 1981.

36. Kroyer JM: Marlex mesh around the channel. Presented at Bariatric Surgical Workshop, Iowa City, May 29–30, 1980.

37. Alden JF: Gastric bypass technique. Presented at Gastrointestinal Disease Course, A.C.S. Meeting, San Francisco, October 12–16, 1981.

38. Luigi LM: Distal gastrostomy and outlet obstruction. Presented at Bariatric Surgery Workshop, Iowa City, May 29–30, 1980.

39. Pace WG, Martin EW Jr, Tetirick T, Fabri PJ, Carey LC: Gastric partitioning for morbid obesity. Ann Surg 190:392, 1979.

40. Martin EW: Gastric partitioning: an update. Presented at Bariatric Surgical Colloquium, Iowa City, June 1–2, 1981.

41. Brolm RE, Ravitch MM: Experimental evaluation of techniques of gastric partitioning for morbid obesity. Surg Gynecol Obstet 153:877, 1981.

42. Printen KJ: Pathology of stapling. Presented at Bariatric Surgical Workshop, Iowa City, May 29–30, 1980.

43. Miller DK: Poster presentation: gastric bypass. Presented at Bariatric Surgical Colloquium, Iowa City, June 3–4, 1982.

44. Fischer MG: Staple line dehiscence in the laboratory. Presented at Bariatric Surgical Workshop, Iowa City, May 28–29, 1980.

45. Mason EE: Vertical banded gastroplasty for obesity. Arch Surg 117:701, 1982.

46. Mason EE: Evaluation of gastric reduction for obesity. Contemp Surg 20:17, 1982.

47. Kirkpatrick JR, Siegel T: Critical determinants of a successful gastric bypass: reservoir versus stoma. Am J Gastroenterol 77:464, 1982.

48. Laws HL: Ring gastroplasty for morbid obesity. ACS Clinical Congress–General Surgery Motion Pictures, Chicago, October 24–29, 1982.

49. Reinhold RB: Critical analysis of long-term weight loss following gastric bypass. Surg Gynecol Obstet 155:385, 1982.

50. Questionnaire. Bariatric Surgical Colloquium, Iowa City, June 2–3, 1983.

CHAPTER 5

Gastric Operations: Specific Techniques

JOHN H. LINNER

In the preceding chapter the important principles of technique, i.e., pouch size, channel size and support, partition strength, and the presence or absence of a gastrojejunostomy, which are common to some degree in all bariatric operations, were discussed. In this chapter the technical details of the operative procedure with which we have had the most experience and found the most effective—a modified Roux-en-Y gastric bypass (GBP)—will be described. A few of the more popular alternative operations will also be outlined.

As pointed out in the preceding chapter, there is no overwhelming evidence to support the unequivocal recommendation of any one bariatric operation at this time, which accounts for the profusion of techniques described in the literature. Several recent reports[1,2] including one of my own[3] have shown that after a 2-year follow-up, the gastric bypass proved to be a more effective weight-reducing operation than the horizontal gastroplasty, (GP) and has become a standard against which newer procedures have been compared.

The operation we currently use evolved over a period of 5 years. We began in 1976 with the Alden loop type GBP (Fig. 4-4),[4] which was revised to a Roux-en-Y GBP (Fig. 4-5), followed by the Gomez type GP (Fig. 4-6)[5] with several modifications, and we have now returned to a Roux-en-Y GBP characterized by a 12 to 15-ml anterior gastric pouch and a 34-Fr. reinforced anastomosis (Fig. 5-1). This may not remain our final choice in such a rapidly changing field but we would not change until one of the newer opera-

tions proved to be superior over at least a 3-year follow-up period.

Because the loop GBP resulted in a troublesome bile reflux gastroesophagitis in six patients it was discontinued after 53 operations. A side-to-side jejunojejunostomy in 11 patients did not prevent bile reflux and was abandoned (Fig. 5-2). The Roux-en-Y configuration was then adopted.

It also became apparent that with the Roux-en-Y gastrojejunostomy, a retrocolic anastomosis was more direct with less tension at the anastomosis, and further, as pointed out by Griffen, a gastrojejunal leak with a Roux-en-Y anastomosis as compared to the loop would not be as disastrous.[6] The additional anastomosis (Roux-en-Y jejunojejunostomy) usually adds less than 20 min to the operation and is rarely the cause of a complication if carefully done.

The GP was discontinued because the failure rate after a 2-year follow-up exceeded 50%.[3] Efforts to reduce this rate resulted in obstructive stenosis in many patients.

The first procedure to be described, and our current choice, is a modified Roux-en-Y GBP and will be designated method I-A (Fig. 5-1). An alternative technique, I-B, first described by Torres,[7] is essentially the same but the anastomoses are made with the EEA (U.S. Surgical) or ILS (Johnson and Johnson) circular cartridge instruments close to the lesser curvature (Fig. 5-3). The third technique, I-C, is identical to I-A except that the anastomoses are made by a hand suture technique without the use of the staple instruments.

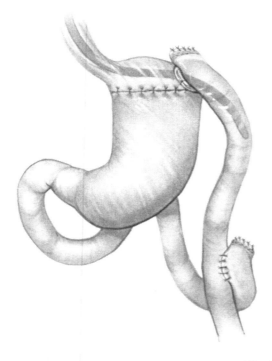

FIG. 5-1. Roux-en-Y gastric bypass with No. 12 Silastic catheter ligated around anastomosis (method I-A).

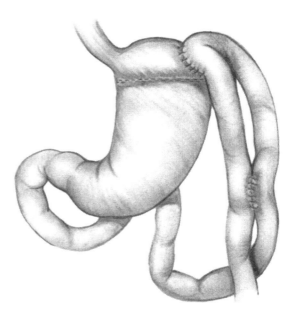

FIG. 5-2. Loop gastric bypass with jejunojejunostomy. This procedure did not prevent reflux of bile in our patients.

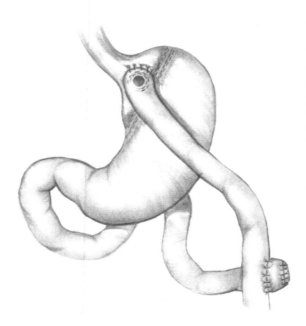

FIG. 5-3. Torres: Roux-en-Y gastric bypass (method I-B).

Modified Roux-en-Y Gastric Bypass (Anterior Pouch Technique, I-A)

The patient is positioned on the operating table with the arms out on padded arm boards. Care must be taken to avoid hyperextension. A foam rubber padded metal foot board is securely fastened near the distal end of the operating table with the patient's feet flush against this support. The patient has support stockings to the knee (Fig. 5-4).

A warming blanket has been placed on the table, and the patient's temperature is monitored throughout the operation. This precaution is of greater importance in revisions and conversions than in shorter primary procedures. Two ground plates are positioned under the patient, one to be used with a bayonet cautery, and the other a cutting-cautery knife unit. The use of two cautery units minimizes blood loss and shortens the procedure.

Intravenous access is usually via one or two arm veins with a No. 16 plastic catheter, or when

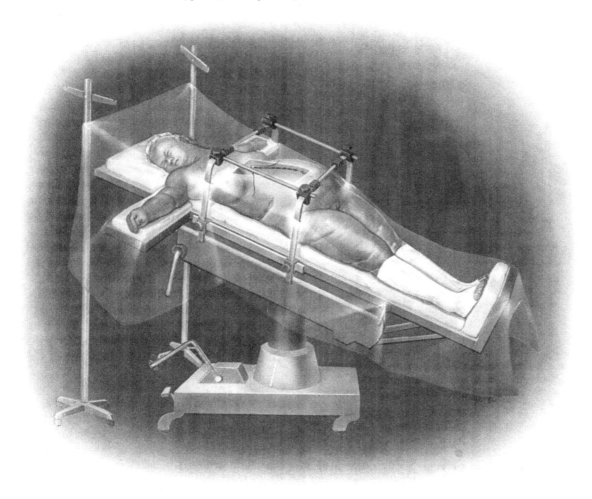

FIG. 5-4. Position of the patient for modified Roux-en-Y gastric bypass technique. Note 20° reverse Trendelenburg position, Poly-Tract retractor, and foot board. By using the upper transverse bar for attachment of the liver retractor, the long bar on the right side can be eliminated from the usual quadrilateral set up, facilitating technical maneuvers in the upper abdomen.

necessary, via a jugular or subclavian catheter. A radial or brachial artery catheter is placed in all patients with cardiopulmonary dysfunction, or whenever there might be reason to monitor blood gases or intraarterial blood pressure (see Chapter 9). A prophylactic antibiotic of choice is started in the preoperative preparation room. [We use cefazolin sodium (Ancef), 1 g, or in patients who are sensitive to penicillin, doxycycline hyclate (Vibramycin), 200 mg in 500 ml of diluent.]

After the patient has been anesthetized and intubated, the abdomen and lower chest are prepared with a povidone-iodine scrub followed by application of a povidone-iodine solution (Betadine). Towels are used to square off the surgical field,

and are held in place with an adhesive plastic skin drape. Drapes are then appropriately placed.

The upright bows of the Poly-Tract retractor are then positioned and a large disposable laparotomy drape is placed over the entire table, pushing the upper ends of the Poly-Tract retractor bows through the paper drape (Fig. 5-4). A newly modified upper bow for the Poly-Tract retractor reduces abduction of the arms. Other self-retaining retractors are commercially available and have been used successfully (Fig. 5-5). A laminectomy straddle table is then brought over the foot of the operating table, and the skin incision is made from the xiphoid to the umbilicus (sometimes below the umbilicus) with a No. 10 scalpel. The subcutaneous

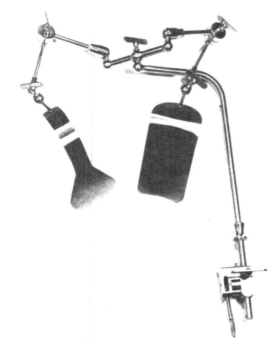

FIG. 5-5. A 2-arm Universal Swiss Automatic Retractor Holder (Hydra/22″) for morbidly obese patients. (Courtesy of Automated Medical Products Corp., 2315 Broadway, New York 10024.)

fat is split by blunt separation down to the fascia by the surgeon with the assistant firmly retracting the tissue from each side. This method of avulsing the fat may seem crude, but actually it is quite bloodless and invariably leads to the fascial midline, which can be difficult to find with a scalpel incision through the fat.

The fascia is then incised to the preperitoneal fat with the cautery knife. We have seldom found it necessary to remove the xiphoid process or extend the incision below the umbilicus unless the patient is unusually short. A midline sternotomy or left lateral thoracotomy has never been indicated in our series of cases. The preperitoneal fat, unless it is quite thin, is excised with the cautery knife to the fascial edges, and the round ligament is divided and ligated during its removal. Wound closure is facilitated by this maneuver.

We then insert a 9-in plastic wound protector with 20–25 ml of .1% Keflin solution instilled between the wound protector and skin edges. The entire celomic cavity is carefully explored, following which the end and side bars of the Poly-Tract retractor are assembled and firmly secured. We no longer use the long bar on the surgeon's side

of the table, which greatly facilitates his access to the upper reaches of the abdomen. The falciform ligament is incised with the cautery knife for approximately 10 cm, and the "upper hand" blade of the retractor is placed with a firm upward pull. A left lateral Mayo blade is positioned in a similar fashion, and the lower aspect of the wound is held apart with a self-retaining Balfour type retractor. The left triangular hepatic ligament is incised only when necessary to gain exposure, taking care to avoid injury to the spleen and the large lateral hepatic vein at the inferior aspect of the left lobe. The lobe is then retracted upward and to the right with a four-pronged liver retractor (Fig. 5-6). A huge fatty liver makes access to the abdominal "attic" extremely difficult. A needle biopsy of the liver is always obtained. The operating table is then tilted into at least 20° reverse Trendelenburg, which together with the "upper hand" affords optimal access. A sterile plastic-covered fiberoptic "snake light" or a head lamp is essential for good visibility during the upper abdominal part of the operation.

A No. 18 gastric suction catheter with a single hole at its distal end is passed down the esophagus and into the fundus by the anesthesiologist, and the peritoneum over the esophagogastric junction is incised, taking care to avoid the anterior vagus trunk. The peritoneal incision is carried to the left down beyond the angle of His for 2 to 3 cm, but always short of the vasa brevia (Fig. 5-6).

The retrogastric space just below the esophagogastric junction is then developed by careful blunt finger dissection from the angle of His to a point on the lesser curvature 2 to 4 cm from the esophagogastric junction. This distance varies depending on the location of the superior branch of the left gastric artery. At least one of these branches to the upper pouch must be left intact (Fig. 5-7). The lesser omentum is incised at the point selected, and with the finger coming up from behind the stomach, an opening adjacent to the lesser curvature is developed. A No. 24 Robinson catheter is passed through this opening and brought out at the angle of His. Care must be taken not to perforate the lesser curvature of the stomach when developing the opening in the lesser omentum (Fig. 5-7).

The lower (anvil) jaw of the TA90 staple instrument is inserted into the open end of the Robinson catheter, and with gentle traction on the catheter and manipulation of the handle, the instrument

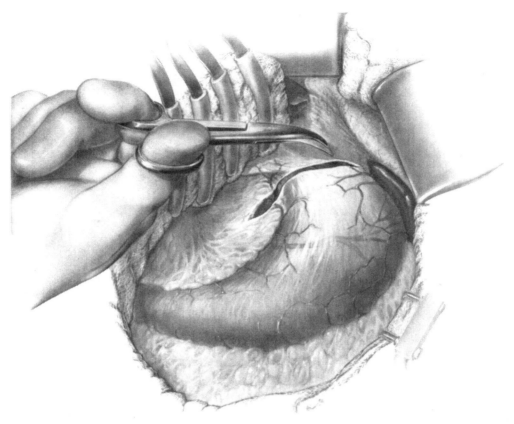

FIG. 5-6. Incising retroperitoneum over esophagogastric junction. It is unnecessary to
ligate any vasa brevia.

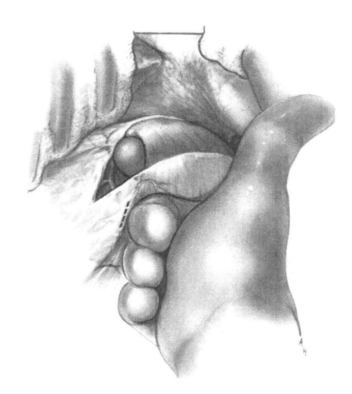

FIG. 5-7. Developing the retrogastric plane
from the angle of His to the lesser curvature.
Great care must be taken to avoid perforating
the posterior gastric wall or lesser curvature
with this maneuver.

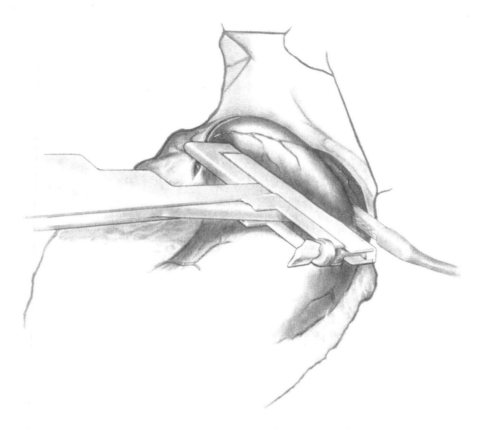

Fɪɢ. 5-8. TA90 staple instrument is guided across anterosuperior gastric wall in an oblique direction with a 24 Fr. Robinson catheter. No vessels are ligated.

is drawn across the upper stomach from right to left (Fig. 5-8).

After removing the catheter and placing the guide pin, the heel end of the staple instrument is moved upward as far as the opening in the lesser omentum will allow, and the pin end is angled downward. The instrument is then turned clockwise on its long axis 45° so that the opening between the jaws is directed anterior-posterior rather than laterally. Using a Babcock forceps a segment of anterior stomach wall is then carefully pulled through the jaws of the instrument, until approximately 2 cm protrudes above the jaws vertically and 5 cm horizontally. The jaws should be cleared of any other tissue, the gastric suction catheter, or sponges, and then approximated by turning the knob. This maneuver, first utilized in our practice by my associate, Raymond Drew, M.D., allows one to create a very small pouch suitable for a gastrojejunostomy without ligating any of the vasa brevia (Figs. 5-8–5-11).

The gastric tube, which had been withdrawn an inch or so prior to tightening the jaws of the stapler, is now reintroduced into the pouch (Fig. 5-9). The pouch is aspirated of any air or fluid by the anesthesiologist, the esophagus is firmly occluded around the suction catheter with the surgeon's right thumb and forefinger, and the anesthesiologist then instills saline from a 30-ml syringe into the gastric pouch in 5-ml increments. The size and distension of the pouch can be easily visualized and palpated. The end point is a moderately distended pouch which should approximate 12 to 15 ml. If a variance of over 5 ml occurs the pouch size can be changed by reapplying the TA90 instrument. After some experience we have seldom found this necessary. Holding the gastric tube 70 cm above the cricoid with an open syringe is a method we used earlier in our experience to measure volume at a given pressure and establish the amount of pouch distension we now use as the end point (Fig. 5-10).

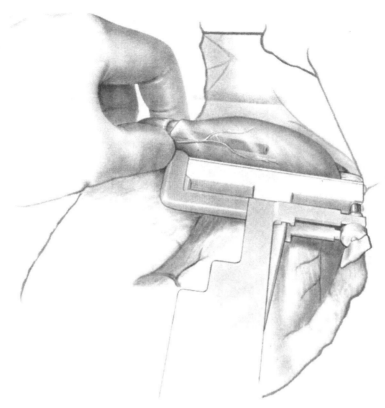

FIG. 5-9. TA90 staple instrument jaws are approximated but not fired, and single-hole gastric suction tube is positioned from above for volume measurement.

After firing, the TA90 instrument is removed and the staple line is inspected anteriorly and posteriorly as far as possible to ensure proper staple formation and complete penetration. Incomplete staple closure is rare, but should it occur, a second staple line must be placed adjacent to the first to prevent staple line failure. Recently we have used two closely adjacent staple applications for revisions and conversions, and are beginning to use this technique in our primary operations as well (Fig. 5-11).

The single staple line is then reinforced with through-and-through interrupted 2–0 silk sutures placed slightly less than 1 cm apart from the lesser curvature to the greater curvature. With double staple lines, the reinforcing silk sutures are placed

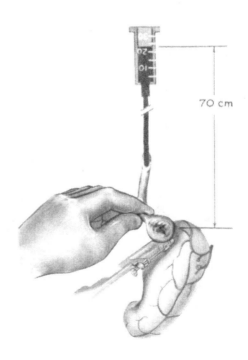

FIG. 5-10. Volume is measured at 70 cm pressure, or at full distension of the pouch as determined by palpation (12–15 ml).

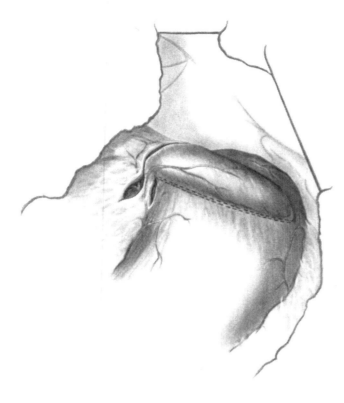

FIG. 5-11. The staple line is fired when correct (12–15 ml) volume is achieved. Note anterosuperior location of pouch with oblique direction of its long axis. No vasa brevia have been ligated (method I-A).

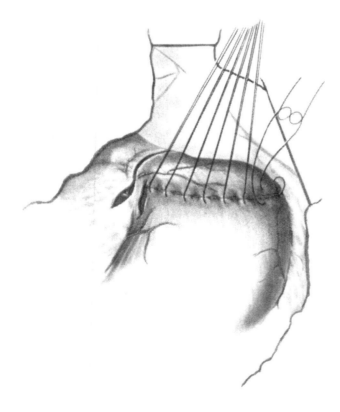

FIG. 5-12. The staple line is reinforced with interrupted through-and-through 2–0 silk sutures. A satisfactory alternative to suture reinforcement is two staple line applications placed less than 1 cm apart (method I-A).

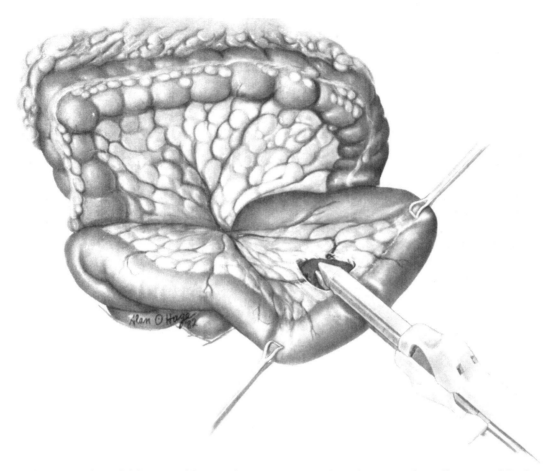

FIG. 5-13. Transection of jejunum with GIA instrument approximately 25 cm from ligament of Treitz. An acceptable alternative is transection between intestinal clamps and suture closure.

1.5 cm apart. All the sutures are then cut except one suture at the greater curvature which is used for traction to facilitate construction of the gastrojejunostomy (Fig. 5-12).

The area is checked for bleeding, a laparotomy pad is placed in the operative area, the operating table is returned to an almost level position, and the upper jejunum at the ligament of Treitz is located. The mesentery of the jejunum, approximately 25 cm from the ligament of Treitz, is carefully incised, visualizing the mesenteric vessels with the aid of translucence from the snake light. One or two mesenteric vessels are ligated and, when necessary, the first vascular arcade vessels (Fig. 5-13). The jejunum is transected using a disposable GIA instrument. A long stitch is placed in the antemesenteric corner of the efferent limb to identify it and to facilitate its passage through

the retrocolic mesocolon. Bleeding points along the transected ends of the jejunum are carefully electrocoagulated or controlled with a stick tie. The Roux-en-Y jejunojejunostomy can either be done at this time, or after the gastroenterostomy. A 3- to 4-cm incision is made in an avascular area of the transverse mesocolon to the left of the midcolic artery (Figs. 5-14 and 5-15). A space is then developed through the transverse mesocolon to the gastrocolic ligament where a second opening is made in an avascular area, usually above or to the left of the left gastroepiploic vessels. Occasionally the most suitable area is between two widely separated vasa brevia above the gastroepiploic vessels (Fig. 5-15).

The operating table is returned to the reverse Trendelenburg position and the efferent limb of the transected jejunum is brought through the

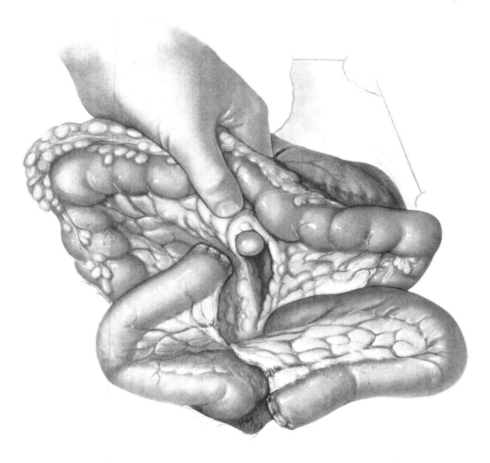

FIG. 5-14. A hiatus is developed in the transverse meso-colon for retrocolic antegastric passage of efferent jejunum to gastric pouch.

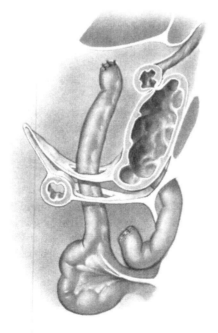

FIG. 5-15. Lateral view showing relative positions of efferent jejunal limb, transverse colon, and gastric pouch.

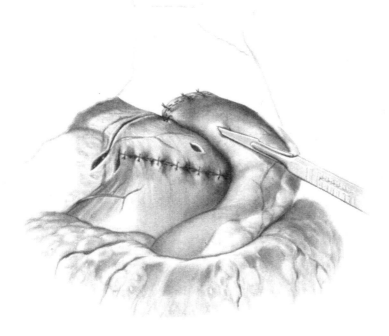

FIG. 5-16. Stab-type incisions are made in the gastric pouch and efferent jejunum for introduction of GIA instrument (method I-A).

mesenteric openings to the gastric pouch. The silk suture left on the pouch is then used to bring the pouch down into view and make it more accessible for the anastomosis. The efferent jejunum is now retrocolic, but antegastric, and should be far enough to the left to not interfere with a distal gastrostomy or a gastropexy should either of these procedures be desired (Fig. 5-15). The efferent and afferent limbs should now be inspected below the transverse mesocolon to make certain that the efferent limb has not been inadvertently rotated.

The efferent jejunum is next anchored to the gastric pouch near its upper aspect, close to the esophagus, with one 3–0 silk suture. It may be necessary to dissect some of the fat pad off the superior aspect of the pouch prior to placing this stitch. Adjacent stab incisions are made in the pouch and efferent jejunum (Fig. 5-16).

The GIA nondisposable instrument is inserted to the 1.5-cm mark and fired (Fig. 5-17). At least two 3–0 silk sutures are placed along the inner aspect of the staple line with additional stick ties placed to control bleeding as needed (Fig. 5-18). The anastomosis is then completed with a TA30 staple instrument as illustrated (Figs. 5-19 and 5-20). Interrupted 3–0 silk sutures are used to reinforce the anastomosis, and it is checked for leaks by simple compression, or by instilling saline into the gastric tube.

The gastric suction catheter is removed and replaced with a 34-Fr. Hurst dilator by the anesthesiologist; the surgeon guides it through the anastomosis into the efferent jejunum.

Using a large right-angle clamp, a No. 1 Prolene suture, which has been threaded through a previously measured and cut 12-Fr. radiopaque Silastic catheter, is brought around the anastomosis between the initial 3–0 tacking suture at the superior pouch and the upper aspect of the anastomosis (Fig. 5-21). The suture is then ligated snugly around the dilator on the gastric side of the anastomosis (Fig. 5-22). The proper length of the Silastic

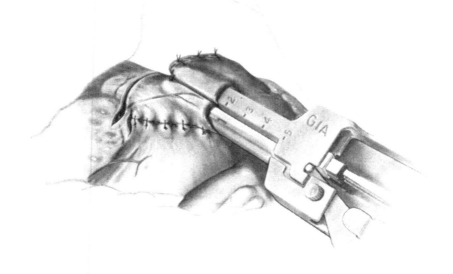

FIG. 5-17. The GIA instrument is inserted to the 1.5-cm mark (method I-A).

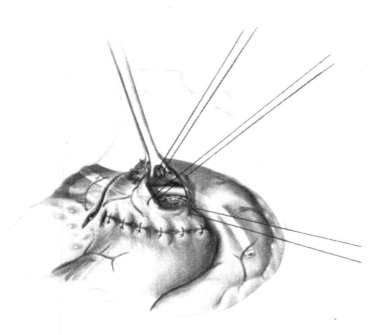

FIG. 5-18. Note hemostatic sutures on posterior wall of anastomosis and guide sutures on anterior wall (method I-A).

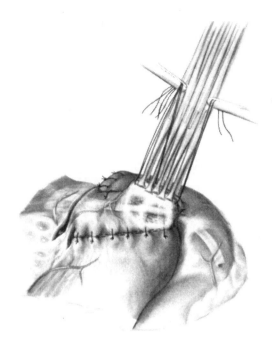

FIG. 5-19. Allis forceps in position for application of TA30 or TA55 staple instrument (method I-A).

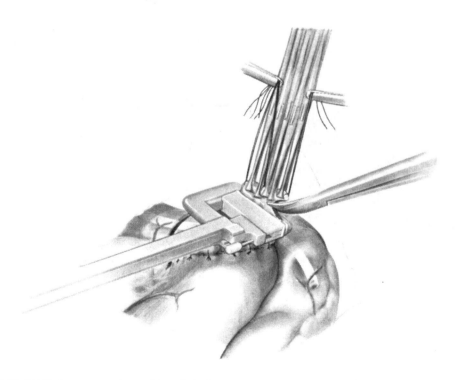

FIG. 5-20. TA30 instrument in position: it is fired and excess tissue is excised (method I-A).

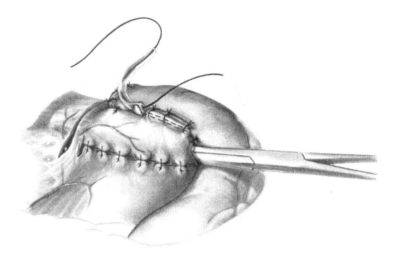

FIG. 5-21. Radiopaque 12-Fr. Silastic catheter with indwelling No. 1 Prolene suture being positioned around anastomosis. Hurst dilator (34-Fr.) is threaded through the anastomosis.

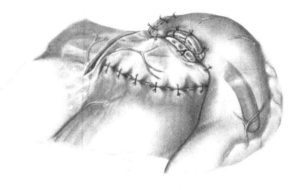

FIG. 5-22. Silastic catheter in place around anastomosis with Prolene suture ligated. Usual length of catheter is 6.3 cm. The dilator is then removed and replaced with a No. 16 nine-hole nasogastric tube. At least two holes should be in the gastric pouch.

catheter using this method is approximately 6.3 cm. One or two 3–0 silk sutures are then placed between the efferent jejunum and the distal stomach to prevent kinking at the anastomosis. The dilator is withdrawn and replaced with a nine-hole No. 16 nasogastric tube with two or three holes positioned in the gastric pouch and the remainder in the jejunum distal to the anastomosis. Adjacent fat is sutured over the anastomosis with interrupted 3–0 silk. Taking care to avoid tension at the anastomosis, four to six tacking sutures are placed between the efferent jejunum and the edges of the transverse mesocolon hiatus.

At 50 cm from the gastrojejunostomy, a Roux-en-Y jejunojejunostomy is performed, usually with the disposable GIA and TA55 instruments. It is extremely important to inspect the inner aspect of the staple line and to place a stick tie on any bleeders (Figs. 5-23 to 5-25). The mesenteric defect of the jejunum is closed with a running 3–0 Vicryl suture.

The operative area is washed with 1 or 2 liter of saline and 100 to 200 ml of 0.1% Keflin solution during the course of surgery. All irrigants are com-

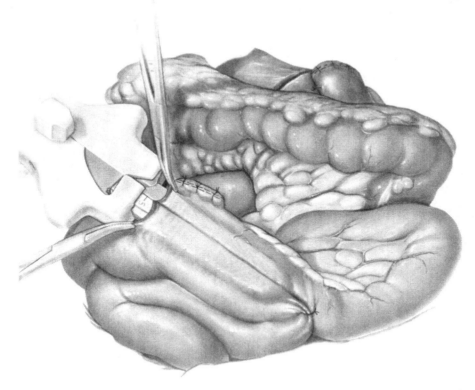

FIG. 5-23. GIA instrument in position for Roux-en-Y jejunojejunostomy (functional end-to-side anastomosis; method I-A). Acceptable alternatives are either suture anastomosis (I-C) or circular staple instrument (I-B).

pletely removed prior to wound closure. The operative area is inspected for bleeding and additional procedures, if any, are performed.

The sponge and needle counts are verified as correct, the Poly-Tract retractor is dismantled, the wound protector is removed, clean towels are placed around the wound, gloves are changed, and closure is carried out using figure-of-eight interrupted No. 0 and/or No. 1 Prolene sutures on the fascia and peritoneum at approximately 1.5-cm intervals (unit method of closure). On extremely heavy patients only No. 1 Prolene sutures are used. In some of the less heavy female patients the fascia is closed with running No. 1 Vicryl suture.

The wound is washed with saline and 0.1% Keflin solution after fascial closure. The subcutaneous layer is approximated with 3–0 Vicryl sutures using the X-L needle in most cases. A 0.25-in Penrose drain is placed above the fascia and brought out from the lower extremity of the

wound, to be removed early on the first postoperative day. The skin is closed with staples. Dressings and a scultetus binder are applied taking care to avoid too tight a wrap around the lower chest that might restrict respiration.

Blood loss is monitored throughout the surgical procedure and replaced on a 3:1 ratio with 5% dextrose in lactated Ringer's solution. In the rare situation when blood loss exceeds 1000 ml, it is replaced in part at least with 5% albumin and/or packed cells, or in some instances, whole blood.

Most patients are extubated in the operating room, but patients with compromised respiratory reserve may require a mechanical respirator for several days. This aspect of patient management is discussed in Chapter 9.

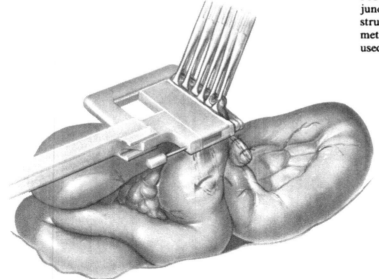

FIG. 5-24. Completion of jejunojejunostomy with TA55 staple instrument (method I-A). Alternate methods I-B or I-C can also be used.

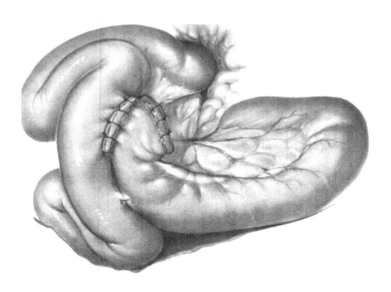

FIG. 5-25. Jejunojejunostomy complete (method I-A). Mesenteric defect is closed with running absorbable suture (Vicryl or chromic catgut). Alternate methods I-B or I-C can be used.

Modified Roux-en-Y Gastric Bypass (Technique I-B)

The second procedure to be discussed, method I-B, was first described by Torres.[7] It is a Roux-en-Y procedure very similar to I-A, but with the following important differences.

1. The anastomoses are made with the 21 mm EEA or ILS circular-type staple instruments.
2. The staple line extends from the angle of His to a point somewhat farther down the lesser curvature, 5 to 6 cm from the esophagogastric junction (Fig. 5-26). (Torres uses a double application of the TA55 staple instrument instead of a single application of the TA90 with suture reinforcement as we have done.)
3. The anastomosis is made on the anterior wall of the stomach, but closer to the lesser curvature. This brings the efferent jejunum further to the right which makes construction of a

gastrostomy more difficult, should that be desired. A Witzel gastrostomy without gastropexy could be used in this situation, however, as described by Johnson et al.[8]

4. The gastrojejunostomy is made with a 21-mm cartridge. Of extreme importance is the very careful placement of the purse-string suture in the anterior wall of the gastric pouch (Fig. 5-27). We use a 2–0 Prolene suture with a curved cardiovascular needle, and take short, deep bites close together to ensure maximum strength. The diameter of the purse-string circle should be approximately 15 mm. A small gastrotomy is made in the center of the circle and the opening is gently stretched just enough to accept the ILS-21 anvil. The purse-string is then snugly tied. If this purse-string tears out, the anastomosis will be extremely difficult to complete (Fig. 5-27).
5. As noted in Fig. 5-27 the rod of the ILS instrument is brought through a small stab-type en-

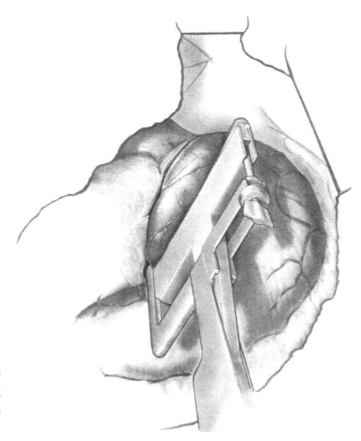

FIG. 5-26. Method I-B: application of TA90 or TA55 instrument, showing an oblique, more vertically placed position from angle of His to further down the lesser curvature (5 cm).

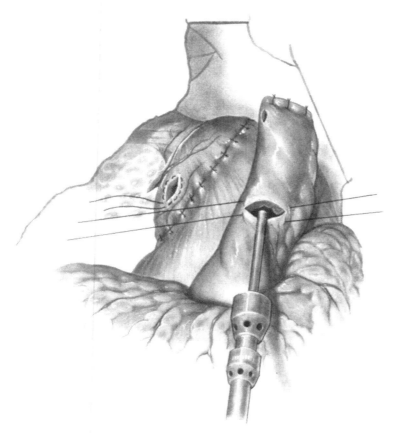

FIG. 5-27. Method I-B: ILS-21 (or EEA-21) rod passed through large (2 cm) and smaller (.5 cm) enterotomy. Note that smaller enterotomy is approximately 1.5 cm from end of staple line, and that purse-string around gastrotomy must have small, deep bites to avoid tearing out.

terotomy 1.5 cm proximal to the staple line on the antimesenteric side of the transected efferent jejunum. (Torres uses a purse-string around the open end of the efferent jejunum.) It is important that the circular cartridge staples do not cross those at the transected end of the efferent jejunum because this can result in jamming. If this occurs the staple instrument cannot be removed without tearing out a large segment of the anastomosis which then has to be repaired. This has happened twice in our practice. The anvil is replaced on the rod and inserted into the pouch through the gastrotomy, and the purse-string suture tied (Fig. 5-28). The cartridge and anvil are then approximated in the prescribed fashion for the instrument used, fired, and carefully withdrawn after partially opening the jaws. The staple line is reinforced with interrpted 3–0 silk. The enterotomy is closed with a TA30 staple instrument. The punched-out tissue rings are inspected for completeness (Fig. 5-28).

6. A No. 1 Prolene suture is ligated around the anastomosis with an 11-mm Hegar dilator in position from below, or a 34-Fr. Hurst dilator passed down from above (Fig. 5-29). This ligature is held in place over the anastomosis with four to six 3–0 gastrointestinal silk sutures and tied down snugly. An alternative method is a purse-string suture of 2–0 Prolene or braided Dacron (Ethibond), taking bites through the seromuscular coats on either side of the anastomosis.

7. The Roux-en-Y jejunojejunostomy is made with the 25-mm EEA or ILS instruments. Although our results have been as good with the I-B as the I-A technique, we have found the I-A procedure to be somewhat simpler, and therefore we are currently using it.

FIG. 5-28. Anvil end of staple instrument has been replaced, passed into gastric pouch, and purse-string tied. A purse-string around small enterotomy is optional (method I-B).

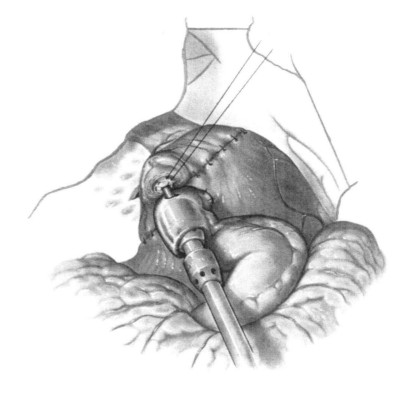

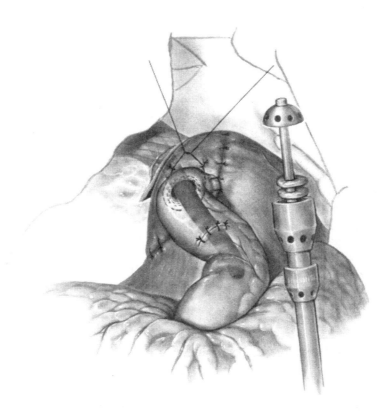

FIG. 5-29. Ethibond or Prolene (2-0) purse-string suture is being tied around a 34-Fr. dilator. Enterotomy has been closed with a TA30 or TA55 instrument. Dilator will be replaced with a No. 16 nasogastric tube. Note intact tissue rings (method I-B).

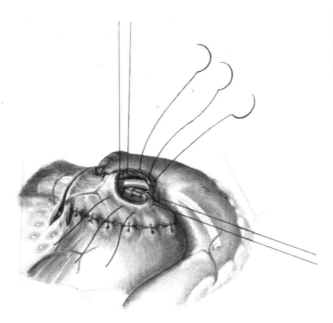

FIG. 5-30. Alternate (suture) method of gastrojejunal anastomosis. This anastomosis is also reinforced with Silastic catheter support (method I-C).

Modified Roux-en-Y Gastric Bypass (Technique I-C)

The third variation on the Roux-en-Y theme, method I-C, is identical to I-A except that all anastomoses are made by a hand-suture technique (Fig. 5-30). The gastrojejunostomy is usually constructed with interrupted 3–0 gastrointestinal silk in a double posterior and a single anterior layer, and the jejunojejunostomy with an inner layer of running chromic catgut suture and an outer layer of interrupted 3–0 silk. The primary advantage in using suture over staple technique is its lower cost. It is also a necessary choice where staple instruments are unavailable. Obviously these various techniques can be combined in any one procedure as long as the essential principles are followed. The gastrojejunostomy is supported by a Silastic catheter in the same way as in I-A (Figs. 5-21 and 5-22).

Other Operative Techniques

Gastroplasty: Horizontal Type

There are many varieties of gastroplasty, and each has its proponents. Our experience with the greater curvature type gastroplasty (horizontal staple line with reinforced greater curvature channel; Fig. 4-6) has been so unsatisfactory that we discontinued its use in 1980. The two principal disadvantages were late weight loss failure and a high incidence of obstructive symptoms with solid foods.

Gomez has also had unsatisfactory results with this procedure, and has changed to the vertical banded gastroplasty.[9] Details of the horizontal GP technique can be obtained from the literature.[5,10]

Gastric Partition

This method was developed at Ohio State University[11,12] and has undergone several changes, particularly the addition of a double row of staples (Fig. 4-7). The reported failure rate of this technique has been too high to recommend its use,[13,14,15,16,17] at least in its initial form, and has been discontinued by its originators at Ohio State University.[18] Whether the addition of external support to the channel will improve the results remains to be seen.

Gastrogastrostomy

LaFave and Alden described this technique in 1979[19] but gave it up after 29 cases because it did not prove to be as effective as the gastric bypass. Buckwalter[20] and Alexander[21] have used this method with apparent success, at least on a short-term basis. Buckwalter has recently changed to the vertical banded gastroplasty.[20] An anastomosis is made between the upper pouch and lower stomach around a single or double staple line, usually with some type of reinforcement around the anastomosis to control size and prevent dilatation (Fig. 4-8 and 4-9).

Gastric Wrap Procedure

Wilkinson has developed a technique in which he wraps the entire stomach with a silicone-impregnated Dacron mesh, more recently Teflon mesh,[38] contracting its lumen to the size of a 36-Fr bougie.[22] Although he has reported encouraging results, the technique cannot be recommended until after a much longer follow-up. The FDA has not approved the use of an equipment manufacturer's model of the gastric wrap as of June, 1983.[23] The management of complications such as bleeding gastric or duodenal ulcer with a total gastric wrap would be difficult. Details of this technique will not be presented here, and the operation should be undertaken only after learning the technique from someone experienced in its use.

Gastric Banding

Several surgeons have adopted variations of a gastric banding procedure originally suggested by Wilkinson, but abandoned by him because of its failure in dogs.[22] Kolle described a technique that involved fastening a lockable nylon band that had been placed within a Dacron arterial prosthesis and tightening it around the upper stomach, with a 12–15 mm bougie within the stomach lumen.[24] A 50 ml proximal pouch was thus created. He reported a series of approximately 85 patients, who had been submitted to this procedure, at the Sixth Annual Bariatric Colloquium at Iowa City. Molina[25] reported his results on 400 patients upon whom he had performed essentially the same operation, and Granstrom[26] reported encouraging results with banding after a one year follow-up comparing gastric bypass, gastroplasty, and gastric banding.

Twelve-month weight losses appeared to be quite satisfactory in these series, but follow-up is too short to recommend this operation at the present time. Pouch dilation, as was found in dogs by Wilkinson,[22] migration of the band into the lumen, or up or down the stomach, and failure secondary to high caloric liquid intake are all possible late complications.

Gastric Bypass with Transection of Upper Stomach

This procedure, developed early in the evolution of gastric reduction surgery, is still being used as the procedure of choice by some surgeons.[27,28] Its two principal advantages are that it prevents staple line disruption with fistulization from the pouch to the lower stomach, and it allows the surgeon to bring the gastroenterostomy up more superficially from its posterior location, thereby facilitating construction of the gastroenterostomy (Fig. 4-5A). The disadvantages are longer operating time and the potential for increased morbidity. Griffen abandoned the transection technique in favor of incontinuity stapling primarily for this reason (Fig. 4-5B).[37] In his experience the leak rate "dropped dramatically, and the operation was done more expeditiously." Miller's leak rate has been 2% with the transection technique,[27] but Reinhold reported no leaks in 38 procedures.[28] The anastomosis is hand-sutured at the greater curvature end of the gastric pouch.

With our present technique, method I-A, there has been no serious technical problem relating to access for constructing the gastroenterostomy, and our leak rate in primary Roux-en-Y procedures has been less than 1%. The staple line disruption rate has been less than 2%.

Vertical Stapling

Tretbar[29] introduced the concept of creating a long narrow tube parallel to the lesser curvature with vertically placed staple lines and no stomal reinforcement (Fig. 4-10). The tubular conduit was thought to serve as both a pouch and a stoma. The number of patients operated upon by this technique has been small and the long-term results have not been published.[30]

Fabito,[31] Eckhout,[32] O'Leary,[33] and Laws[16] have developed somewhat similar procedures, but have added stomal support (Fig. 4-11). In a nonrandomized study, Eckhout reported that in his personal experience the principal advantages of the vertical gastroplasty over the gastric bypass were the following:

1. Less operating time
2. Fewer and less serious complications
3. Lower mortality
4. More rapid recovery after surgery
5. Gastrostomy was unnecessary
6. Elimination of dumping syndrome, marginal ulcer, and afferent loop problems
7. Fewer staple line disruptions
8. Easier access to stoma for gastroscopic examination

The primary disadvantage was vomiting. It was necessary for patients to remain on a liquid diet for at least 3 and sometimes up to 6 months postoperatively in his patients. In my opinion, the other more serious disadvantage is that in the long run this technique may fail, as occurred so frequently in our experience with the horizontal gastroplasty, because many of these patients tend to avoid solid foods and subsist on highly caloric liquids and semisolids with ultimate weight loss failure.

Whether the vertical will prove more effective than the horizontal gastroplasty remains to be seen. The vertical gastric bypass has the pouch outlet directly below the gastroesophageal junction rather than at a sharp angle to the left on the greater curvature, which is a distinct advantage should dilatation of a stenotic stoma be necessary.

Details of various vertical stapling techniques can be found in the references.

Vertical Banded Gastroplasty

Mason[34] developed this operation in 1980, and together with Doherty has performed over 300 of these procedures as of this writing.[35] A window is developed in the mid-stomach close to the lesser curvature, permitting application of two vertical staple lines from the window to the angle of His. A 1.5 × 5.5 cm band of Marlex mesh can then be placed around the inferior aspect of the lesser curvature 22 (Fig. 4-13). Although follow-up has been brief, Mason is enthusiastic enough about the early results to state, "I would like to predict that vertical banded gastroplasty will be the end of the evolutionary line for gastric reduction as a treatment for morbid obesity."[36]

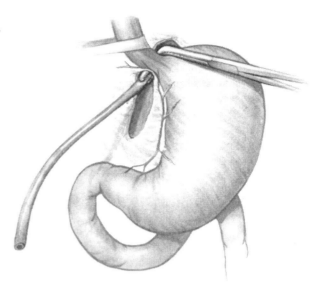

FIG. 5-31. Vertical banded gastroplasty, Right-angle clamp is used to bring catheter around esophagogastric junction for later use. Note Penrose drain around lower esophagus. (Figs. 5-30 to 5-36 were adapted from Mason EE: Vertical banded gastroplasty for obesity. Arch Surg 117:701, 1982.)

Technique of Vertical Banded Gastroplasty
A 32-Fr. Ewald tube is passed into the stomach by the anesthesiologist.[34,36] The abdomen is opened through an upper midline incision and a Penrose drain is placed around the esophagus at the esophagogastric junction. The avascular area of the lesser omentum is incised, and by blunt finger dissection with the left hand the tissue just to the left of the esophagus at the angle of His is exposed. A right-angle clamp is then passed through this areolar tissue from the left side of the esophagus to the opening in the lesser omentum, and a straight catheter is grasped, passed around the esophagus, and clamped for later use (Fig. 5-31).

The anvil of the EEA is placed on the anterior wall of the stomach adjacent to the Ewald tube, approximately 9 cm below the esophagogastric junction and 3 cm from the lesser curvature. The stomach is marked lightly with the electrocautery through the center of the anvil (Fig. 5-32).

The anvil is then placed in the lesser sac adjacent to the Ewald tube and opposite the cautery

FIG. 5-32. The anvil of the EEA-25 is placed on the anterior wall of the stomach, adjacent to the indwelling Ewald tube and approximately 3 cm from the lesser curvature and 9 cm from the angle of His. The stomach is marked lightly with the electrocautery through the center hole.

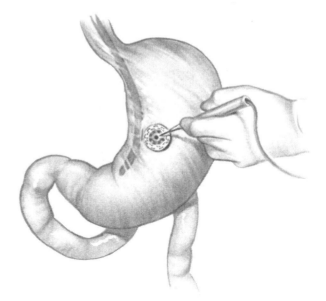

mark, and a Hemovac trocar is pushed through both walls of the stomach into the center of the anvil. One end of a short piece of tubing is attached to the trocar, and the other to the shaft of the EEA instrument. The shaft can now be readily passed through both walls of the stomach (Fig. 5-33). The anvil is then replaced on the shaft, and the EEA instrument is tightened and fired, cutting a stapled window in the stomach adjacent to the lesser curvature containing the Ewald tube (Fig. 5-34).

The flanged end of the straight catheter is brought through this window from the lesser sac and is used to guide the toe of the TA90 instrument through the lesser sac and up to the left side of the esophagus at the angle of His. The pin is placed, and the TA90 is partially closed (Fig. 5-35). A small Penrose drain is then passed from the window around the lesser curvature between the neurovascular bundle and the gastric wall, and the Ewald tube is then positioned with its distal end within the pouch. Both Penrose drains are drawn up tightly and clamped, and the volume of the pouch is then measured holding a syringe containing 60 ml of saline at 50 cm above the cricoid. The volume should measure approximatly 25–35 ml. If necessary, the TA90 can be released and the size altered as indicated (Fig. 5-36).

The TA90 is then closed to the mark and fired. The straight catheter is again attached to the toe of the TA90 and it is backed out to be reloaded. The TA90 should be repositioned just to the left of the first set of staples, and using sponge sticks the pouch is pressed down until the first staple line is approximately 2 mm from the clamp. The TA90 is then fired and removed.

A 7 × 1.5 cm strip of Marlex mesh, marked with one transverse line near the end and with a second line exactly 5.5 cm from the first, is wrapped around the lesser curvature channel through the EEA-created window and the opening between the neurovascular bundle and the gastric wall. The two lines are superimposed and sutured with 3–0 Prolene sutures at each of the overlapped ends and in the middle. [Doherty uses a 5-cm instead of a 5.5-cm circumference (Fig. 5-37)].

The lesser omentum is sutured to the edge of the EEA-created window to cover both the Marlex band and the window, and the Ewald tube is replaced with a nine-hole nasogastric tube with half of the holes beyond the stoma.

Eckhout's[32] and Fabito's[31] techniques are similar to Mason's vertical banded gastroplasty with these differences. In the former two, there is no EEA window, the stoma is smaller (30 Fr. instead of 32 Fr.), the stoma support is a suture-imbri-

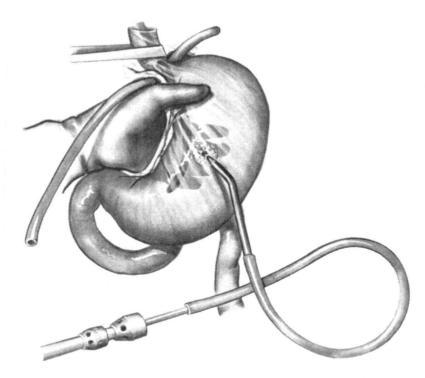

FIG. 5-33. The anvil is placed in the lesser sac, opposite the mark on the anterior wall, and a Hemovac trocar with a tubing attached to the EEA rod is pushed through both walls of the stomach.

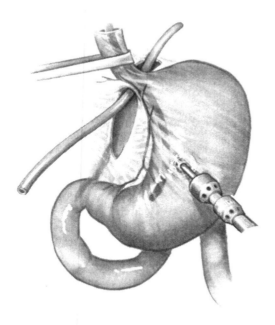

FIG. 5-34. The anvil has been replaced on the rod. The instrument is then tightened and fired, cutting a window through both walls of the stomach. Bleeders around the edge of the EEA window are secured with 3–0 silk stick ties.

cated-pseudopylorus or a 3-mm Silastic catheter instead of a Marlex band, and the double staple line is reinforced with a running 2–0 Prolene suture. The suture within the Silastic catheter support is passed through the gastric walls and ligated around a 30- or 32-Fr. dilator. This may account for the relatively high incidence of migration of the Silastic band into the lumen. Eckhout[32] has had at least two erosions of the Silastic catheter in 90 patients; Laws has had 11.[16] Mason stressed that one of the advantages of the vertical banded gastroplasty technique is that the Marlex band passes through the "gastric window" and remains "totally outside" the gastric walls which should prevent, or at least deter, its migration into the lumen. Our Silastic catheter support around the gastrojejunostomy is also totally outside the anastomosis with no penetrating suture.

To date, in our practice, there have been two band erosions. These bands were removed endoscopically by cutting them with the scissors. Two of our No. 1 Prolene purse string sutures migrated and required cutting.

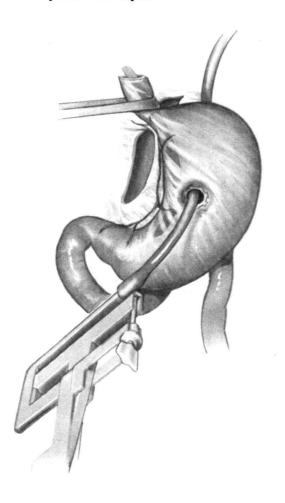

FIG. 5-35. The TA90 anvil is placed in the flanged end of the straight catheter which has been brought through the EEA window; the TA90 is then guided up to the angle of His and the jaws are lightly approximated close to the Ewald catheter.

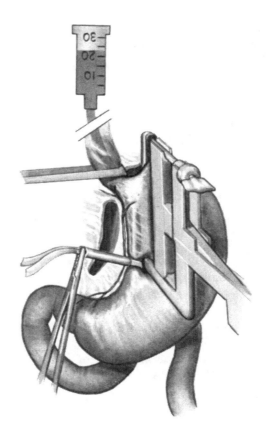

FIG. 5-36. With the TA90 jaws approximated, Penrose drains around the lower esophagus and the lesser curvature of the stomach opposite the window are drawn up tightly for volume measurement (between 25 and 35 ml).

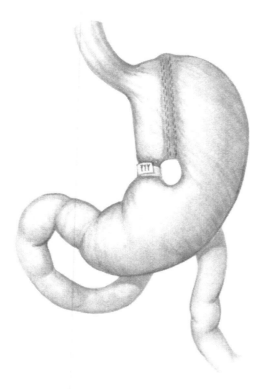

FIG. 5-37. A 7.5 × 1.5 cm strip of Marlex mesh is brought around the lesser curvature of the stomach through the EEA window and sutured at a mark 5.5 cm from a mark near the end of the strip with 3–0 Prolene. The Marlex band and EEA window are then covered with adjacent omentum.

Summary of Specific Techniques

The choice of specific operation is not as important as adherence to the general principles outlined in Chapter 4. We have preferred a retrocolic, antegastric Roux-en-Y operation with a 12- to 15-ml pouch, a 34-Fr. anastomosis supported by a Prolene ligature within a 12-Fr. (4-mm) radiopaque Silastic catheter, and a single 4.8-mm staple line reinforced with interrupted 2–0 silk sutures. A double staple line plus sutures is recommended in revisional procedures and recently in primary procedures as well. The jejunojejunostomy is placed 50 cm distal to the gastrojejunostomy. The anastomosis can be performed in one of three ways: (1) with the GIA plus TA30 or TA55 staple instruments; (2) with the EEA or ILS-21 staple instruments; or (3) by a hand-suture technique.

We have found the GIA plus TA30 or TA55 staple method the most satisfactory, but it is, of course, more expensive than the hand-suture method. The principal advantages of the Roux-en-Y gastric bypass technique over the gastroplasty are its effectiveness and a high degree of patient satisfaction. The disadvantages are that it is a somewhat longer and more complex procedure, and that the distal stomach cannot be examined by conventional means. The horizontal gastroplasty or gastric partitioning procedures have not been sufficiently effective over the long term to justify their use.

The gastrogastrostomy procedure seems to be effective in some hands and is a relatively simple, safe procedure. Follow-up has been short, however.

The vertical banded gastroplasty has been quite successful after a short follow-up (24 months), and could possibly become the procedure of choice. Final assessment must await a longer follow-up period.

References

1. Freeman JB, Burchett HJ: A comparison of gastric bypass and gastroplasty for morbid obesity. Surgery 88:433, 1980.
2. Lechner GW: Subtotal gastric exclusion and gastric partitioning: a randomized prospective comparison of 100 patients. Surgery 90:637, 1981.
3. Linner JH: Comparative effectiveness of gastric bypass and gastroplasty. Arch Surg 117:695, 1982.
4. Alden JF: Gastric and jejunoileal bypass. A comparison in the treatment of morbid obesity. Arch Surg 112:799, 1977.
5. Gomez CA: Gastroplasty in the surgical treatment of morbid obesity. Am J Clin Nutr 33:406, 1980.
6. Griffen WO, Young VL, Stevenson CC: A prospective comparison of gastric and jejunoileal bypass procedures for morbid obesity. Ann Surg 186:500, 1977.
7. Torres JC: Gastric bypass, Roux-en-Y. Presented at Bariatric Workshop, Iowa City, May 29–30, 1980.
8. Johnson WO, Lapez MJ, Kraybell WG, Bricker EM: Experience with a modified Witzel gastrostomy without gastropexy. Ann Surg 195:692, 1982.
9. Gomez CA: Lesser curvature Marlex-banded gastroplasty. Scientific Exhibits. Bariatric Surgery Colloquium. Iowa City, June 2–3, 1983.
10. Mason EE: Surgical treatment of obesity. Major Probl Clin Surg 24:391–400, 1981.
11. Pace WG, Martin EW, Tetirick T, Fabre PJ, Carey LC: Gastric partitioning for morbid obesity. Ann Surg 190:392–400, 1979.

12. Ellison EC, Martin EW Jr, Laschinger J, Majzisik C, Hughes K, Carey LC, Pace WG: Prevention of early failure of stapled gastric partitions in treatment of morbid obesity. Arch Surg 115:528, 1980.

13. Martin EW: Gastric partitioning; an update. Presented at the Bariatric Surgical Colloquium, Iowa City, June 1–2, 1981.

14. Ellison EC: Stapled gastric partition: single vs double row. Presented at the Bariatric Surgical Colloquium, Iowa City, June 1–2, 1981.

15. Laws HL, Piantadosi S: Superior gastric reduction procedure for morbid obesity. Ann Surg 193:334, 1981.

16. Laws HL: Ring gastroplasty for morbid obesity. Presented at the ACS Clinical Congress–General Surgery Motion Pictures, Chicago, October 24–29, 1982.

17. Poires WJ, Flickinger EG, Meelheim D, VanRig AM, Thomas FT: The effectiveness of gastric bypass over gastric partition in morbid obesity. Consequence of distal gastric and duodenal exclusion. Ann Surg 196:389, 1982.

18. Carey LC: Panel discussion. Advances in Gastrointestinal Surgery. 47th Annual Surgery Course. University of Minnesota, Minneapolis, Minnesota, June 15–18, 1983.

19. LaFave JW, Alden JF: Gastric bypass in the operative revision of the failed jejunoileal bypass. Arch Surg 114:438, 1979.

20. Buckwalter JA, Herbst CA Jr: Perioperative complications of gastric bariatric operations. Scientific Exhibit. Bariatric Surgical Colloquium, Iowa City, June 2–3, 1983.

21. Alexander GK: Proximal gastric exclusion (gastrogastrostomy). Presented at the Bariatric Surgical Colloquium, Iowa City, June 1–2, 1980.

22. Wilkinson LH, Peloso OA: Gastric reservoir reduction for morbid obesity. Arch Surg 116:602, 1981.

23. Wilkinson LH: Gastric Wrapping: Observations, changing concepts and results. Bariatric Surgery Colloquium. Iowa City, June 2–3, 1983.

24. Kolle K, Stadaas J: Gastric banding. Scientific Exhibits: Bariatric Surgery Colloquium, Iowa City, June 2–3, 1983.

25. Molina M: Gastric banding. Bariatric Surgery Colloquium, Iowa City, June 2–3, 1983.

26. Granstrom L, Backman L: One year weight loss after gastric bypass, gastroplasty, and gastric banding. Scientific Exhibit. Bariatric Colloquium. Iowa City, June 2–3, 1983.

27. Miller DK: Poster presentation: gastric bypass. Presented at the Bariatric Surgical Colloquium, Iowa City, June 3–4, 1982.

28. Reinhold RB: Critical analysis of long-term weight loss following gastric bypass. Surg Gynecol Obstet 155:385, 1982.

29. Tretbar LL, Taylor TT, Sifers EC: Weight reduction, gastric plication for morbid obesity. J Kans Med Soc 77:488, 1976.

30. Tretbar LL: Vertical stapling updated. Presented at the Bariatric Surgical Workshop, Iowa City, May 29–30, 1980.

31. Fabito DC: Vertical stapling gastroplasty for obesity. Presented at the Bariatric Surgical Workshop, Iowa City, May 29–30, 1980 and June 1–2, 1981.

32. Eckhout GV, Prinzing JF: Surgery for morbid obesity: comparison of gastric bypass with vertically stapled gastroplasty. Colo Med 78:117, 1981.

33. O'Leary JP: Partition of the lesser curvature of the stomach in morbid obesity. Surg Gynecol Obstet 154:85, 1982.

34. Mason EE: Vertical banded gastroplasty for obesity. Arch Surg 117:701, 1982.

35. Mason EE, Lewis JW, Doherty C, Scott DH, Rodriques EM, Blommers TJ: The current status of gastric reduction for obesity. Bariatric Surgical Colloquium. Iowa City, June 2–3, 1983.

36. Mason EE: Evaluation of gastric reduction for obesity. Contemp Surg 20:17, 1982.

37. Griffen WO, Bivens BA, Bell RM, Jackson KA: Gastric bypass for morbid obesity. World J Surg 5:817–822, 1981.

38. Wilkinson LH, Peloso OA, Milne RL: Gastric reservoir reduction for correction of morbid obesity. Fourth International Congress on Obesity. New York, October 5–8, 1983.

CHAPTER 6

Gastric Operations: Postoperative Management and Complications

JOHN H. LINNER

General Considerations

The great majority of our patients are extubated in the operating room or postanesthesia recovery room, depending upon return of respiratory function, which is in turn related to the patient's weight, length of operative procedure, and cardiopulmonary status. Criteria for extubation are discussed in Chapter 9. All of our patients are cared for in the intensive care unit for the first 24 h, and longer if indicated. ICU care is probably unnecessary except for those patients who require ventilator management, or older patients. This determination must also take into account the adequacy of the floor nursing staff.

The nasogastric tube is irrigated intermittently and withdrawn 1 to 2 in on the first postoperative day to prevent perforation by the tip of the tube. It is usually removed on the second postoperative day if a 4-h trial period of clamping is tolerated without distress, and less than 100 ml returns when the tube is opened and placed on suction. We have found it unnecessary to wait for passage of flatus to remove the tube.

A gastrostomy is routinely used for patients who have a JIB takedown, with or without a concurrent gastric bypass, and for patients who have a gastric revision procedure, but not usually for those with a primary gastric bypass unless they are either superobese (over 2.5 times ideal weight) or have cardiopulmonary dysfunction. The gastrostomy tube is left in for at least 1 week, and occasionally for several months if supplemental nutrition is necessary. Recently, in patients who do not have a gastrostomy tube, we have empirically used metoclopramide hydrochloride (Reglan), 10 mg every 4 h for 36 h, to stimulate emptying of the distal stomach and to serve as an antiemetic. This would, of course, not prevent blowout secondary to afferent limb obstruction (ALO), but it would obviate gastric dilatation due to pylorospasm or distal gastric atony. If the primary procedure has been a loop instead of a Roux-en-Y gastroenterostomy, a gastrostomy is recommended because the incidence of ALO is higher with a loop anastomosis. Alden[1] uses a Witzel gastrostomy routinely for primary Roux-en-Y gastric bypass to prevent early staple line disruption as well as blowout. Halverson,[2] who uses a loop-type gastric bypass, routinely employs a Stamm gastrostomy to prevent distal gastric blowout, which occurred in two of his patients without a gastrostomy.

We rarely use a jejunostomy tube, but Bothe et al[3] have found it helpful for feeding purposes when there is delayed stomal function. Early enteric fluid and nutrition can be supplied in this way if the intravenous line is tenuous. A gastrostomy tube can also be used for the same purpose.

Routine Postoperative Orders

Below are listed our routine postoperative orders which are self-explanatory, and can be modified depending upon individual circumstances.

1. ICU.
2. Meperidine (Demerol) 50–100 mg q3h p.r.n. pain—or if sensitive—Levo-Dromoran (plain) 2–4 mg q3h (IM) p.r.n. pain.
3. Compazine 10 mg or Tigan 200 mg q6h (IM) p.r.n. nausea.

4. Metoclopramide hydrochloride (Reglan) 10 mg q4h IV piggyback times 36 h unless patient has a gastrostomy. (This is on a trial basis.)

5. Diazepam (Valium) 5 mg q6h (IM) p.r.n. tension or sleep.

6. Balanced duodenal salt solution (Travert's Electrolyte #2 with 5% dextrose) at 150 ml/h for first 36 h, then at 125 ml/h.

7. Cefazolin (Ancef) 1 g IV piggyback q6h × 4 doses. (If penicillin-sensitive, substitute doxycycline hyclate (Vibramycin) 200 mg in 5% DW 500 ml piggyback once 1st postoperative day.)

8. Soluble multivitamins (M.V.I.) 5 ml in 1 liter q.d.

9. Incentive spirometer and IPPB q2h—alternate × 36 h. After 36 h use disposable incentive spirometer q.i.d. Ambulate patient with help as soon as possible, usually the night of surgery.

10. NG tube to low suction—irrigate p.r.n. after surgery. Maximum 25 ml per irrigation. Withdraw 1–2 in and retape 1st postoperative day only.

11. On 2nd postoperative day start clamping tube 4 h as tolerated. If tolerated, and less than 125 ml returns, remove NG. Then 1–2 oz. H_2O q1h per ora × 3 h. Then clear liquids in small amounts. Start full liquids on 4th postoperative day.

12. Foley catheter to straight drainage. Culture urine and remove Foley 2nd or 3rd postoperative day.

13. If urine output is less than 35 ml/h, give 500 ml flush with D5, lactated Ringer's. If effective, may repeat q8h p.r.n. If not, give 25 g mannitol IV q8h p.r.n. If no response, Lasix 30 mg IV q8h p.r.n. Check urine specific gravity before diuretics are used. D/C order after 3 days.

14. Hgb at 4:00 P.M. and early A.M. (Occasionally, CBC and electrolytes are drawn 1st day. Also arterial blood gases whenever indicated.)

15. CBC and electrolytes 2nd and 5th postoperative days.

16. Ambulate patient with help, if possible evening of surgery, then 3–4 times daily as tolerated with binder on.

17. Encourage coughing, turning, moving legs, and so on at frequent intervals.

18. Larylgan throat spray p.r.n.—occasional ice chips.

19. Heparin 5000 U q12h subcutaneously. Starting 8:00 A.M. day after surgery × days.

20. Dietician to instruct patient on 4th or 5th postoperative day.

21. Upper GI x ray on 5th or 6th postoperative day. Follow radiograph with 1 oz. of M.O.M. or mineral oil.

Respiratory physiotherapy and early ambulation are vital in preventing postoperative pulmonary complications, and minidose heparin, plus support stockings to the knee, are valuable adjuncts in preventing thromboembolism. Thigh-high stockings seldom stay up, and too often are found rolled down in a tight obstructing band just above or at the knee joint. Some patients' legs are too huge for any type of stocking or wrapping.

Prophylactic antibiotics are continued for 24 h in the usual case, and for 36 to 48 h in patients who have had a JIB takedown.

Oral Intake

After the nasogastric tube is removed, which is usually on the 2nd postoperative day, the patient is given 1 to 2 oz. of water every hour for 3 h. If tolerated, clear liquids in small amounts are given, to be sipped slowly, followed on the 4th day by a full liquid diet which includes cooked cereal. Intravenous fluids are discontinued as soon as the patient is taking up to 400 ml of clear liquid per 8-h shift, usually by the 4th postoperative day. When the IV has been discontinued the patient is allowed to shower and shampoo. In patients with gastrostomy or jejunostomy tubes, the IV can be discontinued earlier, and fluids provided by the enteric route.

Usually by the 5th day a soft post–gastric bypass diet is started, and the patient is given thorough dietary instructions by the hospital dietician. This is reinforced by a visit from the office nurse who gives the patient a two-page dietary instruction handout to take home (see Appendix 3).

If there is concern about the integrity of the anastomosis or the blood supply to the pouch, oral intake should be delayed for 5–8 days, and the anastomosis visualized by an upper GI tract x-ray examination using a small amount of Gastrografin prior to starting oral fluids.

Patients are warned against eating apple peelings, citrus pulp, stringy celery, and fibrous meats.

Patients with vertical gastroplasties must be particularly careful with all solid foods the first 3 months postoperatively. All patients must cut their meat into extremely small pieces, and chew it well. Some may find it necessary to either grind or blenderize meats.

Vitamins

An oral multivitamin–mineral tablet or liquid vitamin is started prior to discharge to determine the patient's tolerance for vitamins, and patients are urged to continue its use for their lifetimes. One of our patients manifested clinical evidence of thiamine (vitamin B_1) deficiency with polyneuritis.[4] A Wernicke-Korsakoff type of encephalopathy has also been reported.[5] These complications can be prevented by the administration of vitamins, and by hospitalizing patients with persistent vomiting early for nutritional therapy.

Postoperative Upper Gastrointestinal Radiography

On the 5th or 6th postoperative day an upper GI radiograph is obtained on every patient, which serves as a baseline should subsequent studies be clinically indicated. It is important to give the patient 1 or 2 oz. of milk of magnesia or mineral oil following this examination to eliminate the barium from the colon.

Drains and Dressings

The dressings and the small subcutaneous Penrose drain are removed on the 1st postoperative day, and the staples or stitches on the day of discharge, usually the 6th or 7th day. Steri-strips, 0.5 in wide, are applied to the wound at that time. Dietary and activity instructions are again reviewed with the patients, and they are given a prescription for multivitamin tablets and a mild analgesic and/or soporific as indicated. They are advised not to use aspirin-containing analgesics. Large tablets should be broken up prior to ingestion to prevent stomal obstruction.

Food Bolus Obstruction

Instructions are also given in the management of obstruction of the stoma due to meat or similar protein. A teaspoon of unseasoned meat tenderizer suspended in 4 oz. of water is sipped intermittently—over a period of several hours—which usually causes the meat to break up and pass through. Papase tablets can also be used for this purpose. Kanulase tablets are helpful in breaking up vegetable matter. Occasionally only gastroscopic manipulation can relieve an obstructed stoma; patients should be informed of this possibility prior to discharge from the hospital, which serves as an added incentive to follow dietary instructions.

Ambulation

Patients should be advised not to sit for long periods of time or take long trips without periodic ambulation to avoid thromboembolism. They should be seen in the office at approximately 3 weeks and instructed to call if any problems arise.

Follow-up Visits

Follow-up visits after the first office call are at 3, 6, 9, 12, 18, and 24 months, and then once yearly for their lifetime. A commitment to return for follow-up should be obtained from the patient prior to surgery.

At 12 and 24 months, serum B_{12}, folic acid, magnesium, lipids, and iron, as well as the more common standard laboratory determinations— CBC, SMA-12, and electrolytes—are obtained. Subsequent studies are ordered as indicated. Approximately 30% of our patients have been found to be iron or vitamin B_{12} deficient or both at 2 years and have been given supplemental therapy as indicated. Halverson[6] reported a 30% incidence of anemia following loop gastric bypass at 2 years with 44% B_{12}, 27% folate, and 31% iron deficiencies. Most patients can be managed by oral supplementation, but in some parenteral replacement is necessary.

Complications During the Perioperative Period

The incidence of postoperative complications depends to a large extent upon the experience of the surgeon and the type of operative procedure. A simple gastric reduction operation that involves placement of one or two staple lines across the stomach is attended by fewer early complications than a gastric bypass with one or two anastomoses.

This comparison is deceptive, however, because as we experienced, the simpler gastroplasty was followed by a 50% failure rate and a correspondingly higher revision rate, which greatly increased the overall morbidity of this operation.[7] Complications are generally more common and severe following revisional surgery.

Early postoperative complications can be divided into the following categories, some of which are germane only for the gastric bypass where anastomoses are involved.

I. Wound
   A. Wound infection
   B. Wound dehiscence
II. Gastrointestinal Tract
   A. Leaks: operative trauma, ischemia, perforation, blowout
      1. Pouch
      2. Distal stomach
      3. Anastomoses
      4. Staple line partition
   B. Obstructions
      1. Afferent limb
      2. Efferent limb
      3. Stomal obstruction
         a. Constructed too small initially
         b. Edema
         c. Kink
         d. Bezoar
         e. Functional—apparently due to atony
      4. Colon obstruction: compression by antecolic efferent limb
   C. Distal bowel obstruction
      1. Herniation into mesenteric defects
      2. Adhesive band obstruction
      3. Twist or volvulus
   D. Postoperative hemorrhage
      1. Gastroenterostomy
      2. Jejunojejunostomy
   E. Stress ulcer
      1. Gastric
      2. Duodenal
III. Splenic Injury—Iatrogenic Splenectomy
   A. Most common in procedures that require mobilization of greater curvature and ligation of vasa brevia
   B. Splenic capsule tears can usually be treated successfully with hemostatic agents such as microfibrillar collagen (Avitene) and gentle pressure; the incidence of splenectomy should be less than 1% for any procedure

IV. Subphrenic Abscess
   A. Leak—most common cause
   B. Postsplenectomy abscess—common sequela of splenectomy
   C. Infected hematoma
V. Pulmonary Complications
   A. Atelectasis
   B. Pneumonitis
   C. Adult respiratory distress syndrome (ARDS)
   D. Pulmonary embolism
VI. Cardiac Failure
   A. Fluid overload
   B. Myocardial infarction
VII. Avoidable Technical Errors
   A. Tube caught in staple line (requires reoperation to release if not detected before closing abdomen)
   B. Inadvertent tear of gastric wall or esophagus during mobilization, especially in revisions
   C. Improper staple formation with resultant staple line disruption
   D. NG tube positioned with no holes in pouch, or with tip impinging against bowel wall
   E. Operative injury to diaphragm with subsequent herniation of stomach or bowel; greatest risk occurs when lysing adhesions during revisional surgery
VIII. Early Death
   A. Septic shock—usually due to unrecognized leak or blowout
   B. Respiratory failure; ARDS
   C. Pulmonary embolism
   D. Myocardial infarction; congestive heart failure

The perioperative complications we have encountered in our practice are listed in Table 6-1.

Complications peculiar to JIB takedown and concurrent gastric reduction will be discussed in Chapter 7.

Prevention

More than in any other type of elective surgery, the key to minimizing postoperative complications in bariatric surgery is prevention. This can be accomplished to a large extent by careful patient selection, eliminating those patients who are poor risks from either a psychiatric or physical point of view. Patients with respiratory or cardiac dysfunction should be treated medically prior to surgery as outlined in Chapter 4 or the incidence

TABLE 6-1 Early Complications Following Primary Surgery: 1976–1983

Complication	GBP–Loop (47 cases)		GBP–Roux-en-Y (285 cases)		GP (187 cases)	
Leaks, perforations			(2)		(5)	
Subphrenic abscess					(1)	
Postoperative bleeding			(1)			
Small bowel obstruction			(1)			
Diaphragmatic hernia (operative trauma)					(1)	
Gastric volvulus					(1)	
Stenosis outlet (early reoperation)					(1)	
NG tube stapled	(1)					
Splenectomy, iatrogenic				1		
Thrombophlebitis				1		2
Pulmonary embolism		1				1
Pneumonitis/atelectasis		3		6		6
Temporary outlet obstruction		1		1		2
Wound infection		3		6		2
Antibiotic enterocolitis	0			1	0	
Adult respiratory distress syndrome	0			1		1
Deaths	0		(1)[a]	1[b]	0	
Total	(1) (2.1%)	8 17%	(4) (1.4%)	17 6.8%	(9) (4.7%)	14 7%

[a] Death due to perforation of excluded stomach.
[b] Death due to adult respiratory distress syndrome.
Numbers in parentheses refer to those complications requiring surgery.

of serious complications will be prohibitive. Smoking must be discontinued at least 2 weeks preoperatively, and drug-dependent patients must not be operated upon unless they are 1 year or more into a successful treatment program. Complications tend to increase and to be more serious in patients over 60 years of age.

The experience and knowledge of the surgeon are also extremely important. There is a learning curve in bariatric surgery related to the huge size of these patients and the resultant difficult access to the upper abdomen where the essential technical aspects of the procedure take place. Postoperative management and the diagnosis of complications are also more difficult for the same reason. These are not procedures to be done as an occasional operation. Surgeons with a large experience report a greater number of perioperative complications early in their series, with a drop in the incidence of complications later. Furthermore, management of the more serious complications such as leak or blowout becomes more effective with a lower mortality as experience grows.[8] Awareness of the complications that can occur and learning to appreciate their presence is essential to proper man-

agement, and is one of the primary purposes of this book.

Important Technical Considerations

Most of the serious complications such as anastomotic leaks, leaks of either the gastric pouch or distal stomach, iatrogenic spleen injury requiring splenectomy, afferent or efferent loop obstruction, or hemorrhage from an anastomosis can be minimized, but perhaps not totally prevented, by careful technique.

Good lighting, some type of effective retraction, and reverse Trendelenburg position during the upper abdominal portion of the procedure are minimum requirements for a safe and technically feasible operation. Since we have modified our gastric bypass procedure and no longer need to mobilize the greater curvature of the stomach or ligate any of the vasa brevia, there have been no perforations due to ischemic necrosis, nor have there been any iatrogenic splenectomies.[7] Vertical gastroplasties along the lesser curvature are also attended by a low leakage and splenectomy rate.[9,10]

Withdrawing the nasogastric tube 1.5–2 in on

the first postoperative day has prevented tube perforations, and using a Roux-en-Y instead of a loop-type gastroenterostomy has virtually eliminated afferent loop obstruction as well as reflux gastritis and esophagitis. Routine use of gastrostomy drainage obviates distal stomach blowout and decompresses an obstructed afferent limb. We strongly recommend that a gastrostomy be used in patients who have had a JIB takedown or a gastric stapling revision because they seem more prone to develop postoperative gastric distension. A number of surgeons use it routinely in every case including primary procedures as pointed out earlier.[1,2] The gastrostomy can serve a useful purpose for supplemental enteric nutrition should this become necessary.

Bowel Obstruction: Early

Small bowel obstruction (SBO) is (almost) never a problem following gastroplasty (GP) operations, and it is rare after primary gastric bypass (GBP) procedures. In our experience, SBO was most common following combined JIB reconstitution and loop gastric bypass. In 679 total gastric-type operations, 519 of which were primary and 160 secondary (revisions, conversions, or JIB reconstitution plus gastric reduction), there was a total of 7 (1.%) small bowel obstructions requiring reoperation. Five of these followed JIB takedown plus gastric reduction; three of the five in loop-type GBP, two in Roux-en-Y GBP, and none in either primary or secondary gastroplasties. Of the remaining two small bowel obstructions, one was in a primary and the other in a secondary Roux-en-Y GBP.

Most of the perioperative obstructions were related to either a twist or a kink at or near the gastroenterostomy or the Roux-en-Y jejunojejunostomy. Both loop and Roux-en-Y GBPs were vulnerable to obstruction in JIB conversions because of the discrepancy in size between the large hypertrophied afferent and the small defunctional efferent jejunum. The loop obstructions were corrected by conversion to a Roux-en-Y jejunojejunostomy as will be discussed in Chapter 7. SBO was more common in our early than our later experience.

Proximal bowel obstruction due to a 180 to 360° inadvertent twist of the jejunum (usually in the Roux-en-Y efferent limb) and its mesentery is a preventable cause of SBO that may not be detected until after the gastroenterostomy has been completed, or worse, until the patient develops symptoms of bowel obstruction and requires a second operative procedure. We had one such case early in our experience. Carefully checking the mesentery in every case to avoid a twist prior to starting the gastroenterostomy is essential. In the loop-type of GBP, kinking at the anastomosis can usually be prevented by ensuring gentle curves without tension, and by suturing the efferent limb to the stomach below the anastomosis for a distance of 2–4 cm. Proper placement of the nasogastric tube with at least two holes in the gastric pouch and no kinks in the tubing is another important measure to prevent both pouch dilatation and perforation, as well as afferent limb obstruction at the anastomosis secondary to pouch distension.

Colon Obstruction

There was one transverse colon obstruction due to compression by a too taut, antecolic Roux-en-Y limb. This was in a patient who had a JIB reconstitution with GBP. The transverse colon was large and redundant. We now use only a retrocolic, but antegastric, Roux-en-Y approach, which makes the gastroenterostomy easier and safer, being more direct with no tension at the anastomosis. Closing the transverse mesocolon hiatus around the efferent jejunum takes only a few minutes.

Wound Infection

Our wound infection rate has been low, less than 2%, attributable in part to the use of prophylactic systemic antibiotics, and irrigation of the peritoneal cavity as well as the wound with normal saline and dilute antibiotic (cephalothin) solution.

We have routinely used a plastic wound protector, positioned early in the operation, with dilute cephalothin solution instilled around its edge in all but 75 patients. Because the wound infection rate more than doubled in this latter group of patients (from less than 1% to over 2%), we returned to using the wound protector. This was not a statistically valid study, of course, but it was impressive and we have been reluctant to enter into a randomized study after this experience.

To date we are fortunate in not having had an evisceration which we credit to the "unit" method of closure described in Chapter 5.

Diagnosis of Complications

Despite the most carefully planned and executed operation, complications will occasionally occur, and it is of vital importance that the surgeon maintain a high index of suspicion during the entire postoperative period. As mentioned earlier, leaks, proximal bowel obstruction, iatrogenic splenectomy, bleeding from anastomoses, obstructed anastomoses, wound dehiscence, and wound infection are usually related to surgical technique and can be minimized by adherence to principles outlined earlier. Atelectasis, pneumonitis, and thromboembolic disease are related more to the adequacy of pre- and postoperative care, but will occur occasionally in spite of optimal management.

Leaks

Leaks or obstructions are frequently obscured in these massive patients, and diagnosis can be delayed for days if the surgeon is not alert to their early manifestations. They occur following either gastroplasty or gastric bypass. The most common single sign of leakage, although not specific, is tachycardia—over 120 beats/min—for which no other obvious explanation can be found. Should this finding be present, hypovolemia, for whatever reason, should be corrected, and a chest radiograph taken to exclude pneumonitis or atelectasis. The most common error that delays appropriate treatment is the assumption that the symptoms are caused by pneumonitis or pulmonary infarction. A lower lobe atelectasis, especially involving the left lower lung segments, or a left-sided pleural effusion can be the result of a leak and subphrenic fluid collection. Tachycardia, tachypnea, leukocytosis, fever, and left shoulder strap pain at any time during the postoperative course are very suggestive of leakage, from either an anastomosis or through the wall of the upper pouch or distal stomach.

Ischemic necrosis of the excluded stomach or pouch seldom occurs before the 3rd postoperative day, and a leak at the anastomosis is usually not apparent clinically until the first oral feeding, unless it is large. In one of our patients the diagnosis became apparent early, and she was reoperated within 24 h of the primary procedure. Occasionally a leak does not become manifest for as long as 2 weeks, after the patient has gone home. Symptoms of a leak at the anastomosis with a loop-type gastroenterostomy tend to be earlier and more severe than with a Roux-en-Y type because larger quantities of bile and pancreatic juice escape into the upper abdominal cavity and subphrenic space with the former procedure. Occasionally the extravasated contents descend into the pelvis causing pelvic and/or vaginal pain with dysuria and urgency.

Ketone Test for Infection Both et al[3] have reported a method for detecting the presence of postoperative infection early, sometimes before other symptoms have become apparent. This is based upon ketogenesis and ketonuria that normally occur in obese patients during the postoperative starvation period unless dextrose-containing intravenous solutions are given or the patient develops an infection. These observers use dextrose-free amino acid solutions and check the urine for ketone bodies every 8 h. Ketonuria is consistently found unless infection supervenes, in which case ketonuria disappears, and the presence of an infection is thus strongly suspected. Mason has not recommended this method because it is his belief that the presence of excess free fatty acids (FFA) enhances intravascular clotting and that dextrose-containing solutions are important in decreasing FFA concentration and preventing thromboembolism.[11] We use dextrose-containing solutions so do not utilize this test.

Radiographic Diagnosis of Leak If a leak is suspected, examination of the upper gastrointestinal tract with a water-soluble radiopaque medium (Gastrografin) will often prove diagnostic. The Gastrografin should be swallowed rather than instilled into the nasogastric tube or the leak may be missed. A negative study does not exclude the possibility of a leak, however, because occasionally it becomes temporarily sealed (see Chapter 11).

If, at the time of surgery, we are concerned about the integrity of an anastomosis or the adequacy of the blood supply to the pouch, we place a soft Silastic suction catheter (Jackson-Pratt) in the left upper quadrant through a stab incision to be used as a "leak sentinel," which can be extremely helpful in the early definitive diagnosis of leakage. It is not an infallible leak indicator, however, and in one of our patients gave us a false sense of security. This patient developed a leak 24–48 h postoperatively with tachycardia (pulse, > 120) and left lower lobe atelectasis. The Jackson-Pratt tube drainage was minimal and had the appearance of clear serum. On the 5th postoperative day when the Jackson-Pratt tube was removed, there was a gush of foul-smelling purulent material that had obviously not reached the tube lumen because of fibrin occlusion. A Gastrografin upper GI film revealed a leak, and the patient was reoperated. In this case we were deceived by the tube initially, and would probably have obtained the Gastrografin study a day or two earlier if the tube had not been used. The Jackson-Pratt tube does not provide adequate drainage for collections due to leak, and open drainage should not be delayed in the hope that it will. A 12- to 24-h delay for the patient to achieve a more optimal condition may rarely be indicated, but generally, the earlier open drainage can be established the better. Early surgery occasionally permits suture closure of a leak that would not be possible later. If a Silastic catheter support surrounding the anastomosis has been used, it should be removed at the reoperation.

Clinical Diagnosis of Leak   When a leak cannot be demonstrated radiographically, the decision to reoperate must be made on clinical grounds. Usually patients with a leak manifest pain, anxiety, and seem unable to find a comfortable position in bed. They often prefer to sit up, and occasionally insist on getting into a chair or even standing. If peritonitis has become generalized, however, they resist any movement. This is in contrast to the normal postoperative course which is accompanied by relatively little pain.

The pain of leakage may be epigastric only, or involve the left shoulder strap area, the entire abdomen, or the pelvis. As the leak progresses, the patient's respiratory and cardiac rates increase, breathing becomes more shallow, the patient spikes a fever, and in later stages septic shock with oliguria, anuria, hypotension, and respiratory failure supervenes. At this point, the mortality rate becomes excessive regardless of what is done. Arterial blood gas levels deteriorate progressively. Except for abdominal pain, tenderness, and a spiking fever, most or all of the above clinical signs can be duplicated by a large pulmonary embolism. The assumption that leak symptoms are due to a pulmonary embolism, and failing to reoperate on that account, can be a fatal error.

There can be all degrees of leakage, from a small, rapidly sealing leak that may respond to antibiotic therapy alone, to large leaks that cause rapidly progressive septic shock. A left subphrenic abscess quite commonly follows a splenectomy with or without the presence of a leak.[12]

Distal Stomach Necrosis (Blowout)
Acute afferent limb obstruction, or obstruction of the distal stomach due to pylorospasm or "vagotomy effect" with acute distal gastric dilatation, can be more subtle because signs of peritoneal irritation do not appear until after necrosis and leakage from the excluded stomach have occurred. These patients experience progressive, severe pain and thirst, and become extremely restless. After gastric blowout has occurred signs of peritonitis and shock soon develop, and the mortality rate sharply increases.

Diagnosis of Gastric Distension   A flat and upright abdominal film will usually reveal the distended stomach and afferent limb. Surgical clip markers placed on the greater and lesser curvature opposite each other at the time of surgery facilitate radiographic diagnosis of gastric distension.[13] A Gastrografin upper GI radiograph may further delineate evidence of afferent limb obstruction and occasionally even obstructing pylorospasm. Unless the nasogastric tube can be manipulated into the afferent stoma and the distal stomach decompressed, which can be difficult to impossible, reexploration is essential, and should be done before necrosis has occurred.

Surgical Management

Our usual surgical approach in treating a leak, blowout, or subphrenic abscess is through the operative incision. When possible, leak sites are closed by sutures and/or covered with adjacent fat. If there is necrosis of the wall of the stomach, resection of the involved area, and occasionally the entire distal stomach, is necessary. The presence of a twist or kink of the jejunum would also require surgical correction. Penrose plus sump-suction drains are brought out through separate left and right stab incisions from the left subphrenic and right subhepatic spaces, respectively, in most patients, taking care to avoid immediate contact between suction tubes and the stomach. It is extremely important that at least one of the drainage tubes be placed high and posteriorly enough to drain the posterior superior aspect of the collection, because it is here that most of the leakage gravitates.

A gastrostomy tube is brought out from the distal stomach whenever possible, and occasionally a double jejunostomy tube is placed with one tube extending upward toward the gastroenterostomy for suction, and the other downward for feeding purposes.

More established subphrenic collections without an apparent leak are occasionally drained through a posterior approach. Rarely, two or more subsequent operations are required to achieve a cure. The relationship of the abscess cavity to the spleen and its accessibility to a posterior approach can best be determined by a CAT scan.

Miller[14] has experienced success in ten of 11 leak-abscesses with percutaneous catheter drainage. This approach requires a well-trained interventional radiologist and CAT scan capability.

Spleen Injury

Splenectomy was necessary in one primary (Roux-en-Y gastric bypass) and three secondary operations (two revisions and one conversion). Splenic capsule tears with troublesome bleeding occurred in 15 additional operations (14 primary and one secondary). These were managed by application of Surgicel and/or Avitene hemostatic material. In those with the most active bleeding, Avitene was more effective in our hands. Avitene wrapped within Surgicel facilitated application in some situations.

In our current anterior GBP, and in vertical-type gastroplasties that do not require mobilization of the greater curvature, spleen trauma should almost never occur. Revisions and conversions are more likely to be complicated by injury to the spleen requiring splenectomy. In one of our revision procedures, the spleen was adherent to the gastric pouch, necessitating splenectomy to accomplish the revision.

During the preoperative work-up, especially for revisional surgery, the patient should be informed that a splenectomy may be required to either complete the operation or to control bleeding.

Staple Line Problems

Staple line partition failures usually appear sometime after the first month, and will be considered in the section on late complications. Every staple line should be examined carefully both anteriorly and posteriorly to ensure proper staple formation. The posterior aspect cannot usually be seen in its entirety, but the portion not visualized can be palpated. If there is evidence of improper staple for-

mation a second staple application should be applied closely adjacent to the first. Many surgeons routinely use a double application of staples as discussed earlier.

A faulty staple line at an anastomosis is usually due to improper placement of the staple instrument and not to faulty staples, and can be detected by compression on either side of the anastomosis, or by instilling saline with or without methylene blue dye through the nasogastric tube. Any defect must be closed by interrupted nonabsorbable sutures.

Postoperative Hemorrhage

Early serious postoperative hemorrhage has been rare in our experience. Careful visualization of the posterior anastomotic staple line at the time of surgery with stick tie control of all arterial bleeders will almost always prevent this troublesome complication. Most postoperative anastomotic bleeding will stop within 24 h, but rarely reoperation becomes necessary. We have had three patients with significant postoperative anastomotic bleeding, two of whom required reoperation for control.

Bleeding from a stomal ulceration usually occurs as a late complication, and has become rare with pouches of less than 50 ml volume.

Stress Ulceration

Stress ulceration with hemorrhage involving the gastric mucosa has been extremely rare in our experience, and most of our gastric perforations involving either the pouch or the distal stomach were thought to be due to ischemia and not stress ulceration. Prophylactic cimetidine was not effective in preventing gastric perforations in our experience and is no longer used.[7] Duodenal ulcer perforation due to stress and hyperacidity has been reported in the immediate postoperative period.[15] These are extremely rare, presenting as any large leak or blowout, and require surgical management. We have not encountered this complication.

If a patient has a history of duodenal ulcer, a vagotomy and some type of gastrostomy should be done. Unless pyloric stenosis is present, a pyloroplasty is unnecessary and may be disadvantageous because of bile reflux.[16] Discrete BB shot–type perforations in either the jejunum distal to the anastomosis or the stomach are usually caused by the nasogastric tube.[17]

Avoidable Technical Errors

Inadvertent stapling of the nasogastric tube can be prevented if the tube location is always checked after the jaws of the staple instrument have been approximated, but *prior* to firing. Additionally, after all stapling has been completed, the upward mobility of the tube should be checked.

If the tube has been inadvertently stapled and not detected during the course of surgery, reoperation will be necessary to release it. The staples must be cut out from their gastric attachments, thus locally resecting both anterior and posterior gastric walls.

The only time we encountered this vexing complication was early in our experience, and reoperation was undertaken on the 5th postoperative day, after all other attempts to disengage the tube proved futile. At surgery, after incising through both gastric walls to free the tube, we closed the defects in both anterior and posterior gastric walls with interrupted 3–0 silk, and then reapplied the TA90 staple instrument above the previous staple line. An alternative method would be to place the staple lines above and below the gastric wall defect with or without transection between the lines. Additional suture reinforcement of the staple line is advisable.

Early Death

Perioperative mortality rates have been reported from less than 1% to 4%.[18] Case selection, type of surgical procedure, and experience of the surgeon are the three most significant factors affecting morbidity and mortality. The risk of death is directly related to the patient's age, weight, and physical condition. The most common causes of early postoperative death are (1) leaks of various types with associated sepsis; (2) respiratory failure; (3) pulmonary embolism; and (11) cardiac failure. Our perioperative mortality has been less than 0.4% with two deaths in 519 primary procedures.[7]

One of the deaths following a GBP was due to gastric distension and necrotic ulceration of the excluded stomach in a 37-year-old male who was 167.5 cm tall and weighed 144 kg. He had rheumatic valvular heart disease with congestive heart failure, and was submitted to a gastric bypass procedure to cause him to lose enough weight to have open heart surgery to replace his mitral valve. He had been unsuccessful in many attempts to lose weight by conservative means and the increased surgical risk was accepted by the patient as well as his medical and surgical advisors on this account. Bleeding from the Roux-en-Y anastomosis caused thrombotic obstruction of the afferent limb and ultimately gastric distension and blowout (see Chapter 11). He succumbed following surgery for the gastric perforation.

A gastrostomy tube in the distal stomach at the time of the gastric bypass would have prevented the gastric blowout. We now use a gastrostomy in all revisions, conversions, reconstitutions, superheavy patients (> 2.5 times ideal weight), and those with impaired cardiopulmonary function, as mentioned earlier.

The second death occurred in a 36-year-old female who was a heavy smoker (2 packs/day), and who failed to stop smoking 2 weeks prior to surgery as ordered. She died early in the morning of the 2nd postoperative day of cardiac arrest secondary to respiratory failure. An autopsy revealed pulmonary edema, pneumonitis, and atelectasis. There were no gastrointestinal leaks. Because of the limited pulmonary reserve in most obese patients, care must be taken to avoid overnarcotization in pain control.

Even though the mortality of morbidly obese patients has been reported as 12 times that of the general population in certain age groups,[19] the mortality of surgical management—including revisional as well as primary operations—should be less than 1%. Because of the miserable quality of life many of these patients experience, they are willing to accept a much higher risk to lose weight. Nevertheless, to justify bariatric surgery, the operative mortality should not exceed 1%, in our opinion.

Nutritional Support

Patients whose complications result in prolonged illness, and/or who require multiple surgical procedures, must have adequate nutritional support, either in the form of parenteral hyperalimentation or enteric tube feeding. Satisfactory healing is dependent upon an adequate supply of protein and calories, even though these patients are obese.

The amount of space devoted to complications in this section would suggest they are extremely common. On the contrary, the acute morbidity rate of primary operations in our patient population has been less than 10% and the mortality rate less than 0.4%. Most patients have an uneventful hospital course and are discharged on the 6th or 7th postoperative day.

Late Complications

There are fewer and less serious late complications following gastric-type operations than following intestinal bypass procedures. Most of them relate primarily to either an inadequate weight loss (or regain of weight) for the reasons outlined, or to outlet obstruction with vomiting, dehydration, electrolyte imbalance, and malnutrition. Otherwise, except for avitaminosis B_1, or B_{12}, folic acid, and/or iron deficiency anemias, there are almost no other deficiency syndromes or serious metabolic diseases associated with gastric-type procedures. The deficiency diseases can be prevented or reversed by vitamin and iron supplementation. Laboratory examination for anemia and for deficiency of vitamin B_{12}, folic acid, and iron should ideally be obtained on all patients annually. Stenotic and obstructed outlets must either be corrected early by dilatation, if possible, or by laparotomy later. Provision of gastrostomy or jejunostomy tube

feeding at the time of the primary operation can permit a delay in surgical correction for many months, and occasionally the obstruction may relent during that interval.

Although the list of reported complications noted below is long the incidence of most is very low with the exception of weight loss failure (see Chapter 7 and Table 6-2).

I. Weight Loss Failure
  A. Pouch too large
    1. Created too large initially (over 30 ml)
    2. Dilatation of pouch over time
  B. Outlet too large
    1. Created too large (over 12 mm)
    2. Dilatation of outlet due to stretching, enhanced by lack of adequate external support
  C. Staple line disruption and fistulization into distal stomach
  D. Poor patient cooperation
II. Excessive Weight Loss: Vomiting, Dehydration, Malnutrition
  A. Outlet created too small initially (<10 mm)

TABLE 6-2 Late Complications Following Primary Surgery: 1976–1983

Complication	GBP–Loop (47 cases)		GBP–Roux-en-Y (285 cases)		GP (187 cases)	
Stomal dilation	(7)		(6)	2	(20)	2
Pouch dilation	(8)		(7)		(12)	2
Staple line disruption	(1)	3	(2)	3	(5)	7
"Snacker" failure		0		0	(6)	13
Stomal obstruction		0		0	(8)	2
Gastric ulcer, excluded stomach		0	(1)		0	
Small bowel obstruction		0	(3)		(2)	1
Cholelithiasis	(4)		(7)		(4)	
Ventral hernia	(3)			0	(4)	
Alkaline reflux gastritis	(6)	1		0	(1)	1
Stomal ulcer		3		1		0
Duodenal ulcer		1				0
Upper GI bleeding		0		2		1
Kidney stones		0		4		3
Anemia		2		6		1
Iron deficiency		1		1		0
B_{12} deficiency		1		5		0
Dehydration		0		0		2
Death		1 ᵃ		0		0
Total	(29)	13	(26)	24	(62)	35
	(61%)	27%	(9%)	8.9%	(33%)	18%

ᵃ Death due to accidental carbon monoxide poisoning.
Numbers in parentheses refer to those complications requiring surgery.

B. Stenosis due to edema, fibrosis, kink, marginal ulceration, or bezoar

C. Bile reflux: most commonly seen with loop-type gastric bypass or gastroplasty with a large stoma

D. Dilatation of esophagus: most common with small (<10 mm) outlets

III. Anemia

A. Microcytic: due to iron deficiency and/or occult GI tract bleeding

B. Macrocytic: B_{12} or folic acid deficiency

C. Combined iron/B_{12} deficiency

IV. Vitamin Deficiency

A. B-complex deficiency: thiamine deficiency causing polyneuritis and/or Wernicke-Korsakoff encephalopathy

V. Upper GI Tract Hemorrhage

A. Marginal ulcer (rare if pouch is smaller than 50 ml)

B. Gastritis of pouch (usually related to use of analgesics)

C. Peptic ulceration in distal stomach

D. Duodenal ulcer (usually in patients with duodenal ulcer history)

VI. Peptic Ulceration

A. Gastric ulcer

B. Duodenal ulcer

VII. Cholelithiasis

A. Incidence high in morbid obesity, and possibly increased by weight loss following gastric bypass—not as cholelithogenic as intestinal bypass

VIII. Dumping Syndrome

A. Almost exclusively with gastric bypass operation; usually an advantage as a deterrent to sweets

B. Associated diarrhea in a small percentage of patients

IX. Diarrhea or Constipation

A. Diarrhea related to dumping or postvagotomy effect

B. Constipation: fewer, smaller bowel movements related to marked decrease in food intake

X. Small Bowel Obstruction: usually due to adhesive band

XI. Hypoglycemia

A. Occasionally causes weakness, shaking, sweating, and rarely blackout 2–3 h after a meal

XII. Psychiatric Problems

A. Exacerbation of depression; anxiety state; identity crises (see Chapter 2)

XIII. Hair Loss

A. Temporary: reverses with adequate protein and vitamin intake

XIV. Redundant Skin with Excoriation, Intertrigo (see Chapter 12)

XV. Ventral Hernia

XVI. Late Death

Discussion

In evaluating late complications, the different types of surgical procedures should be considered separately, because each has sequelae peculiar to that operation as discussed in Chapter 5.

Weight Loss Failure

Horizontal gastroplasty or gastric partitioning procedures, for example, have a higher reported weight loss failure rate than gastric bypass[7,20,21] and also a higher incidence of outlet stenosis and obstruction.[7,22] The incidence of esophageal dilatation tends to be higher with these procedures.[22]

Weight loss failure can occur with any of the currently recommended procedures for a number of different reasons, and usually eventuates in some type of revision as discussed in Chapter 7.

Peptic Ulceration of the Excluded Stomach

Anemia from GI tract bleeding or iron deficiency is more apt to occur following gastric bypass. Peptic ulceration of the excluded stomach or duodenum in the GBP procedure is fortunately extremely rare, but when it occurs presents a difficult diagnostic problem.

Anderson[23] reported the case of a 34-year-old woman who required an exploratory laparotomy 3 years after her gastric bypass for persistent pain of undetermined origin, and at surgery was found to have a 1-cm perforated posterior antral ulcer. The ulcer was locally excised, and the gastric bypass taken down with apparent cure. Although no late follow-up was reported, this patient most likely regained all her lost weight within a year or two.

We had a similar case, that of a 52-year-old woman with epigastric pain of unknown origin, present intermittently for over a period of 2 years following a Roux-en-Y GBP. An exploratory laparotomy was performed and we removed a diseased gallbladder and a diverticula-containing ascending colon, believing one of these organs to be the cause of her pain. Unfortunately her symptoms recurred after a brief respite, and a second laparotomy, this time including a gastrotomy, revealed a perforating posterior antral ulcer, approximately 1 cm in diameter, the source of her pain. We elected to resect the entire stomach up to the gastric pouch. Following this second procedure, she was totally relieved of her pain, is in good health, and has maintained an excellent weight loss.

Unless the local inflammatory response is too severe, or the patient's general condition too poor, we recommend subtotal gastrectomy rather than local excision plus takedown of the gastric bypass in this situation.

Bleeding from the Excluded Stomach

In a combined study of 3000 patients who had had a gastric bypass from 3 months to 3 years earlier, Printen et al[16] found significant bleeding from the excluded stomach in eight patients, an incidence of 0.3%. Five patients, four with a duodenal ulcer and one with gastritis, bled massively and required an emergency laparotomy. Three had chronic bleeding, two from a duodenal ulcer and one from a gastric ulcer. The correct diagnosis in the chronically ill patients was suspected after gastroscopy had excluded marginal ulceration or pouch gastritis as the source of bleeding. A trial of cimetidine therapy in the latter group proved ineffective. Definitive diagnosis was made at laparotomy, and all patients were successfully treated by subtotal gastrectomy.

Although this is a rare complication, it must be borne in mind and appropriate management instituted early. We have not as yet encountered this problem in our practice, which may in part be due to the fact that all of our patients with a history of duodenal ulcer were submitted to a vagotomy and usually a pyloroplasty at the time of their gastric bypass. The authors did not suggest that the risk of this complication was sufficiently great to be a contraindication to the gastric bypass operation.

Radiographic Visualization of the Excluded Stomach

In one of our patients with undiagnosed pain 1 year following a Roux-en-Y gastric bypass, the distal stomach was visualized by injecting water-soluble radiopaque media through a skinny needle inserted percutaneously through the gastrostomy scar into the gastric lumen (see Chapter 11). Graduated catheters were then threaded into the stomach which not only yielded the diagnosis (partial afferent limb obstruction), but also permitted decompression of the excluded stomach, duodenum, and afferent jejunum. Gastric distension facilitated the examination in this patient. We plan to use this method in selected patients who have had a gastrostomy or gastropexy when presented with obscure symptoms which have not yielded to conventional diagnostic procedures. McNeely[24] reported a novel technique for visualizing the excluded portion of the stomach and duodenum described in Chapter 11.

Stomal Ulcer

Two of our patients with significant upper GI tract hemorrhage requiring blood transfusions responded to conservative measures. The cause of bleeding in one was a stomal ulcer that responded to a course of cimetidine and has not recurred in 4 years; the cause of the other was hemorrhagic gastritis of the pouch due to an analgesic (Excedrin). Her bleeding has not recurred after 2 years.

Stomal ulcerations in GBP patients are almost always the result of the pouch being too large (>50 ml). If the ulcer does not respond to medical therapy, revision with reduction of pouch size plus vagotomy is probably the best treatment. A pyloroplasty is considered by Alden to be unnecessary, and possibly deleterious.[16]

Bile Reflux Gastritis

Upper GI bleeding can also result from gastritis and/or ulcerations due to bile reflux associated with a loop gastroenterostomy, particularly if the anastomosis is large. This can best be corrected by converting the loop to a Roux-en-Y gastroenterostomy with a 50- to 60-cm efferent limb. Attempting to prevent reflux of bile by a side-to-side jejunojejunostomy proximal to the gastrojejunostomy in 11 of our patients was unsuccessful.[7]

There has been some evidence to suggest that chronic alkaline (bile) gastritis in a Billroth II subtotal gastrectomy increases the incidence of metaplasia and carcinoma of the pouch, which is, at least, a theoretical disadvantage of the loop gastroenterostomy.[25]

Outlet Stenosis

Obstructing outlet stenosis will occasionally respond to endoscopic visualization and dilatation using either Puestow-type dilators or a Gruntzig balloon catheter under fluoroscopic guidance. Both methods have been used successfully in a few of our patients, but the Gruntzig balloon is easier to insert into the more inaccessible gastroplasty outlets. A 9-mm Gruntzig balloon catheter is passed through the outlet by means of a previously placed guidewire and inflated. If additional dilatation is required, the endoscope can be inserted through the outlet alongside of the deflated catheter, and the balloon again inflated. Fluoroscopic as well as endoscopic guidance is required. The patient should be observed carefully for perforation. Persistent obstruction will necessitate surgical correction as will be discussed in Chapter 7.

Stomal obstruction due to food or bezoar formation usually occurs within the first 6 months postoperatively. Its management was discussed earlier. Gastroscopic removal was necessary in five patients when attempts to dissolve the food bolus had failed. Prevention by careful patient education is obviously the key to this problem.

If an outlet is made 9 mm or smaller initially, it should usually be accompanied by a feeding gastrostomy or jejunostomy because many of these patients will require supplemental feeding for 3 to 12 months postoperatively.

Cholecystitis-Cholelithiasis

Cholecystitis with cholelithiasis is a common sequela of morbid obesity, particularly during a period of rapid weight loss. The incidence is thought to be higher following intestinal bypass surgery than gastric reduction operations.[26]

Because of the high incidence of gallbladder disease, reported to be as high as 73.5% by one observer,[27] we have become more liberal in our indications for a concurrent cholecystectomy. These additional indications include the presence of symptoms in the patient's medical history strongly suggesting gallbladder disease, or cholesterosis noted within the wall of the gallbladder at surgery.

Dumping Syndrome

The dumping syndrome occurs primarily in patients who have had gastric bypass, which has the advantage of reducing the intake of carbohydrates (sugar especially) in a significant number of patients. Occasionally dumping occurs with foods other than carbohydrates, apparently due to distension. In over 500 patients we have never found revisional surgery necessary because of dumping.

The diarrhea associated either with dumping or vagotomy usually abates in time, and often responds to eliminating sweets and milk from the

diet. The patient should also be reminded to eat slowly.

Hypoglycemia

Hypoglycemia with weakness, occurring 2 h or so after meals, often responds to eating some form of protein-containing food, such as peanuts or crackers, around the time the attack is expected or immediately after onset.

Small Bowel Obstruction

Late bowel obstruction is usually due to an adhesive band or mesenteric defect. The incidence has been approximately 3% in our series of primary gastric operations.

Constipation

Infrequent bowel movements are a source of anxiety to some patients, but usually an explanation of the cause, i.e., decreased food intake, allays their concern. Seldom are laxatives needed, but Metamucil and/or a stool softener (Colace) have occasionally been used.

Loose and Sagging Skin

Hanging skin folds involving the abdomen, breast, arms, buttocks, and legs are often the mark of a successful weight-reduction operation, but are also a source of great concern and irritation to many patients. Except for an occasional abdominal panniculectomy, we refer patients with extensive or multiple skin deformities to plastic and reconstructive surgeons (see Chapter 12). The results of this type of surgery have been very gratifying to a high percentage of patients.

Hair Loss

Hair loss has been a temporary problem in some of our patients, but has always responded to stabilization of weight loss and adequate protein and vitamin intake.

Ventral Hernia

Ventral hernias should be repaired after maximum weight loss has been achieved—often in conjunction with an abdominal panniculectomy.

Late Death

Late deaths seldom if ever bear any relationship to the operation. One of our patients died following an accident.

Death could, of course, result from untreated

malnutrition or electrolyte imbalance in a patient with outlet obstruction.

Whether gastric reduction surgery will prolong life remains to be determined. It definitely improves the quality of life, however, for most patients.

References

1. Alden JF: Gastric bypass technique. Presentation at the Gastrointestinal Disease Course, A.C.S. Meeting, San Francisco, October 12–16, 1981.
2. Halverson JD, Zuckerman GR, Koehler RE, Gentry K, Michael HEB, Deschryver-Kecskemeti K: Gastric bypass for morbid obesity. A medical-surgical assessment. Ann Surg 194:152, 1981.
3. Bothe A Jr, Bistrian BR, Greenberg I, Blackburn GL: Energy regulation in morbid obesity by multidisciplinary therapy. Surg Clin North Am 59:1017–1031, 1979.
4. Peltier G, Hermreck AS, Moffatt RE, Hardin CA, Jewell WR: Complications following gastric bypass procedures for morbid obesity. Surgery 86:648, 1979.
5. Haid RW, Gutman L, Crosby TW: Wernicke-Korsakoff encephalopathy after gastric plication. JAMA 247:2566, 1982.
6. Halverson JD: Metabolic deficiencies after gastric restriction. Presented to Bariatric Surgical Colloquium. Iowa City, June 2–3, 1983.
7. Linner JH: Comparative effectiveness of gastric bypass and gastroplasty. Arch Surg 117:695, 1982.
8. Mason EE: Surgical treatment of obesity. Major Probl Clin Surg 24:146–147, 1981.
9. Eckhout GV, Prinzing JF: Surgery for morbid obesity: comparison of gastric bypass with vertically stapled gastroplasty. Colo Med 78:117, 1981.
10. Mason EE: Vertical banded gastroplasty for obesity. Arch Surg 117:701, 1982.
11. Mason EE: Surgical treatment of obesity. Major Probl Clin Surg 26:325–328, 1981.
12. Buckwalter JA, Herbst CA Jr: Complications of gastric bypass for morbid obesity. Am Surg 139:55–60, 1980.
13. Alden JF: Personal communication. 1980.
14. Miller DK: Poster presentation: gastric bypass. Presented at the Bariatric Colloquium, Iowa City, June 3–4, 1982.
15. Moore CE, Buerk C, Moore G: Gastric bypass and acute duodenal ulceration and perforation. Surg Gynecol Obstet 148:764, 1979.
16. Printen KJ, LaFavre J, Alden J: Bleeding from the bypassed stomach following gastric bypass. Surg Gynecol Obstet 156:65, 1983.
17. Mason EE: Surgical treatment of obesity. Major Probl Clin Surg 24:180–186, 1981.
18. Mason EE: Surgical treatment of obesity. Major Probl Clin Surg 26:170, 1981.
19. Drenick EJ, Bale GS, Seltzer F, Johnson DG: Excessive mortality and causes of death in morbidly obese men. JAMA 243:443–445, 1980.
20. Lechner GW: Subtotal gastric exclusion and gastric partitioning. A randomized prospective comparison of 100 patients. Surgery 90:637, 1981.
21. Poires WJ, Flickinger EG, Neelheim D, VanRig AM, Thomas FT: The effectiveness of gastric bypass over gastric partition in morbid obesity. Consequence of distal gastric and duodenal exclusion. Ann Surg 196:389, 1982.
22. MacLean LD, Rhode BM, Shizgal HM: Gastroplasty for obesity. Surg Gynecol Obstet 153:200, 1981.
23. Anderson OS, Paine GT, Morse EK: An unusual complication of gastric bypass: perforated antral ulcer. Am J Gastroenterol 77:93, 1982.
24. McNeely F, Macgregor AMC: Distal gastric and duodenal evaluation following gastric bypass by percutaneous transabdominal upper GI series. Scientific Exhibit, Bariatric Surgical Colloquium, Iowa City, June 2–3, 1983.
25. Dahm K, Werner B: Susceptibility of the resected stomach to experimental carcinogenesis. Krebs Forsch Klin Onkol 85:219, 1976.
26. Madura JA, Loomis RC, Harris QA, Grisfeld JL, Tompkins RK: Relationship of obesity to bile lithogenicity in man. Ann Surg 189:106, 1979.
27. Solochek SM: Gallbladder disease in the morbidly obese. Presented at the Bariatric Surgery Colloquium, Iowa City, June 1–2, 1981.

Chapter 7

Revisional Surgery

John H. Linner

General Considerations

Revisional gastric surgery comprises reoperations that are done primarily for weight loss failure, regain of weight, or outlet obstruction. Reoperations for acute complications (leaks, hemorrhage, or certain late complications such as distal bowel obstruction or peptic ulcer, discussed in Chapter 6) are not revisional operations. Revisional intestinal surgery is done primarily for serious metabolic complications or unacceptable side effects.

Revisional surgery embraces these arbitrary categories:

1. *Revision.* The initial operation is retained, but is modified: e.g., altering the size of the pouch or outlet, as in a gastric bypass (GBP) or gastroplasty (GP), or in the case of a jejunoileal bypass (JIB), adding or deleting a segment of small bowel.

2. *Conversion.* The original operation is changed to a different type: a GP to a GBP or a GBP to a gastrogastrostomy (GG). A JIB can also be converted to a GBP or GP, but usually, in this circumstance, the term reconstitution with or without "concurrent" or "concomitant" GBP or GP is used. Seldom is a JIB superimposed on a gastric reduction procedure, or the reverse, as will be discussed later.[3]

3. *Restoration.* Reconstitution, takedown, or "reversing the shunt" are terms applied to restoring the gastrointestinal tract to its normal preoperative state. To shorten the text, JIB takedown (reconstitution) plus a gastric reduction operation will be designated T/G, and a gastric revision or conversion, G R/C.

Revision-Conversion Rate

Whereas restoring (taking down, reconstituting) a JIB with a concurrent gastric reduction procedure (T/G) has become a fairly common operation,[1,2] restoring a gastric reduction operation is rare.[3] We have performed 85 JIB restorations in the past 6 years, and only one gastric restoration. On the other hand, gastric revisions/conversions (G R/C) are common.[4] We have had a G R/C rate of just under 10% over the past 6 years, most of them being conversions from a horizontal GP to a Roux-en-Y GBP, or revisions from a loop to a Roux-en-Y GBP. In our series of 519 primary gastric operations, 50 have undergone revisional surgery of one type or another. There were 25 additional G R/C in patients who had their primary operation elsewhere.

In our experience, the failure rate of horizontal GP was much higher than that of GBP, and the revision rate was correspondingly higher.[5] Not all patients who were failures opted for a secondary operation, and some were lost to follow-up. The G R/C rate roughly parallels, but is only an approximation of, the failure rate of any given operation. Although the ideal of 0% revisional surgery will perhaps never be achieved, the G R/C rate should be less than 2% if the guidelines set forth in Chapters 4 and 5 are observed. Patients who have experienced failure in spite of having retained a small pouch and outlet need close supervision and encouragement to adopt better dietary and exercise habits, and in most cases, should not be reoperated. The only exception to this general rule is a patient with a horizontal GP. Here, conversion from a GP to a GBP may be justifiable because the GBP has proved more effective both as a primary as well as a revisional operation. This has been reported by others as well.[6,7] As pointed out earlier, our experience has been exclusively with the horizontal GP and may not apply to the vertical type.

Indications for Revision

Weight Loss Failure

The most common indication for revisional surgery (excluding JIB, which will be considered later) is weight loss failure, or regain of weight, usually the result of pouch or outlet enlargement. The pouch and/or outlet may have been made too large initially, or dilatation may have occurred over a period of time. A small pouch (10–15 ml) retains its size and effectiveness much longer than a larger pouch, and a small (10–12 mm) externally supported outlet longer than one that is large or has no support. Although it is true that a determined, hyperphagic patient can eventually defeat any of the gastric-type operations, the incidence can be minimized by applying the principles presented in Chapters 4 and 5. These include, in addition to technique factors, patient follow-up with continued patient education. A well-instructed, well-motivated patient will do better with the identical operation than one not so motivated. As pointed out earlier, the operation is only one part (although the most important) of a total behavioral modification attack on morbid obesity.

Correction of Weight Loss Failure

The choice of which secondary procedure to use for weight loss failure depends upon the experience and predilection of the surgeon. We currently favor the Roux-en-Y GBP, and consequently, almost all of our failed GPs are converted to a GBP with a smaller (10–15 ml) pouch and a smaller (10–11 mm) reinforced outlet. Failed Roux-en-Y GBPs with a large pouch and/or outlet are simply revised downward with the addition of external stomal support. In addition to reducing pouch and outlet size, patients with a loop GBP usually undergo revision to a Roux-en-Y GBP.

Gastrogastrostomy   Other surgeons[8] are partial to a GP type of configuration, and prefer to convert a GBP to a gastrogastrostomy (GG) or some other form of gastroplasty. A failed horizontal GP or GBP would usually be reduced in size and converted to an anterior GG in their hands.

A horizontal GP can be converted to a vertical GP by utilizing one or two applications of the GIA instrument, one prong being inserted through a small gastrotomy just above and anterior to the existing staple line on the greater curvature, and the other immediately below through a second gastrotomy. It is essential to apply the GIA a second time if necessary to reach the lesser curvature so that the septum separating the gastric pouch and the distal stomach will be completely eliminated. The gastrotomy defect on the greater curvature can be closed with a TA-55 instrument, and the vertical gastroplasty performed as described in Chapter 5.

Gastric Bypass Revision   When revising a GBP, it is often unnecessary to take down the gastroenterostomy unless it is very low or very large. For many revisions, we have been able to reduce the pouch size by either angling the new staple line high enough above the original one to achieve the appropriate size, or by resecting the fundic portion of the redundant pouch using either the TA90 or TA55 staple instrument.

The outlet is reduced in size by placing a Silastic catheter (12 Fr.) around the anastomosis through which a 34-Fr. Hurst dilator has been passed by the anesthesiologist. The catheter is held in position on the gastric side of the anastomosis by ligating its indwelling No. 1 Prolene suture (see Chapter 5).

Transection   If it is necessary to reduce the pouch size significantly, leaving a large central section, the stomach can be transected, resecting the excess gastric wall between the old and the new staple lines. An anastomosis can then be made between the pouch and the distal stomach or between the pouch and a limb of jejunum. This anastomosis should preferably be made at the greater curvature end of the pouch, resecting a small triangle of tissue at the left extremity of the pouch that is often ischemic after transection, and likely to leak if not resected. The anastomosis is then constructed using the viable gastric wall around the edges of the excised triangle. Suture technique is recommended for this anastomosis. The transected margins of the proximal pouch and distal stomach should be approximated at several points to prevent twisting or kinking at the stoma.[9]

Central Gastric Compartment If a GBP is reduced in size by placing one or two staple lines at some distance above the old staple line, and the stomach has not been transected, it is advisable to create a small gastrogastrostomy between the central gastric compartment and the distal stomach to prevent the blind central section from distending with gastric juice and possibly perforating. If the distance between the old and new staple lines is less than 2 cm this precaution may be unnecessary because in a narrow occluded segment of stomach, the secretory cells apparently undergo pressure atrophy before distension and necrosis occur.

If a horizontal gastroplasty pouch is reduced in size by a more superiorly placed staple line(s), egress from the central compartment through the existing outlet obviates the necessity of a gastrogastrostomy between the central and distal stomach.

Addition of JIB to GBP In failed gastric reduction operations (except in those due to outlet enlargement), Buchwald[10] has recommended the addition of a modified JIB, leaving the GBP (or GP) intact. In this situation, a 65-cm length of functional efferent jejunum, measured from the gastroenterostomy to the point of transection, instead of the usual 40 cm, as in his primary JIB procedure, is used to compensate for the bypassed duodenum. The distal functional ileum length is the same in both: 4 cm. Results of this type of revisional surgery have not as yet been published, but the operation should not be used generally, in our opinion, until long-term results become available. There is no reason to believe that a JIB addition to a GBP will not develop the same excessive morbidity as a primary JIB. The reverse, i.e., adding a GBP to a failed JIB, is probably equally hazardous and not recommended.[11,12]

Outlet Obstruction

Secondary operations for outlet obstruction are simpler than those for weight loss failure since they are usually in patients who have lost weight, and may be quite thin. The obstruction should be managed conservatively as long as possible, because not infrequently the obstruction relents—or the patient learns to eat more slowly—and no further treatment is required. Most of our gastroplasties with outlet obstruction have been converted to a gastric bypass, since in our experience, the ultimate result has been more satisfactory whether the reoperation was for outlet obstruction or weight loss failure.

Overcorrection of Outlet Obstruction
One of our gastroplasty patients, whose outlet stenosis did not respond to dilation, became discouraged waiting for the obstruction to relent, and without notification engaged another surgeon to relieve her symptoms. He was unfamiliar with bariatric surgery and corrected the obstruction by creating a large outlet, which caused her to quite promptly (12 months) return to her preoperative weight.

Refractory obstruction should be corrected surgically, but not overcorrected, and should be either dilated to 12 mm or reconstructed to that size, with added external support. A temporary tube gastrostomy should always accompany revisions or conversions.

Minilaparotomy and Endoscopy
Rank[13] described a novel technique for dilating an obstructed GP stoma using a simultaneous minilaparotomy and endoscopic approach in the operating room. These patients had had gastrostomies with their primary operation.

His technique is as follows: using a short (5 cm) laparotomy incision just under the left costal margin, the anterior wall of the excluded stomach is exposed, and a short gastrostomy created. A sterile rigid sigmoidoscope is then inserted into the stomach to visualize the obstructed stoma from below. At the same time, an endoscopist passes a gastroscope from above into the gastric pouch. A 2–0 silk suture is pushed through the GP stoma from below with a biopsy forceps to be picked up by the endoscopist. Through-and-through string is used to pass a guidewire through the outlet, and graduated dilator modules are gently forced through. The outlet is dilated to 12 mm, and the string left in place should subsequent dilation become necessary. The patient is usually discharged on the second postoperative day.

The advantage of this method is that the difficult and sometimes hazardous dissection of the upper stomach and pouch is obviated. This approach could not be used, of course, for a GBP or in situations where revisional surgery of the pouch is necessary. It may not be a feasible approach for an obstructed vertical GP because the outlet may be too low.

Staple Line Disruption

Another technical cause for failure is staple line disruption. Surgical correction with the addition of one or two staple lines is usually required. Often, at the time of surgery for disruption, the pouch size is reduced and the outlet brought to standard size by external reinforcement around a 32–36-Fr. dilator.

Technique Pointers

Dissecting the upper stomach away from the liver and spleen can be quite tedious and harrowing at times, but a few suggestions may prove helpful.

The superior surface of the liver need be dissected just enough to place the right angle blade of the Poly-Tract retractor under the sternum. Otherwise, only the inferior surface of the left lobe is dissected in most patients, but care must be taken to avoid stripping off Glisson's capsule which can result in troublesome, and sometimes, excessive bleeding. The diaphragm is at times densely adherent to the anterior superior aspect of the stomach, and care must be taken to repair any laceration that may occur to the diaphragm during its dissection.

Spleen
The spleen is the most difficult organ to separate from the stomach without consequential injury, and rarely a splenectomy becomes obligatory. Bleeding from most capsular tears can usually be controlled with hemostatic agents, as discussed in the previous chapter. If a splenectomy is done, a suction catheter is brought out through a stab incision from the left subphrenic space. In dissecting the greater curvature of the stomach, it is helpful to know whether the vasa brevia had been ligated at the previous operation, because mobilization can be facilitated with this knowledge.

Staple Line Application
The previous staple line is usually seen only as a faint depression on the anterior wall of the stomach in most patients a year or more after their primary operation. The new staple application is always above the old when the reoperation is being done

for weight loss failure, unless the pouch is small, and failure is due to outlet enlargement. Occasionally the gastric walls are so thick the staples sink deeply into the tissue, and tend to pull loose even with the 4.8-mm staples. In this situation, it is our opinion that interrupted, through-and-through silk sutures around the new staple line (or lines) is an important adjunct. Transection of the stomach between staple applications plus suture reinforcement is another alternative.

Types of Revision Procedures

GP to GBP

In converting a GP to a GBP, although we usually use the GIA plus TA30 staple technique, in some situations the anastomosis can best be made by the suture method, and occasionally the ILS or EEA-21 circular staple instrument technique is the most satisfactory.

It is not possible in a GBP revision or conversion operation (G R/C) to utilize the anterior wall technique as described for primary operations in Chapter 5, because the existing staple line location or the thickness of the gastric wall does not permit it. The new staple lines usually must be oriented the same as the old, but placed higher as determined by pouch volume. If the pouch is very large technique I-A, set forth in Chapter 5, could be used.

All revisions, conversions, and JIB reconstitutions should be augmented by a distal stomach gastrostomy as emphasized earlier.

Loop to Roux-en-Y GBP

When it becomes necessary to revise a loop GBP because of alkaline reflux gastritis, the most effective method, in our experience, has been to convert the loop to a Roux-en-Y GBP. If dissection around the gastroenterostomy is too difficult to permit resection of a segment of afferent limb from the gastroenterostomy to the point of transection for the Roux-en-Y jejunojejunostomy, a modified Tanner-19 double stoma jejunojejunostomy has been recommended (Fig. 7-1).[14] We have not found this technique applicable or necessary to date in our practice, primarily because we always prefer to dissect out the anastomosis, either to resect it and move it higher, or to place another staple line under it.

In our experience, as well as that of others,[15] a side-to-side jejunojejunostomy done either in conjunction with a GBP, or at a later date, has usually been ineffective in preventing bile reflux.

Rarely, intractable iron deficiency anemia or severe dumping is an indication to convert a GBP to a GG or a GP. This has been unnecessary in our practice to date but has been reported.[16]

JIB Revision

During our experience with JIB surgery from 1954 to 1977, we revised the initial operation in several patients by either adding a segment of defunctional small bowel into the functioning tract to correct excessive weight loss, or deleting a segment of functional small bowel to initiate additional weight loss.

In one patient with calcium oxalate kidney stones, a segment of defunctional small intestine was introduced into the functional stream to decrease oxalate excretion and subsequent stone for-

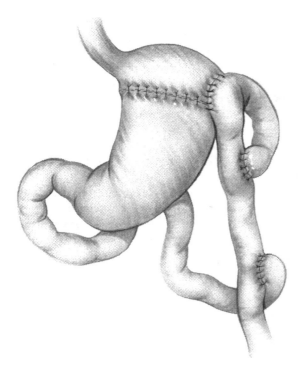

FIG. 7-1. Tanner-19 modification of the conversion of a loop (Billroth II) to a Roux-en-Y type. For use when gastroenterostomy cannot be safely dissected out.

mation. The desired effect was not achieved, however, and unfortunately, the patient regained most of her weight. Because renal function became dangerously impaired, 1 year later it became necessary to submit her to a reconstitution of the entire small bowel and a concurrent gastric bypass. She has done well since, with improvement in kidney function and a good loss of weight.

JIB Reconstitution

Although segmental revisions for a failed JIB are seldom done because of unpredictable and generally poor results, reconstitution of a JIB with conversion to a GBP or GP (T/G) has become a relatively common operation. From 1953 to 1976 we performed 174 JIBs and have found it necessary to submit 56 (36%) of the patients to a small bowel reconstitution. All but six of these had a simultaneous GBP or GP. There were 29 additional T/Gs that had had their JIBs performed elsewhere. The incidence of JIB reconstitution, with or without a gastric reduction operation, has been reported from as low as 2% to over 25%.[1,2,17]

Fifty percent of our JIB patients have done well with minimal morbidity and satisfactory weight loss. There are undoubtedly some patients who would be better served by a JIB than a gastric reduction procedure, but there are no criteria for selection at the present time.[18]

Since T/G is becoming one of the most important of the revision procedures, it is described in detail below.

Indications for T/G

The indications for JIB reconstitution with or without a concurrent gastric reduction in our practice have been the late metabolic complications, and the intolerable side-effects experienced in varying degrees by over 40% of these patients following this operation. Briefly, these have been renal calculi and renal failure, hepatic failure, inanition, dehydration and electrolyte imbalance, immunopathy (arthritis, dermatitis, nephritis), gas bloat syndrome, severe intractable diarrhea, and general malaise (Table 7-1). Many patients have more than one complication or side effect. Additional indications reported in the literature were tuberculosis, neurologic symptoms, alcoholism, and patient unreliability.[19]

The decision to reverse a JIB is easy if any of the above complications are severe or unrelenting.

TABLE 7-1   Indications for Restoring Continuity in Patients with
Jejuno-ileal Bypass—85 Patients.*

	Principle Cause	Secondary Cause
Severe diarrhea	26	38
Gas-bloat syndrome	12	36
Arthritis	11	32
Kidney stones	9	21
Electrolyte disturbance (acidosis, hypokalemia)	10	11
Inanition—hypoproteinemia	3	7
Weakness—Lethargy	5	5
Dermatitis	2	6
Liver Dysfunction—Cirrhosis	4	6
Hypomagnesemia and/or Hypocalcemia	2	2
Anemia	0	5
Neurologic Symptoms	1	0

* 59 from our practice and 26 from elsewhere. Some patients had 3 and 4
complications.

It is more difficult when symptoms are minimal and the risk potential unclear. Two examples of the latter situation are hepatic dysfunction with early cirrhosis and recurrent nephrolithiasis with/or without renal dysfunction. The determination as to which complications or side-effects are of sufficient severity to warrant reanastomosis of the small intestine is moot, and varies widely depending upon the surgeon's personal experience and bias.[1,2,5,17] We tend to recommend shunt reversal earlier than many, because it has been our experience that protracted delay in an attempt to rehabilitate the patient with liver or kidney disease by conservative measures can be dangerous.

Symptoms suggesting liver disease—weakness, ascites, edema, nausea, vomiting, anorexia, jaundice—can best be accurately evaluated by percutaneous liver biopsy (Chapter 3). Technetium sulfa colloid liver scans have occasionally been helpful, and are probably more accurate than most liver function tests in assessing the degree of liver dysfunction (Chapters 3 and 11). When liver disease is suspected, a percutaneous liver biopsy should be obtained, and the decision to reestablish small bowel continuity based primarily upon the histopathology found and the patient's general clinical status. Marubbio[20] reported that the most important histopathologic finding indicating invariable progression of liver disease after JIB is the presence of central pericellular fibrosis. Progression of this lesion results in fibrosis that extends from the cen-

tral lobule to the periportal spaces culminating in micronodular cirrhosis. Fatty metamorphosis and early nonbridging portal fibrosis are reversible lesions, and can be treated by a high protein intake (enteric or hyperalimentation) plus antibiotics, providing the patient is kept under careful surveillance with serial liver function studies and liver biopsies (Chapter 3). Intestinal continuity should be reestablished if there is progression of liver fibrosis or clinical signs of liver failure.

Recurrent urinary tract calculi or nephrocalcinosis are indications for shunt reversal in our opinion, and prolonged delay before small bowel reanastomosis can result in permanent and even fatal renal damage. How many episodes of nephrolithiasis should be permitted prior to undertaking JIB restoration is a matter of judgment, but close observation with repeat intravenous pyelography and renal function studies is mandatory if conservative management is elected. Our patients with nephrolithiasis have been followed by the Hennepin County Medical Center Renal Service (Regional Kidney Disease Program), and the decision to restore small bowel continuity due to kidney involvement has been a joint one (Chapter 3).

For distressing symptoms such as intractable diarrhea, gas bloat, arthralgia, inanition, and general malaise, restoration is often at the patient's insistence.

Patients with dehydration, electrolyte imbalance, inanition, and hepatic dysfunction can occasionally be rehabilitated by parenteral (and enteric) nutrition, and reversal averted, but careful follow-up, as indicated earlier, is essential.

If JIB takedown is elected, patients should be fully informed of the consequences of restoring their small intestine; i.e., regain to pre-JIB weight, unless a concurrent gastric reduction is done. The impact this latter procedure will have on their normal eating habits must also be clearly outlined. The option to convert a JIB to a GBP or GP has made JIB reversal more acceptable to patients who would otherwise prefer to retain their JIB and suffer almost any discomfort or risk rather than revert to their obese state.

Preparation for Surgery

A JIB reconstitution need never be done as an emergency operation, and depleted patients or those with hepatic dysfunction should be hospitalized and given adequate replacement therapy. This usually involves the administration of parenteral hyperalimentation for as long as necessary for the patient to achieve a safe preoperative status. In preparing malnourished patients or those with liver dysfunction, Mason[21] recommends 3 to 4 liters of hyperosmolar amino acid solution daily with one of the liters free of glucose. This type of cycling causes fat to be mobilized from the liver, preventing deterioration of liver function which would otherwise occur by the increasing accumulation of fat. Ideally, serum albumin levels should approach 3 g prior to reconstitution. Additional blood or 5% albumin is administered as needed to restore blood volume or a low hemoglobin. Patients with severe malnutrition or hepatic dysfunction should have their operation staged with the GBP 6 to 12 months later.

Patients who are in generally good condition are usually hospitalized early the day before surgery, and in most, intravenous fluids are begun after the admission process has been completed. Significant electrolyte imbalance, particularly hypokalemia, must be corrected prior to the day before surgery. Patients with fluid and electrolyte deficiencies are either admitted several days earlier or treated as outpatients prior to admission.

Bleeding Associated with Liver Failure

A coagulation survey is particularly important in patients with liver involvement. Coagulopathy should be corrected before surgery if possible. Unfortunately, vitamin K will not correct hypoprothrombinemia

in a patient with severe liver disease. One of our patients with severe liver dysfunction and modestly altered coagulation parameters, died of uncontrollable bleeding following a JIB reconstitution. This case will be presented in more detail later. Prophylactic heparin should never be used in patients with liver failure, and we seldom use more than 3000 units of heparin in any patient undergoing JIB restoration (at least for the initial preoperative dose), because some of them have extensive vascular adhesions.

Preoperative Orders

The immediate preoperative orders are essentially the same as those listed in Chapter 5 for a primary gastric reduction operation with the exception that the heparin dosage is either reduced or eliminated, and the antibiotic coverage is broader and continued longer. We usually use three antibiotics: a cephalosporin, an amino glycoside, and an antianaerobic agent such as clindamycin or metronidazole. A single broad-spectrum antibiotic such as cefoxitin could be used instead, perhaps just as effectively.

Unless the patient has poor nutrition or liver dysfunction, as mentioned earlier, we combine the JIB reversal with a concurrent gastric bypass. Even if a combined T/G procedure is planned it is important to inform the patient that because of certain exigencies that may develop during the course of surgery, it may not be safe or feasible to do both procedures in a single stage, and the gastric reduction would have to be done at a later date. We have had three of 85 patients who required staged operations.

Operative Technique

The abdomen is prepared and draped as previously described (Chapter 5) and entered through an upper midline incision. The Poly-Tract retractor bows are positioned, but the end and side bars are not added until the gastric bypass portion of the operation is begun.

The *proximal end of the defunctional bowel,* the *anastomosis of the functional jejunum and ileum,* and the *defunctional ileocolic anastomosis* are exposed by sharp dissection. In the case of an *end-to-side JIB,* there is, of course, no ileocolic anastomosis.

End-to-end Anastomosis

The *functioning end-to-end anastomosis* is resected, placing a TA55 or TA90 staple instrument on the proximal side and either a TA55 or, if the circular-type staple instruments are to be used, a 2–0 Prolene purse-string suture on the distal side. Occasionally we resect 10–20 cm of the jejunum proximal to the functional anastomosis to prevent kinking of this afferent limb at the Roux-en-Y anastomosis. If suture technique is planned, an intestinal (Dennis) clamp is used on the transected ends of the small bowel instead.

End-to-side Anastomosis   With an *end-to-side JIB* the TA90 staple instrument is placed parallel with the long axis of the terminal functional ileum, making sure that it is into viable ileum, but not so

deeply as to cause obstruction (Figs. 7-2 and 7-3). If the functional ileum is too small, the resection should be made transversely to avoid obstruction. The staple lines are reinforced with 3–0 silk.

A TA55 or TA90 staple instrument is placed on the proximal (functional jejunal) side of this anastomosis (or it can be held with an intestinal clamp if suture technique is preferred) to be used as the afferent limb of the Roux-en-Y jejunojejunostomy. A functional *end-to-end* anastomosis instead of a *Roux-en-Y* is made if the JIB restoration *alone* is done *without* a concurrent GBP, or if the gastric reduction is either a *loop GBP* or a *GP of any type* (Figs. 7-4 and 7-5).

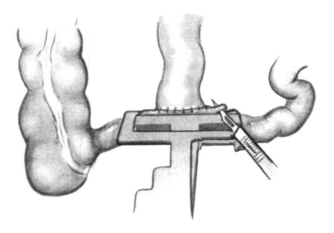

FIG. 7-2. Transecting functional jejunum at end-to-side anastomosis using a TA90 instrument. If the lumen is too narrow, the transection should be done transversely.

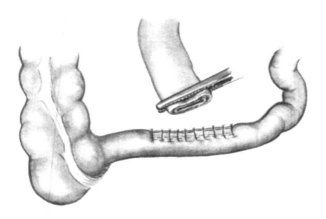

FIG. 7-3. Dismantled end-to-side JIB. Transected functional end is anastomosed to the proximal defunctional end only if a JIB conversion or a loop-type gastroenterostomy is planned. Otherwise, for a Roux-en-Y GBP, it is anastomosed to the side of the defunctional jejunum 50 cm distal to the proximal end.

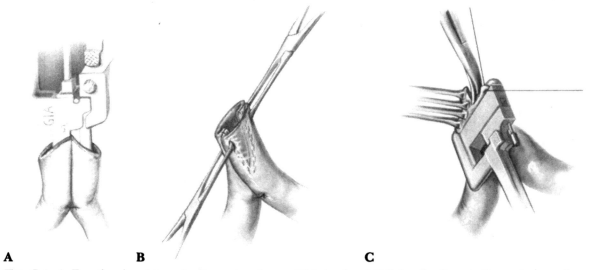

A   B   C

FIG. 7-4. **A** Functional end-to-end enteroenterostomy. GIA is placed full length along antimesenteric walls. This technique is best if there is discrepancy in lumen size. **B** Staple lines are drawn apart by Allis forceps for application of TA55 or TA90 instruments. Additional Allis forceps are placed across the end prior to placing staple instrument. **C** Completing anastomosis with TA55 or TA90 in place.

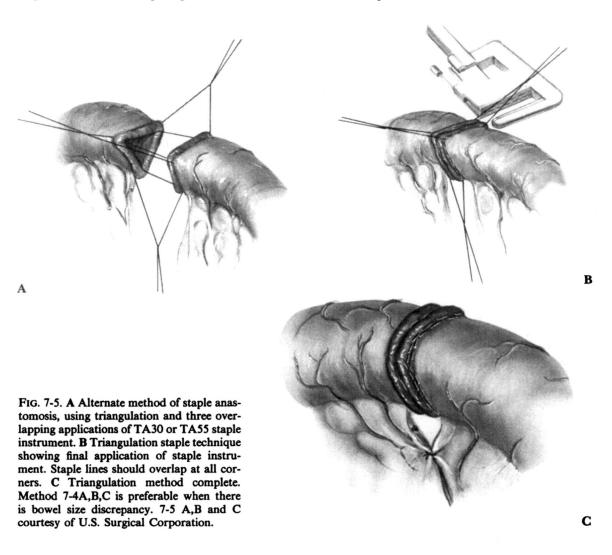

FIG. 7-5. **A** Alternate method of staple anastomosis, using triangulation and three overlapping applications of TA30 or TA55 staple instrument. **B** Triangulation staple technique showing final application of staple instrument. Staple lines should overlap at all corners. **C** Triangulation method complete. Method 7-4A,B,C is preferable when there is bowel size discrepancy. 7-5 A,B and C courtesy of U.S. Surgical Corporation.

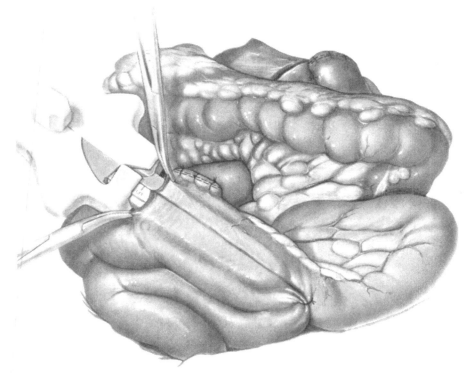

FIG. 7-6. GIA instrument in position for Roux-en-Y jejunojejunostomy (functional end-to-side anastomosis, method I-A). Acceptable alternatives are either suture anastomosis or circular staple instrument.

Ileocolic Anastomosis In the end-to-end JIB, a TA55 or TA90 staple instrument is placed on the colon side of the *ileocolic* anastomosis and a TA55 staple instrument or a 2–0 Prolene purse-string suture on the proximal or small intestine side. Usually a 10- to 12-cm segment of the defunctional bowel adjacent to the colon is resected for pathologic examination. Ulcerations have been present in two of our patients and nonspecific ileitis in several others. Pathology involving the distal defunctional ileum has been reported by Gourlay[22] as well.

Reconstruction Reconstruction is as follows: When an *end-to-side* JIB is restored and combined with a *Roux-en-Y GBP,* the functioning jejunum, which has been separated from the side of the terminal ileum, is anastomosed to the side of the *proximal nonfunctional jejunum,* 50–60 cm distal

to its proximal end (Figs. 7-6 to 7-8). We have usually resected 2–4 cm of the proximal nonfunctional jejunum for bacteriologic and pathologic examination using a TA30 or TA55 staple instrument.

In the case of an end-to-end JIB takedown, the distal end of the defunctional ileum, which had been removed from the colon, is anastomosed to the transected end of the functional terminal ileum (Figs. 7-9 and 7-10). When the terminal ileum is short (4 cm or less) we often construct this anastomosis with the EEA or ILS 25-mm circular staple instrument. If the lumen of the defunctional bowel will not accommodate the 25-mm instrument, or if the length of terminal ileum is over 4 cm, we either do a functional end-to-end anastomosis using the GIA *plus* TA55 (or TA90) instruments, or an end-to-end anastomosis using either staple or suture technique (Figs.7-4 and 7-5).

FIG. 7-7. Completion of jejunojejunostomy with TA55 staple instrument (method I-A).

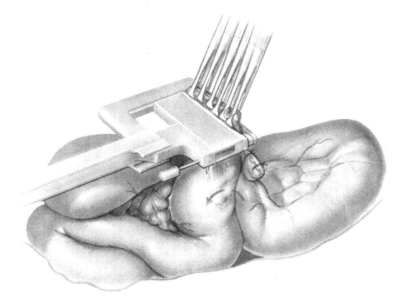

FIG. 7-8. Jejunojejunostomy complete (method I-A). Mesenteric defect is closed with running absorbable suture (Vicryl or chromic
catgut).

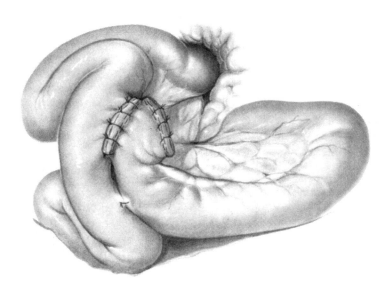

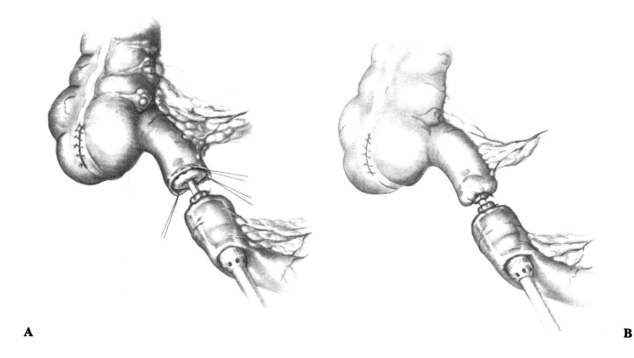

A   B

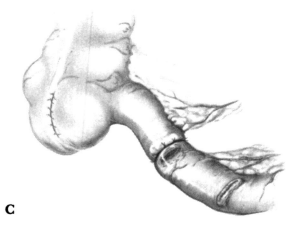

C

FIG. 7-9. A Anastomosis of distal defunctional ileum
to terminal functional ileum, using the EEA- or ILS-
25 or -28 instruments. This anastomosis can also be
made by the triangulation or suture technique. B Purse-
strings are tied and anvil approximated to cartridge.
C Anastomosis completed. Enterotomy closed with
TA30 or TA55 instrument.

Bypassing Terminal Ileum   In reconstructing an
end-to-end JIB with a short (4 cm) distal (functional) ileum, Buchwald[10] prefers to turn in the
short terminal ileum, and allow the ileocecal anastomosis to serve as the functional connection for
the restored small intestine. This eliminates constructing one anastomosis and dismantling the
ileocecal anastomosis, which shortens operating
time and simplifies the operation. We prefer, however, to resect a short segment of the *defunctional*
ileum at the ileocecal anastomosis, and anastomose
the distal defunctional to the *terminal functional*
ileum, for the reasons noted earlier. We have never
found the terminal ileum to be too short for an
end-to-end anastomosis, but in one case dense adhesions precluded dissecting out the ileocecostomy
and we opted for the simpler method which proved
helpful in this case.

Roux-en-Y Anastomosis   Because of the disparity
in size between the large afferent jejunum and
the small defunctional efferent jejunum, careful
construction of the Roux-en-Y anastomosis is essential to avoid obstruction, especially of the efferent limb. We commonly use a GIA and TA55
for this anastomosis (Figs. 7-6, 7-7, 7-8), taking
great care to avoid incorporating too much of the

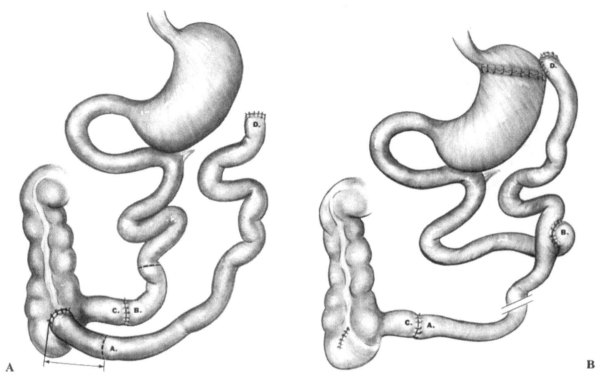

FIG. 7-10. A End-to-end type JIB. Distal 4 to 6 cm of defunctional ileum is usually resected. B Takedown of JIB with concurrent gastric bypass.

efferent jejunum into the anastomosis which results in excessive narrowing and possible obstruction. Two applications of the TA55 or TA30 instrument in a V-fashion, as illustrated, creates a larger anastomosis and is occasionally used (Fig. 7-11). The anastomosis can also be done with suture technique, but again care must be taken to avoid turning in too much tissue. The anastomosis must be carefully checked for leaks.

We have had no problems associated with using the proximal end of the small defunctional efferent jejunum for the gastroenterostomy in our Rouxen-Y technique, except partial obstruction due to a kink 4–5 cm distal to the gastroenterostomy in one patient. This was an avoidable technical error.

The mesenteric openings are closed with running 3–0 Vicryl to prevent herniation and the operative area is washed with 1 or 2 liters of warm saline and dilute antibiotic solution. Gloves are changed and the Poly-Tract retractor is assembled.

The gastric bypass procedure is done as previously described in Chapter 5. The efferent jejunum is brought up in a retrocolic but antegastric fashion for the anastomosis. Care must be taken to avoid twists or kinks.

Staple Line Because of the higher incidence of staple line disruption in T/G operations, we currently place two closely adjacent staple lines instead of one with interrupted silk sutures along the staple line.

Gastrostomy In all reconstitutions and revision operations, as stressed before, a tube gastrostomy should be added with an anterior gastropexy. A gastrostomy allows earlier removal of the NG tube, and can be used for prolonged enteric nutrition if necessary. A needle biopsy of the liver is always performed.

Gloves are again changed and closure is made in layers as previously described in Chapter 5.

Postoperative Care
Postoperative management is essentially the same as that following the primary procedures presented in Chapter 6, with a few differences outlined below.

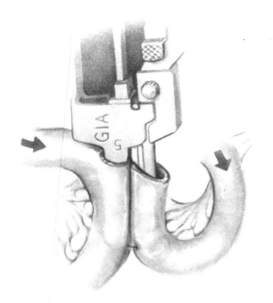

A

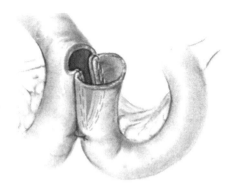

B

FIG. 7-11. **A** Alternate technique for Roux-en-Y anastomosis, showing GIA insertion. **B** Staple lines should
be inspected for bleeding. **C** Staple lines are drawn apart
using Allis forceps. **D** Two overlapping applications of
TA30 or TA55 instrument to complete anastomosis.
E A complete anastomosis with alternate Roux-en-Y
method. From Chassin JL: *Operative Strategy in General
Surgery,* Vol. 1. New York, Springer-Verlag, 1981.

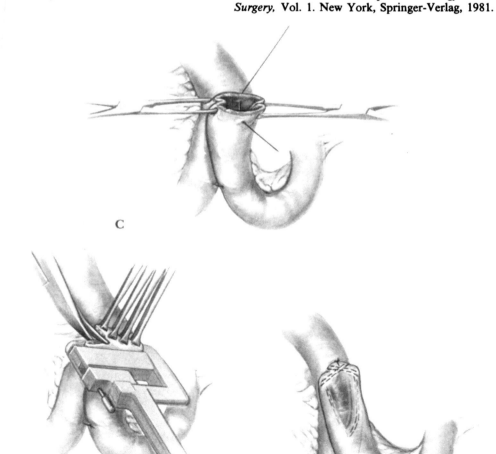

C

D

D

E

If the patient has been severely depleted, hyperalimentation started some time preoperatively (1–3 weeks) is continued for as long as necessary postoperatively to ensure adequate healing. Gastrostomy drip feeding is usually started by the 4th or 5th postoperative day, and when established, parenteral hyperalimentation is discontinued. Although small bowel function may be delayed following restoration, in our experience it has always eventually returned to normal, even though in a few patients it has taken a month. Several patients had had their JIB over 10 years earlier. Transit delay can be the result of adynamic (atrophic) ileus, partial mechanical obstruction, or rarely, complete obstruction at one of the anastomoses.

Antibiotics are continued for 72 h, or longer if significant spillage had occurred during surgery.

An upper GI radiograph to evaluate pouch and stoma size and a small bowel follow through to determine transit time to the colon are obtained on the 6th or 7th postoperative day. Transit time has been as long as 22 h in one patient and is often over 4 h. Visualization of the distal stomach and duodenum to the Roux-en-Y anastomosis by instilling contrast media into the gastrostomy tube is an important part of this examination.

The gastrostomy tube is not removed until oral alimentation is assured—usually 3 to 4 weeks postoperatively—when it is removed at an office visit.

Most patients are discharged from the hospital on the 7th to the 9th postoperative day.

Complications of Revisional Surgery

As would be expected, the perioperative complication rate is somewhat higher following revisional surgery than that following primary gastric reduction surgery (Tables 7-2 and 7-3). The risk of injury to the spleen and diaphragm is greater in gastric revisions, and the leak rate is also usually higher. There were three iatrogenic splenectomies in 160 revisional operations, and only one in 519 operations of the primary group. Otherwise the type and management of complications are much the same as discussed in Chapter 6.

Small Bowel Obstruction

The incidence of small bowel obstruction following T/G was higher than in our series of primary gastric operations, as expected. Most of these were early in our experience when we were using a loop instead of a Roux-en-Y.

TABLE 7-2   Early Complications Following Revisional Surgery: 1976–1983

Complication	G R/C (75 patients)	JIB T/G (85 patients)
Leaks, perforations	(1)	(1)
Subphrenic abscess	(2)	(1)
Postoperative bleeding	0	(1)
Colon compression-obstruction	0	(1)
Small bowel obstruction	(1)	(5)
Prolonged adynamic ileus	2	2
Cholestasis-cholangitis	(1)	0
Outlet obstruction (early reoperation)	(1)	0
Wound infection	(1)	(1)
Thrombophlebitis	1	0
Pulmonary embolism	2	0
Atelectasis/pneumonitis	2	0
Adult respiratory distress syndrome	0	1
Splenectomy, iatrogenic	3	0
Death[a]	0	1
Total	(7) 10 (9%) 13%	(10) 4 (11%) 4.4%

[a] Death due to hemorrhagic diathesis related to liver failure.
Numbers in parentheses refer to complications necessitating surgery.

TABLE 7-3   Late Complications Following Revisional Surgery: 1976–1983

Complication	G R/C (75 patients)		JIB T/G (85 patients)	
Stomal dilation		0	(4)	4
Pouch dilation		0	(3)	3
Staple line disruption	(2)	3	(3)	5
Stomal obstruction	(3)	1	(1)	
Small bowel obstruction	(2)	4	(2)	2
Cholelithiasis		0	(3)	
Ventral hernia	(2)		0	
Kidney stones		1		2
Anemia		1	0	
B$_{12}$ deficiency		4		1
Iron deficiency		1	0	
Dehydration		1	0	
Death[a]		—	(1)	
Total	(9)	17	(17)	17
	(11.7%)	18.3%	(19%)	21.3%

[a] Death due to suicide in depressed patient 2 months post-T/G.
Numbers in parentheses refer to complications necessitating surgery.

Staple Line Disruption

Staple line disruption (SLD) has been reported to be higher following revisional surgery, up to 16% in one series of JIB takedown plus GBP.[1] Our SLD rate in a group of 160 patients with T/G has been 8% compared to 2% for primary operations where the staple line has been reinforced with interrupted silk sutures. Protein malnutrition has been considered the probable cause, but patient gorging has also been indicted.[1] Our SLD rate has improved since adding suture reinforcement of the staple line, and there have been no disruptions since using double staple lines plus sutures (Table 7-2).

Deaths

There were two deaths following revisional surgery, one a late death in a 47-year-old male patient who had had a T/G operation six weeks earlier. He had recovered from his operation but was depressed and committed suicide just before being admitted to the hospital for electroshock therapy.

The second death occurred following a JIB restoration (without a GBP) in a 48-year-old patient from outside our practice with advanced cirrhosis and liver failure. She had a 5-day period of preparation in the hospital, and seemed to be in satisfactory condition for surgery. Her coagulation profile was abnormal with a bleeding time of 10 min (normal, 9 min), a prothrombin time of 15.3 s (control, 11.5 s), and a PTT of 49.6 s (normal, 36 s). The platelet count was 85,000, clot retraction 30%, and there was no evidence of clot lysis. We did not believe that additional preparation would improve her clotting factors.

At surgery, adhesions were unusually extensive and vascular, and after approximately 1.5 h, bleeding became brisk from all raw surfaces and could not be stopped. She continued to bleed after the operation had been completed and died in shock 6 h later. Over 50 units of blood and blood products were used including cryoprecipitate, platelet transfusions, fresh frozen plasma, and fresh whole blood. The possibility of disseminated intravascular coagulation was not excluded, but coagulopathy due to liver failure was the presumptive diagnosis. Liver biopsy showed advanced cirrhosis with small and large pseudolobules. Whether a longer period of preoperative preparation would have prevented this death will never be known. Had the patient been seen and operated on earlier before liver failure supervened, this hemorrhagic diathesis would undoubtedly not have occurred.

Results of Revisional Surgery

G R/C

Generally, gastroplasty revisions have not proved successful for the same reasons they were unsuccessful initially. If stomal obstruction was corrected, the patient would tend to regain too much weight. Pouch size reduction seemed to be of temporary benefit, because the patient would consume too many calories in semisolid or liquid form.

On the other hand, conversions from a GP to a GBP were usually very successful, especially those done after we inaugurated the use of the very small (10–15 ml) pouch and the externally supported 11-mm outlet.

Bile gastritis was effectively controlled in almost every instance following revision of a loop to a Roux-en-Y GBP. In one patient where the jejunojejunostomy was made 35 cm instead of 50 or 60 cm from the gastroenterostomy, only partial relief was obtained.

JIB Reconstitutions

Almost all patients who have JIB reconstitutions are relieved of the symptoms or side-effects for which the operation was done. The relief is prompt and dramatic for those suffering from arthritis, dermatitis, diarrhea, and gas-bloat syndrome. If the patient has hepatic cirrhosis, the return of normal hepatic function may be delayed, and may never return completely to normal. Oxalate excretion usually returns to normal, and the tendency to form additional calcium oxalate stones is minimized after T/G. In one patient reported in Chapter 3, calcium oxalate stones were dissolved using a dilutional technique after JIB reconstitution.[23]

Most patients note an improvement in general well being and strength following T/G.

The effect of reconstitution on weight is variable. If a concurrent gastric reduction is not done, 100% of the patients will gain weight, most to reach or exceed their pre-JIB weight.

Others, who are overweight at the time of the T/G, will lose weight, often to their "goal" weight, and malnourished patients who are below ideal weight will gain, but there is no standard pattern. It is advisable to create a standard small pouch and stoma even in a malnourished patient, supplementing the patient's nutrition via the gastrostomy

tube rather than making a large pouch to compensate for the poor nutritional status.

One of our patients, frustrated with the constriction of food volume, wished to have the GBP taken down and the JIB reinstated. Because she had hepatic dysfunction this could not be safely done, unless she were willing to have only the GBP taken down and accept the inevitable weight gain. She rejected this course of action, and has gradually adjusted to the intake limitations of her GBP.

Summary

Revisional surgery has become an important aspect of surgery for morbid obesity. It is more demanding than primary surgery and the morbidity is somewhat higher. It is therefore important to select as the primary operation one that has the least chance of requiring a revision, and to apply to whatever operation is selected the important principles of a small measured pouch and outlet, with outlet support as outlined earlier.

The T/G rate for JIB will vary depending upon the experience and bias of the surgeon. In my opinion, every effort should be made to ameliorate the patient's symptomatology by conservative means outlined in Chapter 3, but JIB reconstitution should not be delayed to the point of irreversible liver or kidney damage.

References

1. LaFave JW, Alden JF: Gastric bypass in the operative revision of the failed jejunoileal bypass. Arch Surg 114:433, 1979.
2. Yale CE: Gastric bypass combined with reversal of intestinal bypass for morbid obesity. World J Surg 4:723, 1980.
3. Mason EE: Surgical treatment of obesity. Major Probl Clin Surg 26:433, 1981.
4. MacArthur RI, Smith DE, Hermreck AS, Jewell WR, Hardin CA: Revision of gastric bypass. Am J Surg 140:751, 1980.
5. Linner JH: Comparative effectiveness of gastric bypass and gastroplasty. Arch Surg 117:695, 1982.
6. Freeman JB, Burchett HS: A comparison of gastric bypass and gastroplasty for morbid obesity. Surgery 88:433, 1980.
7. Lechner GW, Callender AK: Subtotal gastric exclusion and gastric partitioning. A randomized

prospective comparison of 100 patients. Surgery 90:637, 1981.

8. MacArthur RI, Jewell WR, Hardin CA, Smith DE: Managing morbid obesity. J Kansas Med Soc 82:113, 1981.

9. Mason EE: Surgical treatment of obesity. Major Probl Clin Surg 26:443, 1981.

10. Buchwald H: Surgical approaches for failed jejunoileal bypass and failed gastric bypass. Surg Clin North Am 59:1121, 1979.

11. Mason EE: Surgical treatment of obesity. Major Probl Clin Surg 26:444, 1981.

12. Alden JA: Personal communication, 1982.

13. Rank DC: Management of gastric stomal stenosis. Presented at the Bariatric Surgical Colloquium, Iowa City, June 1–2, 1981.

14. Tanner NC: Observations on ulcer disease. Surg Clin North Am 56:1358, 1976.

15. Cooperman AM: Postoperative alkaline reflux gastritis. Surg Clin North Am 56:1453, 1976.

16. Mason EE: Surgical treatment of obesity. Major Probl Clin Surg 26:215, 1981.

17. Schwartz MZ, Rucker RD, Schneider PD, Coyle JJ, Guzman IJ, Varco RL, Buchwald H: Management of morbid obesity by jejunoileal bypass. World J Surg 5:807, 1981.

18. Griffen WO Jr, Young VL, Stevenson CC: A prospective comparison of gastric and jejunoileal bypass procedures for morbid obesity. Ann Surg 186:500, 1977.

19. Halverson JD, Wise L, Wazna MF, Ballinger WF: Jejunoileal bypass for morbid obesity. A critical appraisal. Am J Med 64:461, 1978.

20. Marubbio ET, Rucker RD Jr, Schmeider PD, Horstmann JP, Varco RL, Buchwald H: The liver in morbid obesity and following bypass surgery for obesity. Surg Clin North Am 59:1079, 1979.

21. Mason EE: Surgical treatment of obesity. Major Probl Clin Surg 26:422, 1981.

22. Gourlay RH, Evans KG: Jejunoileal bypass and the defunctional bowel syndrome. Surg Gynecol Obstet 148:844, 1979.

23. Smith C, Linner JH: Dissolution of calcium oxalate renal stones in patient with jejunoileal bypass and after reanastomosis. Urology 19:21, 1982.

CHAPTER 8

Results of Gastric Reduction Surgery

JOHN H. LINNER

In evaluating any surgical procedure designed to treat morbid obesity, the following must be considered: the effectiveness of the operation with respect to the extent and duration of weight loss, the cost in terms of early and late complications, and the net effect these factors have on the patient's quality of life. Whether longevity will be increased appreciably cannot be determined until actuarial studies have been completed on a significant number of patients. This kind of information is essential in arriving at a valid conclusion as to which surgical approach is best, and more importantly, whether surgery for obesity is a justifiable method of treatment.

Measured only in terms of weight loss, intestinal bypass operations have proved to be very effective. The considerable late complications and side-effects as previously discussed, however, have caused most surgeons in the United States to abandon its use.

Gastric reduction surgery, on the other hand, has relatively few long-term complications, but the operation is technically more difficult than the JIB, the early complication rate is higher, and except for the high JIB reconstitution rate, the revision rate is considerably higher as discussed in Chapter 7. Very few long-term (3 years or more) weight loss results have been published, and those published are usually for procedures that have been either abandoned or extensively modified. A final judgment concerning the long-term effectiveness of the newest generation of gastric reduction operations, therefore, cannot as yet be made. We have been very encouraged with the results of our latest version of the Roux-en-Y gastric bypass as described in Chapter 5, but the follow-up for this

operation, except for relatively few patients, has been less than 2 years. Experience gathered from our earlier GBP procedures followed for up to 4 years, however, causes us to be optimistic about the anticipated long-term results.

Our experience with gastric reduction surgery began in 1976 after we discontinued the JIB procedure in favor of the gastric bypass. A historical tabulation of our procedures can be seen in Table 8-1. The first operations had large pouches and outlets, and the 1- and 2-year results were not as good as those for GBPs done in the last 2 years. The 2-year period from 1978 to 1980 during which 187 horizontal gastroplasties were done yielded the poorest results, and that operation was also abandoned. For the past 2.5 years the early results of our modified Roux-en-Y GBP have been significantly better than those following any previous 2-year period.

Data will be presented for the three types of gastric reduction operations employed from May 1976 to January 1983, i.e., the loop GBP, Roux-en-Y GBP, and the horizontal gastroplasty. The

TABLE 8-1 Historical Data on 693 Patients

Dates	Procedures	No. of Cases
1954	JIB,E-E	1
1969–1976	JIB,E-S;JIB,E-E	173
1976–1977	GBP–loop	47
1977–1978	GBP–Roux-en-Y	106
1978–1980	GP	187
1978–Jan. 1983	GBP–Roux-en-Y	179

JIB, jejunoileal bypass; GBP, gastric bypass; GP, gastroplasty; E-E, end to end; E-S, end to side.

TABLE 8-2   Patient Data for 519 Consecutive Primary Gastric Bariatric Operations, May 1976–January 1983

	Mean (Range)		
Variable	GBP–loop	GP–horizontal	GBP–Roux-en-Y
Sex ratio (F:M)	4:1	8:1	7:1
Age range (years)	(21 to 51)	(17 to 63)	(16 to 64)
Height range (cm)	(150 to 193)	(140 to 185)	(147 to 191)
Ideal body weight (kg)	66(53 to 89)	64(47 to 82)	64(57 to 86)
Preoperative weight (kg)	127(74 to 174)	119(84 to 200)	126(85 to 206)
Preoperative excess weight (kg)	61(21 to 103)	55(25 to 123)	62(27 to 129)
Preoperative excess weight (%)	93(40 to 191)	86(42 to 186)	96(48 to 218)
	(47 patients)	(187 patients)	(285 patients)

TABLE 8-3   Weight Loss Results for Most Recent Follow-up, 1 Year or More Postoperative

	Mean (Range)		
Variable	GBP–loop	GP–horizontal	GBP–Roux-en-Y
Weight loss (kg)	29(0 to 86)	23(−20 to 89)	45(0 to 117)
Weight loss (% preoperative weight)	22 (0 to 57)	19(−17 to 51)	35(0 to 62)
Weight loss (% excess weight)	47(0 to 101)	44(−37 to 113)	74(0 to 168)
Final weight (kg)	99(58 to 136)	95(57 to 151)	82(51 to 145)
Final excess weight (kg)	33(−1 to 75)	31(−5 to 86)	18(−11 to 78)
Final overweight (% excess weight over ideal weight)	51(−1 to 139)	49(−8 to 133)	29(−18 to 120)
Expected follow-up[a]	43 patients	179 patients	223 patients
Actual follow-up	41 patients	155 patients	193 patients
% follow-up	95	87	87

[a] Follow-up was not expected for those patients whose surgery was less than 1 year ago, who died, or whose gastric surgery was revised or converted prior to 1 postoperative year.

loop procedures, our earliest, with the largest pouches and anastomoses, were discontinued primarily because of the relatively high incidence of alkaline reflux gastritis, as pointed out earlier. The revision rate for failed gastroplasties continues to grow, and accounts for our reluctance to adopt any form of gastroplasty, including the vertical banded gastroplasty, until these have proved to be effective for a period of at least 3 years.

The patient population comprising our experience can be found in Table 8-2.

Follow-up

Unfortunately, long-term follow-up is difficult at best, particularly if patients are referred from a distance. A commitment from the patient prior to surgery to participate in a lifetime follow-up is extremely important. An interested staff that will call or write to patients encouraging them to return for evaluation is paramount. One of the problems of obtaining data, such as current weight, at yearly intervals is because a few patients do not return at all, and many do not return annually. Out of a group of 100 patients, 20 may not return for their annual visit at all, but may show up at 2 years or 3 years, and out of the group of 80 that do return at a year, 40 may miss their second anniversary visit to show up at the third or fourth anniversary or sometime in between. Patients do not return for follow-up for different reasons. Some live too far away and simply cannot make a return visit. A few are unhappy about the results of their surgery or its effect on their eating habits, and will not return on that account. Some are ashamed to come in because they have failed to follow instructions.

Writing and telephoning patients has proved helpful, but there still is a group of patients who were lost to follow-up during the first year. Of 519 patients who underwent a primary GBP or GP prior to January 1, 1983, 457 did so prior to January 1, 1982 for a 1-year or more follow-up. Two patients died and 10 had revision of their surgery prior to its first anniversary, so weight results could not be evaluated. Of 445 patients who could have a 1-year or greater follow-up, 56 were lost to follow-up prior to 1 year, resulting in an 87% follow-up.

Weight Loss

The use of a microcomputer has greatly facilitated record keeping and the evaluation of weight loss results, as will be more completely discussed in Chapter 10. Our most recent weight loss results, 1 year or more postoperatively, expressed as *percent preoperative weight loss, percent excess weight loss, final excess weight in kilograms,* and *final percent excess weight over ideal weight,* can be found in Table 8-3. The loop GBP was our earliest

type, and both pouch and stoma were considerably larger than those of our Roux-en-Y GBP of the past 2 years. Given the same size pouch and stoma there should be no difference in weight loss between a loop or a Roux-en-Y GBP. The comparison between the GP and the Roux-en-Y GBP procedure is sound because there were Roux-en-Y procedures done before, during, and after the 2-year GP period (Table 8-1), and pouch and stoma sizes were quite similar. It is only in the Roux-en-Y procedures of the last 2 years that the pouch measurements have been appreciably smaller.

Weight loss results plotted against follow-up interval can be seen in Figs. 8-1–8-6, which compare the three types of gastric reduction operations. It will be noted that in each category of results, the Roux-en-Y GBP was the most effective operation.

Reinhold, in an excellent analysis of long-term weight loss,[1] stressed the value of expressing final results as final percent excess weight over ideal weight (percent overweight), which we have also

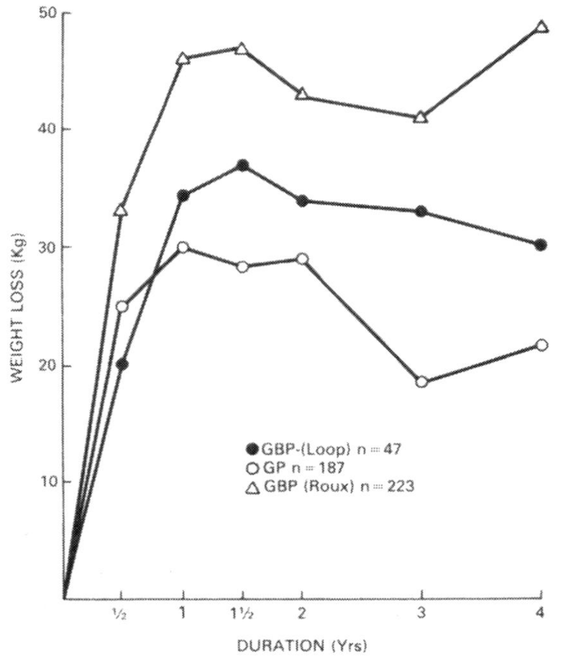

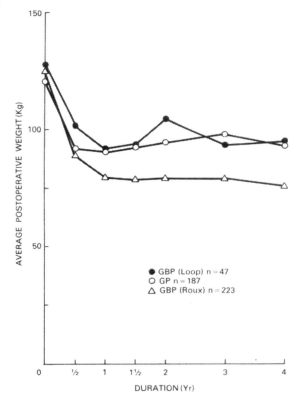

FIG. 8-1. Weight loss in kilograms for three types of procedures.

FIG. 8-2. Average postoperative weight in kilograms for three types of procedures.

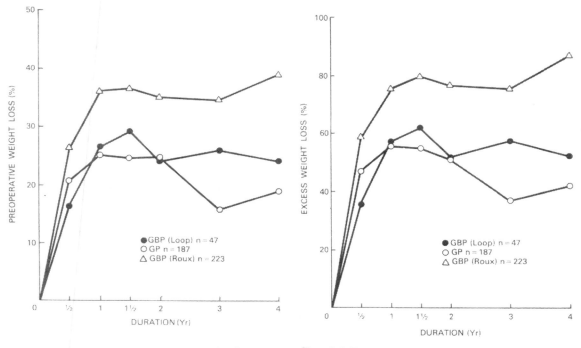

FIG. 8-3. Percent preoperative weight loss for three types of procedures.

FIG. 8-4. Percent excess weight loss for three types of procedures.

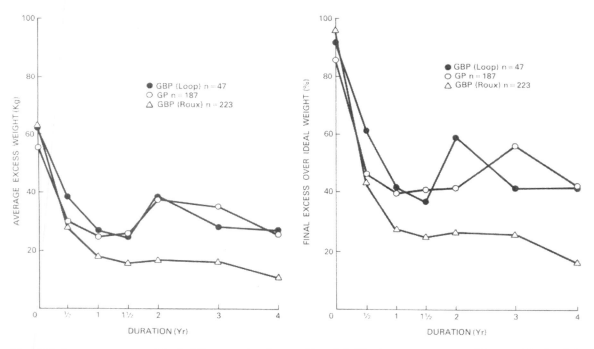

FIG. 8-5. Average excess weight in kilograms for three types of procedures.

FIG. 8-6. Final percent excess weight over ideal weight for three types of procedures.

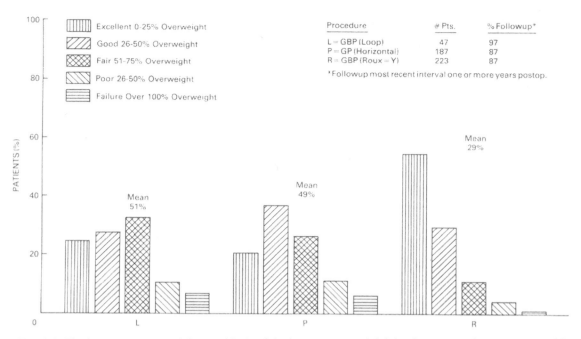

FIG. 8-7. Final percent excess weight over ideal weight (percent overweight) for three types of procedures, distributed in quartiles and graded from excellent to failure.

found to be a useful number. Alone, this statistic reveals nothing about how much weight the patient has lost, nor the percentage of excess weight lost, but it does indicate where the patient is relative to his ideal weight. A final weight of less than 25% over ideal weight is considered excellent, and other categories from "good" to "failure" on a quartile percentage basis can be seen in Fig. 8-7. The superiority of the Roux-en-Y GBP within our own comparative series is apparent.

Ideal weight, however, should not be the ultimate target weight in bariatric surgery because it is often unrealistic, and for many patients even undesirable. It is better to establish a "goal weight," usually 10–20% over ideal weight.

Failure

In evaluating failures (Fig. 8-8), the following factors have been included: (1) failure to lose enough weight (we have arbitrarily used 20% or less); (2) need for a revision or conversion operation (which is an expression of failure); and (3) perioperative deaths.

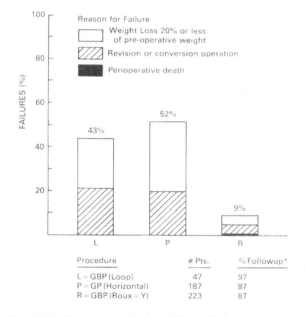

FIG. 8-8. Percent cumulative failures for three types of procedures with follow-up from 1 to 4 years, and reasons for failures (2 perioperative deaths).

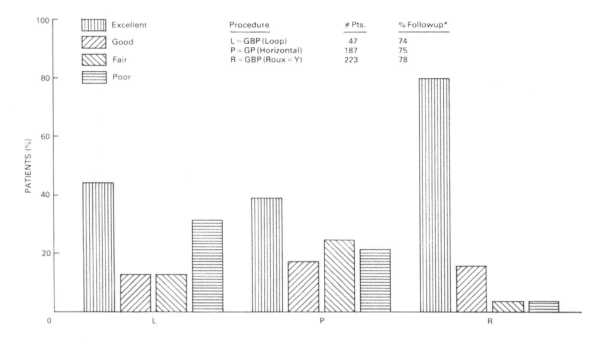

FIG. 8-9. Patient's own evaluation (1–4 years of follow-up) for each of three types of operations.

Satisfaction

Patients were asked to assess their general satisfaction with surgical results, grading themselves "excellent," "good," "fair," or "poor" (Fig. 8-9). The superiority of the Roux-en-Y GBP in our patient series is again demonstrated. This assessment was not obtained with the same uniformity as follow-up weights, so the percentage follow-up was not quite as good.

Summary

Our weight loss results for Roux-en-Y GBP compare favorably with the best reported results of other series,[1-7] and have strengthened our belief that the Roux-en-Y GBP is the most effective of the various gastric reduction operations, and a standard against which other procedures should be compared.

The other criteria of success, e.g., quality of life, interpersonal relationships, job opportunities, blood pressure, pulmonary function, diabetes, varicose veins, and peripheral edema, are affected positively, but are, of course, dependent upon significant weight reduction. Against these positive attributes of gastric reduction surgery must be weighed the morbidity and mortality as discussed in Chapter 6 and addressed in a recent article by VanItallie and Kral.[8] The list of potential complications as presented in this article is long, but fortunately, with knowledge, care, and experience morbidity is low.

References

1. Reinhold RB: Critical analysis of long-term weight loss following gastric bypass. Surg Gynecol Obstet 155:385, 1982.
2. Alden JF: Gastric and jejunal bypass. Arch Surg 112:799, 1977.
3. Halverson JD, Koehler RE: Gastric bypass. Surgery 90:446, 1981.
4. Lechner GW, Callender AK: Subtotal gastric exclusion and gastric partitioning. A randomized prospective comparison of 100 patients. Surgery 90:637, 1981.
5. Buckwalter JA: A prospective comparison of the jejunoileal and gastric bypass operations for morbid obesity. World J Surg 1:757, 1977.
6. Mason EE: Surgical treatment of obesity. Major Probl Clin Surg 26:193–199, 1981.
7. Freeman JB, Burchett HJ: A comparison of gastric bypass and gastroplasty for morbid obesity. Surgery 88:433–444, 1980.
8. VanItallie TB, Kral JG: The dilemma of morbid obesity. JAMA 246:999, 1981.

CHAPTER 9

Anesthesia for the Morbidly Obese Patient

JAMES M. GAYES

General Considerations

The anesthetic management of the morbidly obese patient presents a number of perioperative challenges to the anesthesiologist ranging from the initial preoperative evaluation of an anxious patient to the operative and postoperative management of respiratory and hemodynamic disturbances. Additional anesthetic concerns include (1) securing a patent airway and adequate intravascular access; (2) preventing pulmonary aspiration of gastric contents; (3) choosing appropriate monitoring devices; and (4) selection of anesthetic technique and agents.

The anesthetic risk is higher for morbidly obese patients, and the commonly associated diseases such as hypertension, diabetes mellitus, thrombophlebitis, pickwickian syndrome, heart disease, and impaired hepatic function further increase the risk.[1,2] This chapter will evaluate these concerns in detail.

Cardiopulmonary Considerations

Even under ideal resting conditions, there is an enormous physiologic strain on the cardiovascular–respiratory systems of morbidly obese patients which is compounded by the stress of anesthesia, surgery, and the supine position. An increased cardiac output is needed for both the pulmonary and the systemic circulation.[3] An increase in pulmonary blood volume, heavy smoking, and chronic lung disease add to the work of the right ventricle.

The left ventricle, subjected to both an increased blood volume and frequently systemic hypertension, is exposed to a chronic increase in afterload causing an increase in total myocardial oxygen demand which is not easily met in obese patients, particularly those with cardiac dysfunction. Alexander[4] and Kaltman[5] have shown that the average resting left ventricular end-diastolic pressure (LVEDP) is frequently elevated, or at best, high normal, in obese patients. Biventricular hypertrophy exists in many morbidly obese patients, but most frequently in those with pickwickian syndrome[6] with its associated cor pulmonale.[7] Optimal care of these patients requires hemodynamic monitoring of intracardiac and pulmonary artery pressures via a pulmonary artery catheter.

Diaphragmatic movement accounts for approximately two-thirds of quiet ventilation.[8] An increase in abdominal contents (fat) minimizes the movement of the diaphragm, pushing it cephalad, with further decreases in functional residual capacity (FRC) and total lung capacity (TLC).[9] When in the Trendelenburg position (Fig. 9-1) there is an additional decrease in FRC, which leads to a ventilation-perfusion mismatch and arterial hypoxemia (Fig. 9-2).[10]

Vaughan and Wise[11] studied obese anesthetized patients during surgery and found that an inspired oxygen concentration of 40% did not uniformly produce adequate PaO_2 values. Furthermore, the use of subdiaphragmatic packs and a slight (15%) head-down position decreased the PaO_2 (Fig. 9-3). Fortunately, during most of the gastric bypass

133

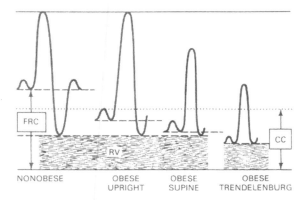

FIG. 9-1. The effect of position change on various lung volumes in nonobese patients compared with obese patients. From Brown BR: Anesthesia and the Obese Patient. Philadelphia, Davis, 1982, p 26. Reproduced with permission of the publisher.

procedure, the operating table is tilted 20–25° in the head-up (reverse Trendelenburg) position to facilitate the surgeon's access to the upper abdomen, which improves ventilation. The total effect of position, surgery, retractors, and laparotomy packs, however, may lead to a decrease in venous return and hence a decrease in cardiac output, and further adding to venous admixture and hypoxia. PEEP has been found to be unpredictable in terms of improving oxygenation in obese patients because of the resulting fall in cardiac output.[12]

With this brief introduction into the principal pathophysiologic problems inherent in dealing with the morbidly obese patient, consideration will now be given to their safe management.

Preanesthesia Visit

The preanesthesia visit should include the following:

1. Educating and preparing the patient psychologically
2. Assessing the history, physical examination, and laboratory data
3. Performing a physical examination pertinent to anesthesia concerns
4. Evaluating the need for preanesthetic medication
5. Deciding which physiologic parameters to monitor intraoperatively

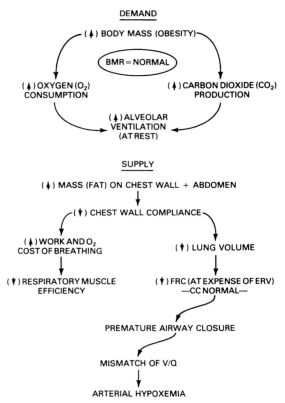

FIG. 9-2. A diagramatic presentation of pulmonary dysfunction in morbid obesity. From Brown BE: Anesthesia and the Obese Patient. Philadelphia, Davis, 1982, p 21. Reproduced with permission of the publisher.

Education and Psychologic Preparation

Optimally the morbidly obese patient should be visited by the anesthesiologist 12–48 h prior to operation. This establishes a good rapport, allows time for discussion between the anesthesiologist and surgeon about any potential concerns, and also allows time for the ordering of additional preoperative laboratory tests. The preoperative visit should instill patient confidence and encourage cooperation. A careful description of the preoperative sequence of events usually allays anxiety and hence may reduce the need for preoperative narcotics.

Patients with cardiopulmonary dysfunction should be seen much earlier than the day before surgery in cooperation with the cardiologist, pulmonary medicine specialist, and internist. These patients must receive appropriate intensive medical treatment to achieve optimal physical status

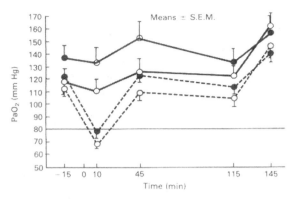

FIG. 9-3. Arterial oxygen tension in morbidly obese patients during anesthesia and surgery. All values were obtained at 40% inspired oxygen concentration. Solid lines represent Pa_{O_2} values with time for Group 1 patients (i.e., no change in operative position); interrupted lines are comparable values for those patients in Group 2 (i.e., position change to 15° head down at "O" time). Operative incision is indicated by circles: closed circle, transverse; open circle, vertical. Change in operative position (interrupted lines) resulted in a statistically significant ($p < 0.001$) fall in Pa_{O_2} values independent of the operative incision. From Vaughan RW, Wise L: Intraoperative arterial oxygenation in obese patients. Ann Surg 184:35–42, 1976. Reprinted with permission from J.B. Lippincott/Harper & Row.

prior to operation, even though this may require several weeks or even months.

History, Physical Examination, and Laboratory Data

A history of longstanding hypertension or angina, and a family history of coronary artery disease are presumptive evidence of heart disease.[13,14] Of the many risk factors requiring evaluation in a patient with coronary artery disease, the most important is a history of previous myocardial infarction, especially the interval between infarction and the date of surgery. Tarhan and Steen[15,16] found the incidence of reinfarction to be 37% in patients operated on within 3 months following myocardial infarction; 16% in those undergoing surgery between 3 and 6 months postinfarction; and 4–5% when the interval was greater than 6 months. Reinfarction was most common on the 3rd postoperative day and was associated with a high mortality (54%). It is wise, therefore, to delay elective surgery at least 6 months following a myocardial infarction. Very few of our patients have had a myocardial infarction, and symptomatic arterio-

sclerotic heart disease, depending upon its severity, can be a contraindication to surgery.[17]

Pulmonary status is as important as the cardiovascular state. A history of smoking, asthma, chronic cough, sputum production, or dyspnea on mild exertion may suggest underlying intrinsic pulmonary disease and require spirometry to document the presence of either obstructive and/or restrictive pulmonary constituents.

Patients who have been on steroids within the preceding 6 months should have steroid replacement therapy starting the night before surgery. Cortisone acetate, 50 mg, is administered intramuscularly the evening before surgery, and at 6:00 A.M. the following day. Hydrocortisone is given intravenously during the operation and continued for an appropriate period postoperatively.

It has been established that patients who smoke more than ten cigarettes a day have an increased postoperative morbidity.[18] Even asymptomatic smokers have significant increases in closing lung volume[19] and abnormalities in mucociliary transport.[20] Recently, Aronson et al.[21] studied the association of cigarette smoking with the occurrence and severity of acute respiratory tract illness. Smokers had a statistically significant greater likelihood of having a lower respiratory tract illness and longer duration of cough. Discontinuing smoking for 2–3 weeks preoperatively is important and results in a smoother induction and safer emergence from anesthesia, as well as decreasing secretions, coughing, and nausea postoperatively.

Systolic and diastolic blood pressure determinations recorded on the chart deserve special attention, and establish a reference point for the management of either hypertension or hypotension perioperatively. One should keep in mind that blood pressure values recorded on the surgical floor may be misleading if an ordinary-sized sphygmomanometer cuff is used. Floor nurses should be instructed in the use of the large (thigh) cuff for obese patients. Based on studies comparing cuff sizes while measuring interarterial pressure,[22] a cuff width 20% greater than the diameter of the arm (about one-third the circumference) is recommended. The American Heart Association still recommends a width two-thirds the length of the upper arm. If the cuff is too narrow, excessive pressure must be applied to compress the vessel and false high readings are obtained. Essential hypertension should be under optimal medical control to help avoid the extreme variations in systolic and diastolic values often encountered in obese patients.

Electrocardiogram

The electrocardiogram and chest roentgenogram complement each other in the diagnosis of left ventricular enlargement secondary to systemic hypertension. "Biphasic" P waves suggest either right or left atrial hypertrophy seen in smokers and in patients with either systemic or pulmonary hypertension or valvular heart disease. Changes in the Q-T interval and T wave occur in patients with calcium or potassium disorders. ST segment changes or the presence of Q waves is evidence of myocardial ischemia or infarction.

Pulmonary Function

Preoperative laboratory evaluation of pulmonary function is essential in any morbidly obese patient, especially those exhibiting alveolar hypoventilation (pickwickian syndrome). Lee et al.[23] reviewed 294 morbidly obese patients who underwent jejunoileal bypass surgery and correlated pulmonary function in these patients with progressive increase in weight and age. This study showed that expiratory reserve volume (ERV), maximum breathing capacity (MBC), and vital capacity (VC) decreased and Pa_{CO_2} increased with progressive increase in obesity.

Preoperative arterial blood gases drawn in the supine position on room air provide an acceptable base for monitoring ventilation during surgery, as well as for evaluating the optimal time for extubation and for monitoring postoperative respiratory care. Hemoglobin and hematocrit values are usually normal in the obese patient, but may be elevated in a patient with the pickwickian syndrome, causing an increase in blood viscosity and an increased tendency to develop thrombophlebitis.[24]

Diabetes Mellitus

Diabetes mellitus should be controlled preoperatively and blood sugar levels should be monitored intra- as well as postoperatively. In a recent study, Walts et al.[25] suggested that insulin-dependent diabetics should not be given insulin immediately preoperatively, but rather glucose or insulin should be administered hourly intraoperatively, as indicated, to prevent hyper–hypoglycemic swings. We have successfully managed a few of our more severe diabetics in this fashion.

Hypokalemia

Obese patients with hypertension who are on diuretics often have a reduction of plasma volume.[26] Most diuretics also cause a depletion in total body potassium which affects peripheral nerve conduction and the activity of neuromuscular blocking agents.[1] Hypokalemia influences electrical conduction and contractility of the myocardium, favoring digitalis toxicity, rendering the heart more likely to develop arrhythmias.[1,27,28]

Clinically, potassium ion variations are determined by the serum concentration. Serum potassium, however, normally represents only $\frac{1}{39}$th of the intracellular potassium, which is the primary concern.[27] Scribner and Burnell[29] have estimated that a fall in serum potassium from 4.0 to 3.0 mEq/liter, if pH remains constant, may reflect a 200 mEq deficit of total body potassium. More recent work suggests that this estimate is conservative,[30] and Wong and associates[27,31] have shown that this decrease in serum potassium represents a total body loss of greater than 1000 mEq of potassium! This deficit cannot be corrected overnight with a few oral doses of KCl elixir. Theoretically at least, 6 days are needed to replace this deficit at a dose of 240 mEq/day. (This includes daily potassium losses of 50–100 mEq.) An attempt to replace serum potassium more quickly should be done only when the electrocardiogram can be monitored closely and serum potassium levels checked frequently.

Liver Function

Fatty liver infiltration occurs commonly with severe obesity,[32] and mild elevations of SGOT and SGPT are frequently seen. This may be accompanied by low serum albumin or total protein levels which decrease the concentration of protein-bound thiopental and increase the amount of free thiopental available for pharmacologic action. Body pH can also diminish the protein-binding of drugs, and low protein combined with acidosis, as occurs with CO_2 retention, leads to an increase in free drug cell penetration and a corresponding increase in anesthetic depth.[1]

Physical Examination Pertinent to Anesthesia Concerns

A physical examination involving the extremities, head, neck, heart, and lungs is important to detect potential problems in preparation for anesthesia and surgery.

Examination of the upper extremities will reveal the adequacy of the peripheral veins for intravenous access. The lower extremities should be evaluated for the presence of thrombophlebitis or pitting edema.

Determining the range of motion of the temporomandibular joint, the status of the teeth, and the extension-flexion ability of the neck will facilitate the intubation process.[33] Inspection of the nares, noting the presence of septal deviation or nasal polyps and the relationship of the trachea to the midline, is essential to facilitate an atraumatic nasal-tracheal intubation using topical local anesthesia in an awake patient. Although at times auscultation of an obese chest may be difficult, it is worth attempting because inspiratory or expiratory wheezes occasionally indicate the need for perioperative bronchodilators.

An obese, hyperinflated chest and a short thick neck may make adequate visualization of the larynx via direct laryngoscopy difficult. A pediatric laryngoscope handle used with the patient in a slight reverse Trendelenburg position occasionally serves as a useful maneuver. In anticipation of a particularly difficult intubation, a fiberoptic laryngoscope or bronchoscope should be available to facilitate visualization of the vocal cords and passage of the endotracheal tube.

*Evaluation of the Need for
Preanesthetic Medication*

When the patient has been prepared carefully during the preoperative visit with appropriate education and emotional support, preoperative medication may be unnecessary. If a preoperative sedative is required, a common choice is diazepam (Valium), given orally, with a small sip of water, which is better absorbed via the gastrointestinal tract than when given intramuscularly.[38] A frequently used alternative is an intramuscular dose of lorazapam (Ativan) 2.5–3 h prior to surgery. Preoperative intramuscular narcotics are frequently avoided because of their respiratory depressant effects. Often an intended intramuscular injection never reaches the muscle because of the thick layer of subcutaneous fat. If indicated, intravenous narcotics or sedatives are administered in the anesthesia preparation room, which permits a more immediate evaluation of the respiratory response.

Monitoring

The history and physical examination together with the preoperative evaluation of the patient's cardiopulmonary status will determine how comprehensive patient monitoring needs to be.

Several basic monitoring techniques such as continuous electrocardiography, urine output, systolic and diastolic blood pressure, and pulse rate are essential for all patients. Those with cardiopulmonary dysfunction, or who weigh in excess of 190 kg, also require an intraarterial cannula to accurately monitor both arterial blood pressure and blood gases. A Swan Ganz* pulmonary artery catheter is used in patients who manifest alveolar hypoventilation (pickwickian syndrome) or significant cardiac dysfunction. Hemodynamic monitoring is essential to assess both right and left ventricular function, to determine the intravascular volume and volume replacement, to evaluate the cardiac and circulatory response to pharmacologic agents, and to manage the course of anesthesia based on initial hemodynamic measurements.[34] This is, of course, particularly important in patients with severe coronary artery disease or evidence of cardiac failure.

It is essential to record both systolic and diastolic blood pressure values. The diastolic blood pressure is an important indicator of the perfusion pressure for the coronary arteries.[35,36] Obtaining the diastolic blood pressure enables one to calculate the pulse pressure (difference between systolic and diastolic blood pressure). Acute changes or trends in the pulse pressure can add information regarding the intravascular volume status. Frequently, a narrowing pulse pressure is indicative of hypovolemia, hypothermia, or other sympathetic stimuli (e.g., inadequate depth of anesthesia).

Korotkoff sounds may be difficult to hear by auscultation, and under these circumstances, a Doppler monitor may be necessary. Prior to insertion of an intraarterial line, the Allen test, which assesses adequacy of the ulnar collateral flow through the palmar arch, should be performed. The morbidity of intraarterial cannulation increases with the size of the cannula used and the time it is left in place.[35] When excess subcutaneous fat prevents cannulation of the radial or femoral

* Trademark of American Edwards Laboratories, Santa Ana, California 92711

artery, either the brachial-axillary, or rarely the dorsalis pedis, artery provides a suitable alternative. Using the Seldinger technique, a 6- to 8-in intraarterial cannula can be placed where it will be affected least by movement. Its length must be adequate to penetrate the heavy layer of overlying fat.

Continuous electrocardiographic display is essential to monitor cardiac rate and rhythm. Ventricular irritability frequently progresses through a spectrum of electrocardiographic findings, from an occasional premature ventricular contraction to ventricular tachycardia and fibrillation. Immediate diagnosis of cardiac arrhythmias and recognition of myocardial ischemia intraoperatively are imperative. Frequently, hypoxia and/or hypercarbia are manifested early by premature ventricular beats. Traditional limb leads are used routinely and have particular value for determining electrical activity of the atria. The precordial V_4 lead is more useful than lead II for detecting ST segment changes which are indicative of myocardial ischemia.[14]

In the obese patient, placing an intravenous catheter in a peripheral upper extremity vein can be extremely difficult and occasionally impossible. Often, placing the arm in the dependent position and applying warm packs will help to identify obscure veins. Placing venous cannulas in the lower extremities should be avoided whenever possible to minimize the risk of thrombophlebitis.[24] Occasionally, a central venous catheter via the internal jugular or subclavian vein is the only means to secure an intravenous line. Rarely, a cutdown is needed.

Hourly urine output indirectly reflects the adequacy of renal perfusion and cardiac output. Urine specific gravity can be helpful in assessing intravascular volume in patients who have not been on diuretics.

Intracardiac pressures can be obtained from either a right atrial (CVP) or pulmonary artery catheter. The latter measures right heart pressures directly and left heart pressures indirectly. In the obese patient with borderline cardiac function, a Cordis introducer can be placed in the internal jugular vein which allows CVP measurement with fluid infusion.[37] A Swan Ganz catheter can then be quickly passed through the Cordis introducer intraoperatively should the need arise. Hemodynamic monitoring makes it possible to obtain mixed saturated venous samples, cardiac outputs, and pulmonary and systemic vascular resistances, which are essential to manage cardiorespiratory problems properly.

Anesthetic Management

Aspiration of Gastric Contents

Obese patients have an increased incidence of hiatal hernia.[26] Vaughan and associates[39] have demonstrated that nearly 90% of obese patients have a gastric juice pH below 2.5 and a gastric volume greater than 25 ml, which exposes them to the risk of the gastric acid aspiration syndrome, first described by Mendelson[40] and later by Teabeaut[41] and others.[42] To avoid aspiration of gastric contents, either a rapid intravenous induction–intubation sequence with cricoid pressure, or an awake intubation of the trachea under topical anesthesia, is suggested, as advanced by Donlon[43] and others.[44] Prior to nasal-tracheal intubation, vasoconstriction of the nasal mucosa with 4% cocaine or Neo-Synephrine is important to avoid epistaxis, which can further complicate airway management. Elective tracheostomy, although rarely necessary, offers a relatively safe alternative in an obese, aspiration-prone patient. Patients with the obstructive type sleep apnea syndrome usually have an established tracheostomy.[45]

Positioning the Patient

In positioning the patient on the operating table, care is taken to avoid any points of pressure, and extremity pulses are checked prior to sterile draping. Arms extended at the sides of the table should not interfere with mechanical retracting devices, and should be available during surgery to permit sampling of arterial blood gases and to gain an additional intravenous or intraarterial line should this become necessary. The arms must not be hyperextended (greater than 90°) to avoid brachial plexus injury. Mason recommends suspending the arms vertically from the elbows using skin traction, and hanging them from lithotomy leg holders to prevent hyperextension.[17]

Choice of Anesthetic Technique

General anesthesia is currently the most popular method employed for surgery of the morbidly obese. Regional anesthesia either alone or combined with a light general anesthesia is recommended by some.[46]

Regional Anesthesia

Subarachnoid block (spinal) anesthesia or epidural anesthesia are the two forms of regional anesthesia most commonly used. Bromage,[47] and later Gelman,[46,48] have effectively used a combination of thoracic epidural anesthesia with nitrous oxide–oxygen (N_2O–O_2) endotracheal anesthesia. A regional anesthetic technique should be used with caution, or not at all, in a patient who has received prophylactic heparin preoperatively.[47]

Many anesthesiologists prefer not to use a regional anesthetic technique in the morbidly obese patient for the following reasons: (1) it is technically difficult; (2) maintaining a desired dermatome level can be inconstant; (3) frequently these patients are unable to ventilate adequately or to cough and clear secretions, even when awake, which can result in severe respiratory complications; and (4) the need for additional sedation or narcotics in an awake, obese patient under prolonged regional anesthesia makes respiratory suppression likely. With the general anesthetic agents currently available, there appears to be very little practical clinical advantage in the use of regional anesthetic techniques in the morbidly obese patient.

Intraspinal and epidural narcotics, e.g., morphine, for pain relief are under current investigation. Pruritus, urinary retention, delayed respiratory depression, and technical difficulty in the obese patient are reasons for concern when considering intrathecal narcotics for postoperative pain relief in the morbidly obese patient.[49-51]

General Anesthesia

There are individual preferences for certain anesthetic agents for induction and maintenance of general anesthesia, but the principles and objectives of management are universal: (1) obtain a safe, secure, patent airway; (2) maintain adequate tissue perfusion and oxygenation; (3) monitor carefully; (4) maintain optimal anesthetic depth with adequate muscle relaxation to facilitate surgical exposure; and (5) extubate early when possible.

Thiopental (Pentothal), plus a narcotic and sedative technique, is the most common choice for induction, and dosage is based on lean body weight. Maintenance may then be accomplished

with a balanced nitrous oxide–oxygen (N_2O–O_2), sedative, narcotic, and muscle relaxant technique, and if desired, a potent inhalation anesthetic may be added.

Recently Lebowitz et al.[52] demonstrated that the combination of pancuronium (Pavulon) and metocurine (Metubine) offers several advantages over the use of pancuronium alone. First, neuromuscular blockage is potentiated by their use in combination, and they cause a similar depth of block at roughly half the dose of either of these drugs if given alone. This low drug dose also reduces the deleterious autonomic and cardiovascular effects of larger doses, an important consideration in the hemodynamically stressed morbidly obese patient.

Potent Inhalation Agents

When sympathetic tone or intraoperative hypertension is not satisfactorily controlled by the balanced N_2O–O_2 technique, or when high inspired oxygen concentration is required, the addition of one of the more potent inhalation anesthetic agents—halothane (Fluothane), enflurane (Ethrane), or isoflurane (Forane)—is indicated.

Halothane One of the major concerns with halothane (Fluothane) is the biotransformation to reactive intermediates that may be hepatotoxic,[53] especially in obese females and in the presence of hypoxia. Epidemiologic studies suggest an association between obesity and unexplained jaundice following the use of halothane.[54] Bentley[55] has recently shown, however, that postoperative rises in SGOT and SGPT in obese patients anesthetized with halothane are not significantly different when compared to N_2O–O_2–fentanyl technique. The relationship between obesity, postoperative liver impairment, and halothane metabolism has not as yet been established. Halothane does, however, provide an adequate level of anesthesia with high inspired oxygen concentrations as well as a bronchodilating property which is extremely useful in obese patients who are asthmatic, who smoke, or who have chronic lung disease.[36]

Enflurane The inhalation anesthetic enflurane (Ethrane) offers the benefits of potentiating neuromuscular blockade as well as possessing inherent neuromuscular blocking properties of its own.[36] This agent thus provides additional muscle relaxation which is helpful in obtaining maximum expo-

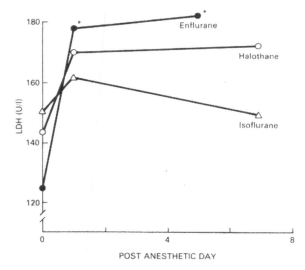

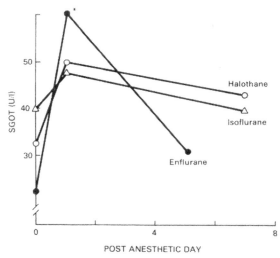

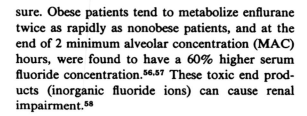

FIG. 9-4. Serum levels of liver enzymes. A Serum lactate dehydrogenase. B Serum glutamic-oxaloacetic transaminase. Asterisks indicate significant increase from control

From Eger EI: Isoflurane (Forane): A Compendium and Reference. Chicago, Airco, 1981, p 79. Reproduced with permission of the publisher.

sure. Obese patients tend to metabolize enflurane twice as rapidly as nonobese patients, and at the end of 2 minimum alveolar concentration (MAC) hours, were found to have a 60% higher serum fluoride concentration.[56,57] These toxic end products (inorganic fluoride ions) can cause renal impairment.[58]

Isoflurane Isoflurane (Forane), a recently released inhalation anesthetic, is one of the most extensively researched drugs in use today.[59] It differs significantly from enflurane and halothane in many respects. The biodegradation of isoflurane is one-tenth that of enflurane and one-hundredth that of halothane.[60] Studies have shown that prolonged and/or repeated isoflurane anesthesia does not produce hepatorenal injury.[60] Isoflurane plus hypoxia and hypercarbia does not cause hepatic necrosis.[59] Increases in hepatic enzymes and bilirubin postoperatively are not different from those following N_2O–O_2–narcotic anesthesia.[60] Repeated anesthesia with isoflurane was not associated with subsequent liver injury (Fig. 9-4 and 9-5).

The increase of serum inorganic fluoride after isoflurane anesthesia is one-tenth that occurring after enflurane and does not interfere with renal function (Fig. 9-6).[60] Catecholamine-induced tachyarrhythmias are much less frequent with isoflurane than with other inhalation agents.[60] Isoflurane, however, can cause a slight increase in heart rate which is usually of little clinical

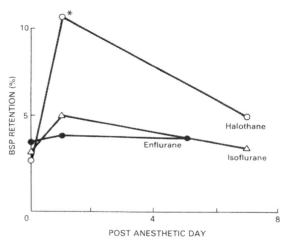

FIG. 9-5. Bromsulphalein (BSP) retention after 11.7 MAC-hours of halothane, 8.8 MAC-hours of Florane, and 9.6 MAC-hours of Ethrane. From Eger EI: Isoflurane (Forane): A Compendium and Reference. Chicago, Airco, 1981, p 78. Reproduced with permission of the publisher.

significance, but must be kept in mind when using this agent.

Muscle Relaxation and Extubation

The addition of these inhalation agents to a balanced anesthesia–narcotic technique is desirable because it avoids the use of large doses of narcotics and muscle relaxants while still providing adequate

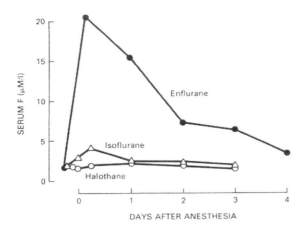

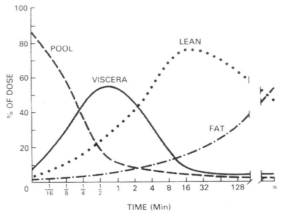

FIGURE 9-6. Serum inorganic fluoride levels after 4.7 MAC-hours of halothane, 2.7 MAC-hours of Ethrane, and 4.1 MAC-hours of isoflurane. From Eger EI: Isoflurane (Forane): A Compendium and Reference. Chicago, Airco, 1981, p 71. Reproduced with permission of the publisher.

FIG. 9-7. Distribution of thiopental in different body tissues and organs at various times after intravenous injection. Blood volume is central pool; viscera, including CNS; kidney, liver, and intestine are lean tissues; and fatty tissues. From Price HL: Clin Pharmacol Ther 1:16, 1960. Reproduced with permission from the C.V. Mosby Company.

anesthetic depth and muscle relaxation. Adequate muscle relaxation during surgery can be judged clinically by the surgeon, but more accurately and definitively with a neuromuscular blockade monitor, which also is extremely helpful in the assessment of paralysis-reversal and preparation of extubation.

Once paralysis has been satisfactorily reversed, the criteria for extubation set forth by Pontoppidan et al.[61] are used, which include evaluation of inspiratory force, respiratory rate, tidal volume, Pa_{CO_2}, and Pa_{O_2}. In the event that the criteria for extubation are not met, mechanical ventilation is continued until the patient is awake, cooperative, and able to adequately ventilate and protect his airway following extubation. The patient should be in a 30–45° semirecumbent position to provide better ventilation and prevent aspiration. Postoperative somnolence may be prolonged because of the delayed release of thiopental from fat absorption (Fig. 9-7).[62]

Narcotic and Inhalation Anesthesia Compared

Recently, Cork et al.[63] compared the outcome of balanced (narcotic) anesthesia and inhalation anesthesia. The time from the last skin stitch until tracheal extubation was not significantly different when comparing either anesthetic technique. In

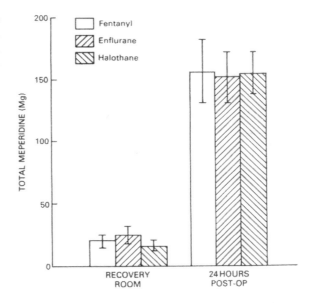

FIG. 9-8. Comparison of postoperative narcotic requirements in three groups of morbidly obese anesthetized patients. (From Brown BR: Anesthesia and the Obese Patient. Philadelphia, Davis, 1982, p 81. Reproduced with permission of the publisher.

addition, recovery room 24-h postoperative narcotic requirements were studied. The data suggest that inhalation anesthetics produce neither delayed awakening nor prolonged postanesthetic recovery time in obese patients (Fig. 9-8).

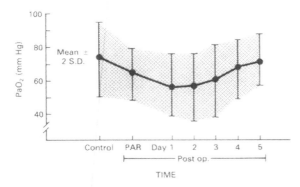

FIG. 9-9. Representation of the fall in Pa_{O_2} with time postoperatively. From Vaughan RW, Engelhardt RC, Wise L: Postoperative hypoxemia in obese patients. An Surg 180:877–882, 1974. Reproduced with permission of J.B. Lippincott/Harper & Row.

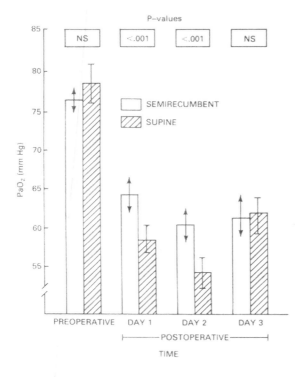

FIG. 9-10. Arterial oxygen tension in the semirecumbent compared with the supine position preoperatively and days postoperatively. From Vaughan RW, Wise L: Postoperative arterial blood gas measurement in obese patients: effect of position on gas exchange. Ann Surg 182:705–707, 1975. Reproduced with permission of J.B. Lippincott/Harper & Row.

Postoperative Hypoxia

Vaughan and Wise[64] have presented data which document a significantly lower preoperative mean PaO_2 in obese compared with nonobese patients matched for age, and in addition, a reduction in arterial oxygen content on the 1st through 3rd postoperative days (Fig. 9-9). This is the time during which myocardial reinfarction is most likely to occur.[15,16] In a subsequent study, Vaughan and Wise[65] demonstrated that during this critical period, the semirecumbent (head-up) rather than supine position improved oxygenation appreciably (Fig. 9-10). Supplemental oxygen should be administered for at least 48 h postoperatively in the largest patients and in those with impaired cardiopulmonary function.

All patients must be ambulated early (starting the evening of surgery whenever possible), and narcotics should be used sparingly. Respiratory physiotherapy, to include deep breathing and coughing, should be conducted frequently. The adjunctive use of the incentive spirometer and/or intermittent positive pressure breathing (IPPB) is helpful in restoring normal pulmonary function and preventing complications.

Summary

Preoperative education to encourage cooperation and allay anxiety is of great importance in the anesthetic management of the obese patient. In addition, these patients must be in optimal medical condition prior to surgery, especially with respect to their cardiorespiratory systems and electrolyte status. Appropriate monitoring is essential.

A balanced N_2O–O_2–narcotic–muscle relaxant–anesthetic technique, with the occasional addition of certain potent inhalation agents (isoflurane, halothane, enflurane), has been our method of choice. It is extremely important to extend supplemental oxygen for 48 h postoperatively for most morbidly obese patients, and to encourage early postoperative ambulation with active respiratory physiotherapy.

References

1. Dripps RD, Eckenhoff JE, Vandam LD: Introduction to Anesthesia: The Principles of Safe Practice. Philadelphia, Saunders, 1977, pp 14, 23, 89, 129.

2. Metropolitan Life Insurance Company: New weight standards for men and women. Stat Bull 40:3–6, 1959.

3. Barrera F, Reindenberg MM, Winters WL: Ventilation-perfusion relationships in the obese patient. J Appl Physiol 26:420–426, 1969.

4. Alexander JK: Obesity and cardiac performance. Am J Cardiol 14:860–865, 1964.

5. Kaltman AJ, Goldring RM: Role of circulatory congestion in the cardiorespiratory failure of obesity. Circulation 48:135–140, 1973.

6. Rochester DF, Enson Y: Current concepts in the pathogenesis of obesity—hypoventilation syndrome. Am J Med 57:402–419, 1974.

7. Backman L, Freyschuso V, Hollberg D: Cardiovascular function in extreme obesity. Acta Med Scand 193:437–446, 1973.

8. Martin JT: Positioning of Anatomy in Surgery. Philadelphia, Saunders, 1978, pp 85–110.

9. Chemiack RM, Guenter CA: The efficiency of the respiratory muscles in obesity. Can J Biochem Physiol 39:1215–1222, 1961.

10. Brown BR: Anesthesia and the Obese Patient. Philadelphia, Davis, 1982, p 21.

11. Vaughan, RW, Wise L: Intraoperative arterial oxygenation in obese patients. Ann Surg 184:35–42, 1967.

12. Vaughan, RW: Obesity: implications in anesthetic management and toxicity. Refresher Course Anesthesiol 9:196, 1981.

13. Kannel WB, LeBauer EJ, Dawber TR: Relation of body weight to development of coronary artery disease. Circulation 35:734–744, 1967.

14. Emerson CW, Davis RF, Philbin DM: Anesthetic management of the patient with coronary artery disease. In Philbin D (ed): Anesthetic Management of the Patient with Cardiovascular Disease. Int Anesthesiol Clin 17:97–124, 1979.

15. Tarhan D, Moffett E, Taylor WF: Myocardial infarction after general anesthesia. JAMA 220:1451–1454, 1972.

16. Steen PA, Tinker JH, Tarhan S: Myocardial reinfarction after anesthesia and surgery. JAMA 239:2566, 1978.

17. Mason EE: Surgical treatment of obesity. Major Probl Clin Surg 26:42, 1981.

18. Norton HJV: Tobacco smoking and pulmonary complications after operation. Fawcett 1:368–370, 1944.

19. McCarthy DS, Spencer R: Measurement of closing volume as a simple and sensitive test for early detection of small airway disease. Am J Med 52:747–753, 1972.

20. Lourenco RV, Klinek MF, Borowski CJ: Deposition and clearance of two-micron particles in the tracheobronchial tree of normal subjects—smokers and nonsmokers. J Clin Invest 50:1411–1419, 1971.

21. Aronson MD, Weiss ST: Association between cigarette smoking and acute respiratory tract illness in young adults. JAMA 248:181–183, 1982.

22. Geddes LA: The Direct and Indirect Measurement of Blood Pressure. Chicago, Yearbook Medical 1970, pp 101–106.

23. Lee JJ, Larson RH, Buckley JJ: Pulmonary function and its correlation to the degree of obesity in 294 patients. Anesthesiol Rev 2:28–32, 1981.

24. Postlethwait RW, Johnson WD: Complications following surgery for duodenal ulcer in obese patients. Arch Surg 195:438–440, 1972.

25. Walts LF, Miller J, Davidson M, Brown J: Perioperative management of diabetes mellitus. Anesthesiology 55:104–113, 1981.

26. Fox GS: Anesthesia for intestinal short circuiting in the morbidly obese patients with reference to the pathophysiology of gross obesity. Can Anesth Soc J 22:307–315, 1975.

27. Wong KC: Cations in anesthesia. 29th Annual Refresher Course Lectures. Am Soc Anesthesiol 195:1–9, 1978.

28. Sack D, Kim ND, Wong KC: Contractivity and subcellular calcium metabolism in chronic potassium deficiency. Am J Physiol 226:756–762, 1974.

29. Scribner BD, Burnell JM: Interpretation of the serum potassium concentration. Metabolism 5:468–479, 1956.

30. Endomnds CJ, Jasani BM: Total body potassium changes with prolonged diuretic therapy. Am Heart J 85:569–571, 1973.

31. Wong KC: The effect of acute hypokalemia and respiratory changes in cardiac excitability. Abstracts of Scientific Papers. Park Ridge, Ill., American Society of Anesthesiologists, 1974, pp 419–420.

32. Westwater JO, Fainer D: Liver impairment in the obese. Gastroenterology 34:686–693, 1958.

33. Hamm CW, Koehler LS: The implications of morbid obesity for anesthesia. Anesthesiol Rev 6:29–35, 1979.

34. Lappas DG, Gayes JM: Intraoperative monitoring in anesthetic management of the patient with cardiovascular disease. Int Anesthesiol Clin 17:157–173, 1979.

35. Kaplin JA: Cardiac Anesthesia. New York, Grune & Stratton, 1979, Chap 2, 4, 5.

36. Churchill-Davidson HC: Wylie and Churchill-Davidson: A Practice of Anesthesia. Philadelphia, Saunders, 1978, pp 507, 517, 558.

37. Brown CQ: Cordis introducers: CVP measurement with fluid infusion. Anesthesiology 55:485, 1981.

38. Gamble JAS, Dundee JW: Plasma diazepam levels after single oral and intramuscular administration. Anesthesia 30:164–169, 1975.

39. Vaughan RW, Bauer S, Wise L: Volume and pH of gastric juice in obese patients. Anesthesiology 43:686–689, 1975.

40. Mendelson CL: Aspiration of stomach contents during obstetric anesthesia. Am J Obstet Gynecol 52:191–205, 1946.

41. Teabeaut JR: Aspiration of gastric contents: An experimental study. Am J Pathol 28:51–63, 1952.

42. Wynne JW, Modell JH: Aspiration of stomach contents. Ann Intern Med 87:466–474, 1977.

43. Donlon JV: Anesthetic management of patients with compromised airways. Anesthesiol Rev 2:22–31, 1980.

44. Lee JJ, Larson RH, Buckley JJ: Airway maintenance in the morbidly obese. Anesthesiol Rev 1:33–36, 1980.

45. Sukerman S, Healy GB: Sleep apnea syndrome with upper airway obstruction. Laryngoscope 89:878–887, 1979.

46. Gelman S, Patel K, Dintzman L: Clinical aspects of thoracic epidural analgesia in morbid obesity. Anesthesiol Rev 6:12–17, 1980.

47. Bromage PR: Epidural Analgesia. Philadelphia, Saunders, 1970, pp 449–454, 456–457.

48. Gelman S, Laws HL, Polzick J: Thoracic epidural vs. balanced anesthesia in morbid obesity: an intra- and postoperative hemodynamic study. Anesth Analg 59:902–908, 1980.

49. Behar M, Olshwang D, Magora F: Epidural morphine in treatment of pain. Lancet 1:527–529, 1979.

50. Wang JK, Nauss LA, Thomas JE: Pain relief by intrathecally applied morphine in man. Anesthesiology 50:149–151, 1979.

51. Bromage PR: Intraspinal narcotics: State of the art. Refresher Courses in Anesthesiology 10:27–36, 1982.

52. Lebowitz PW, Savarese JJ, Ramsey FR, Ali HH, deBros FR: Combination of pancuronium and metocurine: Neuromuscular and hemodynamic ad-

vantages over pancuronium alone. Anesth Analg 60:12–20, 1981.

53. Brown BR, Sipes IG: Biotransformation and hepato-toxicity of halothane. Biochem Pharmacol 26:2091–2094, 1977.

54. Walton B, Simpson BR: Unexplained hepatitis following halothane. Br Med J 4:1171–1176, 1976.

55. Bentley JB, Vaughn RW, Cork RC: Hepatorenal indexes among general anesthetics in obesity. Anesthesiology 53:5259, 1980.

56. Leehning RW, Mazze RI: Possible nephrotoxicity of enflurane in a patient with renal disease. Anesthesiology 40:203–205, 1974.

57. Bentley JB, Vaughan RW, Miller MS: Serum inorganic fluoride levels in obese patients during and after enflurane anesthesia. Anesth Analg 58:409–412, 1979.

58. Young SR, Stoelting RK, Peterson C: Anesthetic biotransformation and renal function in obese patients. Anesthesiology 42:451–457, 1975.

59. Eger EI: Isoflurane, a Compendium and Reference. Chicago, Airco, 1981.

60. Eger EI: Isoflurane, a review. Anesthesiology 55:559–576, 1981.

61. Pontoppidan H, Laver MB, Geffin B: Acute respiratory failure in the surgical patient. Adv Surg 4:163–254, 1970.

62. Collins VJ: Principles of Anesthesiology. Philadelphia, Lea & Febiger, 1972, p 389.

63. Cork RC, Vaughan RW, Bentley JB: Best general anesthetic agent for morbidly obese. Anesthesiology 53:5258, 1980.

64. Vaughan RW, Wise L: Postoperative hypoxemia in obese patients. Ann Surg 180:877–882, 1974.

65. Vaughan RW, Wise L: Postoperative arterial blood gas measurement in obese patients: effect of position on gas exchange. Ann Surg 182:705–707, 1975.

CHAPTER 10

Use of a Microcomputer for Data Management

RAYMOND L. DREW

Before acquiring a microcomputer, our relevant data including complications were kept on long "master sheets" with the most recent weight recorded in pencil to be erased when a new weight was entered. Individual "flow sheets" in each patient's chart were used to record all weights and other more detailed information. Analysis of these data, especially comparison of one operation with another, became increasingly difficult, and prompted us to investigate the application of a computer to our data.

Telephone access to a mainframe computer was first considered but the costs of software development plus time sharing seemed excessive and accessibility limited. Approximately 2 years ago, after extensive investigation, we selected a microcomputer system that has proved very satisfactory. We continue to use individual patient flow sheets as before but, in addition, now enter preselected relevent data into our microcomputer.

For readers who are not familiar with computer technology, a brief explanation of some of its fundamental aspects, and how we applied a microcomputer to our data, may be of value.

General Information

A computer system consists of hardware (the computer and its attached devices) and software (the programs of encoded instructions that tell it what to do). At the present time it is more difficult to find the right software for a specific job than the hardware capable of doing it. Every model of computer is different, and a program that works for one may not work for another, without considerable transposition. The software available for a specific job narrows the choice to compatible hardware. Computer storage and retrieval of data is termed data base management (DBM). Other possible computer applications in a medical office such as billing, accounts receivable, word processing, and so on should also be considered when selecting a computer, but they are beyond the scope of this discussion. Location of the computer, both in terms of the amount of space it occupies, and convenience to all personnel using it, should be considered. Our installation required modification to be used for word processing as well as data base management. The personnel requirement for data entry is another consideration.

Hardware

Computers range considerably in size and complexity. The three main classifications are mainframe, minicomputer, and microcomputer. The mainframe computer is very large and fast and is designed to handle a network of multiple terminals, disk memory storage devices, and printers. A minicomputer is suitcase to file-cabinet size, and is designed to handle up to six terminals, disk storage devices, and a couple of printers. A microcomputer is designed to support a single terminal and single printer (and is often inside the terminal). With the progressive miniaturization of memory circuit boards, microcomputers of today often have more power than minicomputers of a few years ago. For a one- to three-man office, a single terminal microcomputer is adequate. For larger offices requiring several terminals, the options are a single minicomputer supporting several terminals vs. networking several microcomputers onto one large disk drive memory unit.

Central Processing Unit

A computer's capability is related to the size of number (bits), quantity of memory locations (RAM), and speed with which it calculates. Computers store and transfer information as digital binary numbers. A *bit* is a binary digit, either 1 or 0 (representing on or off). A *byte* is eight bits, representing an eight-digit binary number such as 10011011. Most microcomputers process information in their circuits 8 bits at a time, but some 16-bit microprocessors are now available. The more bits a computer uses per step the fewer steps it takes to compute, so the faster it is. A computer's calculating memory is called random access memory (RAM). These are the silicon chip memory locations where the machine simultaneously holds information while it is computing. For business or data base management, the minimum size is 64,000 bytes, abbreviated 64K (kilobytes). Microcomputers with 128–256K capacity are becoming more common and handle larger programs faster. The computer has an internal clock which pulses at a set frequency and keeps the information flow through the circuits synchronized. The faster it runs, the faster the computer can carry out calculations. Home computers run at a frequency of 1–2 megahertz (million cycles per second), office computers 4–6 megahertz (Mhz).

Our microcomputer uses an 8080A Central Processing Unit (CPU), which is an 8-bit, 4-Mhz processor with 64K RAM. This does the job very adequately, but it would be more pleasant to use if it were faster. The time required for a program to process a data file depends upon the number of steps the program performs on each record, and the number of records to be processed in the file. Our present 690-operation data file has required an hour or more to be processed by some of our complex programs. Some programs required revision because they exceeded available RAM. Presently, if equivalent software were available, we would prefer a 16-bit processor with 128K RAM.

Disk Memory

Disk memory is storage memory. The magnetic disks hold information, just as tape does for a tape recorder. All the programs, and the data files, are stored on disk. When the computer is turned on, the programs and data files for the requested job are loaded from the disk into the computer's RAM. As the program is run, any data changes made in the file are saved back onto the disk. When the computer is turned off, RAM is erased. The computer also has read only memory (ROM), which is preserved when the power is turned off. It is used for internal operating instructions for the computer itself. Other information cannot be written on it, so it is not available to outside programs or data.

There are two types of disks, floppy and rigid. Floppy are less expensive, hold considerably less data, are slower, and come in two sizes, 5.25 in or 8 in. The mini-floppy, 5.25 in, holds 90–700K. The 8-in floppy holds 500K to 2MB (megabytes, million bytes). When used, floppy disks are inserted into a disk drive, like a cassette tape into a recorder. Rigid disks rotate much faster so more data can be found more quickly, and have a capacity of 5–70MB. They are usually sealed units, but some have removable disk cartridges.

A rigid disk is essential for managing a large data file. Our main data file now uses 432K or essentially fills our 596K-capacity floppy disk. The control files that sort and report the data would require a second floppy drive, and the data base management programs, a third. There would be no room for output files, and constant shuffling of disks in and out of the drives would be necessary. The rigid disks are also more reliable regarding possible occurrences of spontaneous data errors. With a rigid disk system, one floppy drive is still needed for program entry and transfer, and may be used for backup of data. One adequate rigid drive costs much less than two smaller ones, so the original purchase should suffice for 5 years. A rule of thumb is to buy double the size of anticipated need. Our 10-megabyte rigid disk is now 60% full.

Terminal

The video screen, or cathode ray tube (CRT), through which the computer communicates to the operator can be in color, black and white, green on black, or amber on black. Color is expensive and unnecessary for business. Green is easier on the eyes than black and white, and amber is said to be better yet.

Printer

A printer is essential for a readable, permanent record. There are three basic types: dot matrix, daisy wheel, and thermal. The thermal printers are the slowest, cheapest, and quietest, but require special paper and do not make multiple copies, so are unsuitable for an office.

Daisy wheel printers type characters from the spokes of a spinning wheel. Their excellent print quality, equal to an electric typewriter, makes them superior for word processing. They are slow by computer standards at 25–55 characters per second (CPS), but are faster than an electric typewriter at 10 CPS. They require a moderate amount of maintenance.

Dot matrix printers are faster, from 80 to 250 characters per second. The print quality is proportional to the density of dots comprising the letters, with 5×7 being quite coarse, and 9×9 fairly dense and also allowing the tails on letters to go below the line (called true descenders). Some offer a "correspondence quality" feature which halves the printing speed but overlaps the dots to improve print quality. Dot matrix printers are best for a high output of data.

We have a 40-CPS daisy wheel printer and have been happy with that choice. Its speed has been adequate for our purposes, and the print quality is excellent.

Software

Data base management system (DBMS) programs are available for microcomputers, and the selection is increasing. There are no DBMS ready "off the shelf" to track our specific data or calculate weight loss results. The programs have to be customized, either by a computer programer or the user himself. A "turn key" system is one already set up by a programer, ready to turn on and use. Although initially expedient, this makes the user dependent on the programer for revisions, as unforeseen new reports are requested. Many of the DBMS are designed for a user to adapt to his requirements, and this was our choice.

The programs were supplied on a floppy disk and were transferred onto a rigid disk. To use the programs for our data, files were set up defining our data, selection, sorting, and report requirements. This was facilitated by the program's use of menus (screens with numbered choices) and a prompting editor, with fill-in-the-blank responses. Familiarization with the DBMS manual and building sample data and report files were also necessary before undertaking the actual project.

The software system that evolved became quite complex, but it developed in simple steps. The heart of it is one large data *file*. The data file contains one *record* for each surgical procedure, whether a primary operation or a revision or conversion of a previous one. Each record contains biographical patient data, operative technique, associated surgery, operative and interval postoperative weights, laboratory data, and complications. Each of these data items in a record is termed a *field*. The characters (letters or numbers) in a field are each represented in the computer by one byte. A patient's weight, a three-digit decimal number, requires three bytes. A name of up to 25 letters requires 25 bytes. The computer stores the information in the same order in every record in the file, to find it and compare it. The first step in setting up the file was to define each of the fields to be stored in each record: its label, how many characters in it, and whether the characters are letters or numbers. Ours has 177 fields of 1–25 bytes each, totalling 624 bytes in each record.

The screen format which prompts for data entry was next defined. A RAM shortage occurred when the computer was unable to hold all the program, file definition, and screen definition information simultaneously. Splitting the screen definition into three categories, each one accessing only a part of the one data file, resolved the memory limitation. The three categories were biographical and operative, complications and lab, postoperative weights and patient satisfaction.

Data entry of records into the file was accomplished by two regular office employees, a secretary and a nurse. Data entered was checked by one of us for accuracy, from a printout of each record entered. Patients whose follow-up was not current were recontacted by phone and mail, and encouraged to return in person.

The weight results were generated with a separate report for each follow-up interval. A selection criterion chose only those records with a follow-up weight entered at that interval. (The program derives averages, and a weight of 0 from a person without follow-up would invalidate the average.) The selected records were indexed and sorted into categories: Roux-en-Y, loop gastric bypass, or plasty; and as primary procedures, in conjunction with a reconstitution of a JIB, or as revision or conversion of previous gastric operation. The weight report format was defined.

The report generator program then calculates from each patient's ideal, preoperative, and present weights what his excess weight was and is, what percentage of ideal weight he was and is, and his weight loss expressed in kilograms and as percentages of his preoperative weight and preoperative excess weight. Each of these weight results was also averaged and printed for each category of operation. The data file was accessed in the index-sorted order, for all patients of each operation type, to be tabulated and averaged together.

The complications report was more complex. There were provisions for 15 early and 35 late complication categories. Using the report generator program would have required 50 report definition files, each with a selection and index file. The 150 additional files would have overloaded even the rigid disk. Each report would have gone through the data file once, in about 20 to 30 min. Fifty passes would have required about 20 h of computer time.

Instead, four custom programs go through the data file four times. Each time seven to 15 specific complication files are built, printed, and erased. The programs are run in sequence from a batch file requiring 6 h total.

Additional report files were written for percentage of follow-up at each interval, pooled latest weight results at 1 year or beyond, failure to lose 20% of ideal weight, most recent patient acceptance, and most recent patient satiety. In each instance the data file was selected and index sorted for a specific report.

All the data input and report output functions have been placed as numbered selections on *menus,* for ease of use.

Costs

In considering the expense of the system there are supply and maintenance costs, as well as the initial cost of the hardware and software. Floppy disks are needed to back up data from the hard disk. Paper and ribbons will be needed for the printer. The monthly maintenance contract cost for the hardware is usually 1% of the initial cost. Software may need servicing by a programer as well, if needs change, and the user is unable to make the changes himself. So far, there have been no hardware failures, and the software has worked, once the initial frustrations of learning it were overcome.

Data Protection

One frequent source of irritation in a dry climate is inadvertent static discharge from a person to the terminal, causing a "crash" with loss of whatever is in RAM at the time. It has not yet altered files in disk storage. An antistatic mat on the floor to ground the operator's feet, and care by those walking by not to touch the computer or operator, have decreased this annoyance. To protect the investment in time building up files and programs, all should be duplicated, and storage of one or two copies off premises is recommended in case of fire.

Summary

A good data base management system will make medical data more readily retrievable. Today's microcomputers are powerful enough for quite ambitious data management. Setting up such a system oneself is a full-time hobby for a year or more. If a programer is engaged to set it up, define carefully for him all data to be stored, and the exact format of all data reports desired, so programing time (and costs) can be kept to a minimum.

CHAPTER 11

Radiographic Examination of the Obese Patient

JOSEPH MILO MELAND

Successful radiographic examination of morbidly obese patients is difficult because of their immense size and body habitus. This is true whether conventional radiographic imaging or isotope technique is used. By the inverse square law, the intensity of radiation is inversely proportional to the square of the distance from its source. Because the anterior-posterior diameter of an obese patient can be three times that of a normal-sized patient, the obese patient may require nine times the radiation to achieve the same film exposure and diagnostic information as his normal-sized counterpart.

This chapter will present some important aspects of diagnostic technique with radiographs to illustrate common early and late complications associated with surgery of the morbidly obese. A detailed discussion of complications may be found in Chapter 6.

Preoperative Evaluation

The radiographic equipment must have at least a 600-mA generator to develop sufficiently powerful x rays for the obese patient.[1] Some patients are so large they will not fit between the fluoroscopic tower and the x-ray table which limits the examination to overhead films without fluoroscopy.

New fast film–screen combinations significantly decrease the patient's radiation dose and improve the clarity of the diagnostic images. These should be used if possible when dealing with obese patients. Currently available systems include the Lannex System by Eastman Kodak, the Trimax System by Minnesota Mining and Manufacturing Company (3M), and the Cronex System by Dupont.

Routine preoperative diagnostic radiography usually includes a PA chest radiograph, an upper gastrointestinal tract examination, an oral cholecystogram, and in selected patients, a barium enema. A cholecystogram in a patient who has had a jejunoileal bypass requires cholecystographic tablets for 2 consecutive days to visualize the gallbladder adequately because of limited absorption from the short small bowel.[2] Ultrasound examination of the gallbladder is occasionally unsuccessful in the morbidly obese patient because of the degradation of sound waves by increased body size.

Double contrast upper GI tract examination is recommended for the preoperative evaluation because it will reveal better mucosal detail at a lower radiation dose. The preoperative upper GI examination in patients having a gastric bypass (GBP) operation is particularly important because radiographic visualization of the distal stomach postoperatively is, under ordinary circumstances, impossible.

Postoperative Radiography

All patients should have an upper GI examination between the 5th and 7th postoperative day unless a complication precludes this procedure. This is important for two reasons: to diagnose any immediate abnormalities, and to provide a basis for comparison in patients who develop complications or

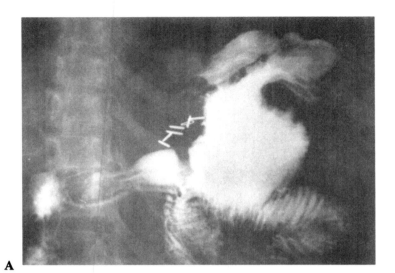

A

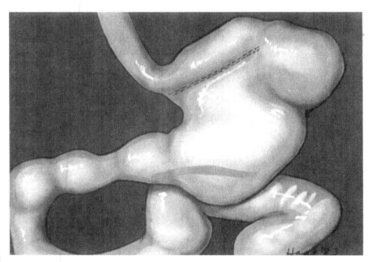

B

regain weight. Double contrast technique is not recommended for postoperative studies.

An initial supine scout film is obtained which reveals the gas pattern in the small and large bowel, and also the location of the staple lines. After the scout film, the patient is given a swallow or two from a 6-oz. cup of barium, and careful attention is paid to the lower esophagus and upper stomach. The patient is then instructed to drink additional barium and to stop when a full feeling is experienced. Fluoroscopic examination is conducted in the AP and left posterior oblique positions. Multiple spot films are taken during the first few swallows of barium and after satiety is reported. The amount of barium required to achieve satiety, and measurements of the pouch and chan-nel size, are noted and included in the x-ray report. The shortest and longest dimension of the pouch and the maximum size of the outlet are used for measurement. Evidence of obstruction, esophageal dilatation, and time required to empty the pouch are also recorded. The barium is followed at least to the Roux-en-Y anastomosis in patients with this type of GBP to note any evidence of obstruction there (Figs. 11-1 and 11-2).

In some patients, the barium passes so quickly through the area of interest that good films of the pouch are impossible to obtain. We then use a paste of powdered natural bran and barium. The mixture is fed to the patient in tablespoon quantities. This simulates semisolid food and gives additional information about pouch and outlet size.

FIG. 11-2. **A** Normal gastric bypass. The pouch and channel sizes are normal. The Roux-en-Y anastomosis is obscured on this oblique view, but was well seen on the AP view. **B** and **C** Examples of gastric bypass with small (10–15 ml) pouches and radiopaque Silastic catheter support around anastomosis.

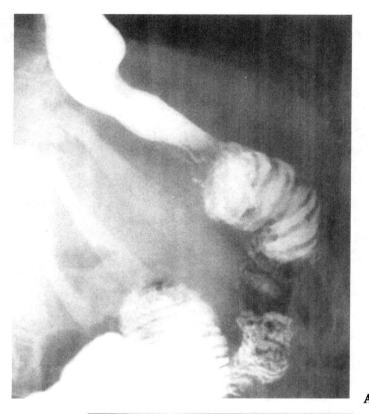

A

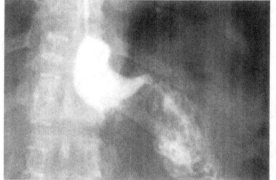

B

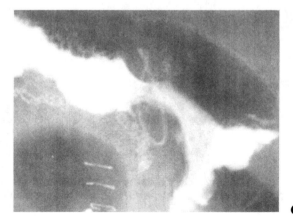

C

Bran–barium paste preparations should be used only after the outlet is seen to be patent. If the outlet is too narrow, the paste can cause complete obstruction. Also the thickened material should not be used in patients who have had conversion of JIB to gastric bypass because of the danger of small bowel obstruction.

In one patient with a distended distal stomach, we were able to instill water-soluble media into the distal stomach through a percutaneously placed catheter, with excellent visualization. This patient had had a gastrostomy with gastropexy, and the radiographs were obtained using a skinny needle technique through the gastrostomy scar. After locating the lumen of the stomach by aspiration and instillation of a few milliliters of Gastrografin, increasing catheter sizes were inserted until a satisfactory conduit was obtained (Fig. 11-3).

McNeely[3] has developed a method for visualizing the excluded stomach and duodenum that will become extremely valuable if it proves to be generally applicable and safe. This technique is as follows. A plain film of the abdomen is first taken, and a point on the patient's abdomen 3–4 cm below the transverse staple line separating the gastric

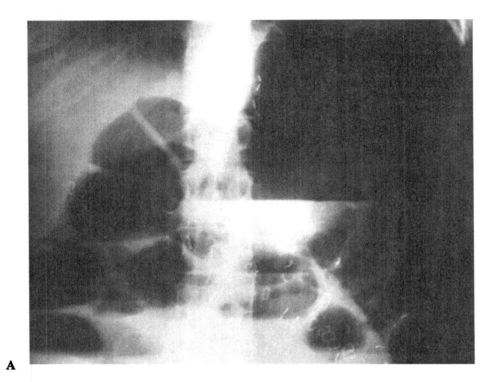

A

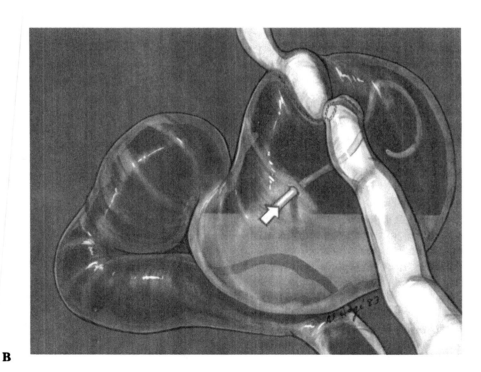

B

FIG. 11-3. Successful treatment of distal stomach distension using percutaneous catheter placement. **A** Gaseous distension of the distal stomach with air–fluid levels in the stomach and distal duodenum. **B** Successful placement of a percutaneous drainage catheter. See text for details. (*Continued*)

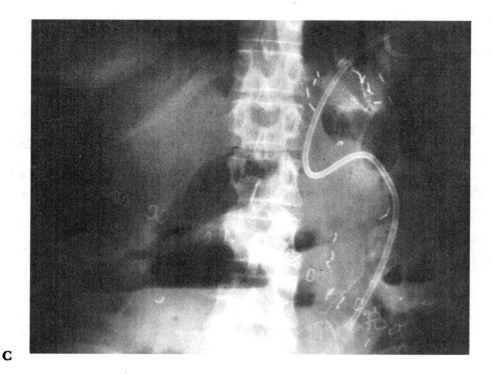

C

FIG. 11-3. C Follow-up film showing clearing of the gastric distension.

pouch from the excluded stomach is selected for introducing a skinny needle. The needle, attached to a syringe containing Gastrografin radiopaque contrast material, is introduced posteriorly, directly through the abdominal wall and deep enough to ensure its passage through both the anterior and posterior walls of the underlying stomach. It is then slowly withdrawn, a centimeter or less at a time, instilling ½–1 ml of Gastrografin at each interval during its withdrawal. The lumen of the stomach, once entered during the withdrawal process, will become apparent. At this time additional contrast is introduced until the amount necessary to complete a satisfactory examination has been injected.

Through the use of this method they were able to visualize an antral and a duodenal ulcer that otherwise could not have been definitely diagnosed except at laparotomy. Further refinement of this method by means of passing a silastic catheter over the needle into the stomach, similar to the method we used on our patient described above (Fig. 11-3), would enhance the diagnostic potential of this technique. We were able to decompress a dilated stomach by this means, the catheter serving as a small tube-gastrostomy.

Pouch Size Measurements

Other methods have been described to determine the volume of the gastric pouch. Koehler and Halverson[4] have utilized pouch size measurements to determine pouch volume by assuming the pouch to be an ellipsoid and applying the following formula: volume $= 0.3 \times S^2 \times L$ where S and L are the short and long diameters of the pouch measured in centimeters on the x-ray film. A magnification factor of 1.2 has been incorporated into the above formula. We seldom use this method of volume measurement because it is only an approximation at best. Pouch size and distensibility vary considerably depending upon outlet size and speed of emptying. A more accurate measurement of pouch size can be obtained by inserting a nasogastric tube with a balloon or condom affixed to its distal end into the gastric pouch, then filling the balloon with barium. No barium escapes using this technique, and the true volume can be measured.[5] We have had no experience with the balloon technique, and believe its usefulness would apply principally to a clinical research study. The actual pouch volume is measured by the surgeon during the operative procedure at our institution.

Late Diagnostic Studies

In late diagnostic studies (months to years postoperatively) the radiologist should be informed prior to the examination of the type of gastric stapling procedure that was done to better evaluate the nature of any defect present. Comparison with old films, and measurement of pouch and channel size as well as volume at satiety, are important parameters to be included in the report. A scout film offers a good opportunity to assess the location and condition of the staples. If the patient is allowed to swallow several ounces of barium before the upper stomach is visualized fluoroscopically and spot films taken, the most important aspect of the study is lost—i.e., pouch and channel size, or even whether any stapling procedure has been done at all. The latter is particularly true if the patient has had a gastroplasty or gastric partitioning procedure, because the barium can flow rapidly into the lower stomach totally obscuring the outlet.

Complications of Bariatric Surgery

Complications are divided into early and late and the use of diagnostic imaging is important in both phases.[6]

Early Complications

The early complications are usually quite severe and the patient may be very ill when sent to the radiology department for evaluation. The surgeon and radiologist must work in close cooperation in this situation to support the patient, to minimize the length of the procedure, and to prevent shock.

The early complications include (1) anastomotic leak (Figs. 11-4 and 11-5); (2) abscess formation with or without a leak (Fig. 11-5); (3) distal stomach distension with or without leakage (Figs. 11-3, 11-6); (4) obstruction of either the gastric channel in the gastroplasty-type procedures, or the gastroenterostomy in the GBP type (Fig. 11-11); and (5) obstruction of the afferent or efferent limb of the small bowel at the Roux-en-Y anastomosis (Figs. 11-6, 11-12).[7,14]

Differentiating pulmonary embolism from anastomotic leakage often necessitates a lung scan as well as an upper GI study.

If an anastomotic leak is suspected, an upper GI examination is performed with a water-soluble radiopaque medium such as Gastrografin used at either half or full strength (Figs. 11-4, 11-5, 11-7A). The presence of extraluminal gas with a fluid level, and a pleural effusion on the left side, is strongly suggestive of a subphrenic abscess. An anastomotic leak may or may not be demonstrated, because the leak may have sealed off. Gastrografin can cause hyperosmolar hypovolemic shock, and the patient should have an intravenous line with fluid running and be as close to normovolemic as possible. Very little contrast is needed to demonstrate most leaks. To reveal a more distal bowel obstruction considerably more contrast is required which increases the risk of hypovolemic shock.

Isotopic scanning with gallium-67 citrate and indium-111 is valuable in localizing abscesses. In the less obese patients, ultrasound studies can also prove helpful. In a late mature abscess, abdominal CT scanning can provide more precise anatomic detail (Fig. 11-7). The patient's girth must be measured before transfer to the radiology department to be sure he will fit through the aperture of the scanner. With computerized imaging of an abscess cavity, it is possible to drain the abscess percutaneously in some patients.[8–10]

Distension and blowout of the distal stomach in a patient who has had a gastric bypass can be an extremely difficult diagnosis to make either by clinical or radiographic means (Fig. 11-6).

Late Complications

Late complications include (1) staple line disruption between proximal gastric pouch and distal stomach (Figs. 11-8 and 11-9); (2) pouch or channel enlargement with failure to lose or to gain weight (Fig. 11-10); and (3) outlet obstruction caused by foreign body (usually food), bezoar formation, stenosis due to scarring, or twisting at the anastomosis or channel (Fig. 11-11).

Stenosis of the outlet occasionally responds to dilatation using a Gruntzig angioplasty catheter over a guidewire that has been passed through the stoma endoscopically. Peustow dilators can also be used (see Chapter 6). The simultaneous use of endoscopic and fluoroscopic techniques is essential for these maneuvers.

Examples of late complications[11,12] are shown in Figs. 11-8–11-14.

FIG. 11-4. Gastric stapling with leak. Water-soluble contrast medium is used for this examination and should be given by mouth rather than through the tube. Note the sliver of contrast extending from the suture line into the left subphrenic space outlining the inferior aspect of the diaphragm.

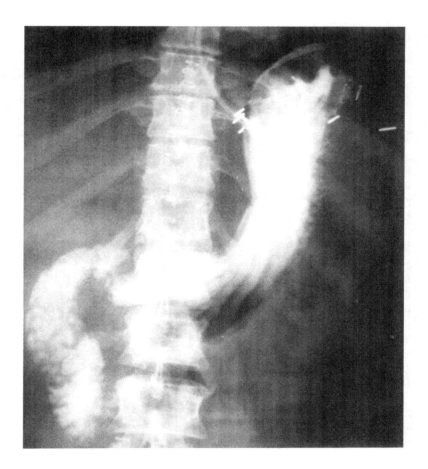

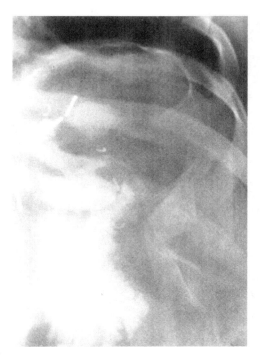

A

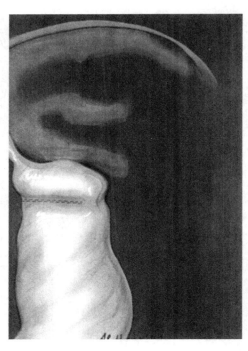

B

FIG. 11-5. **A** and **B** Subphrenic abscess with leak demonstrated. The leak of water-soluble contrast can clearly be seen extending into the left subphrenic space and filling loculations in the subphrenic abscess cavity.

155

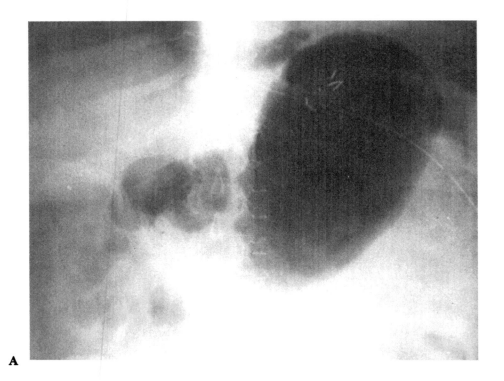

A

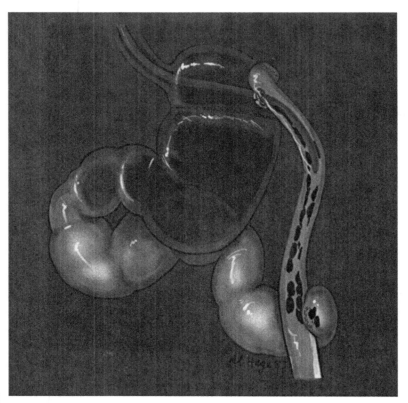

B

FIG. 11-6. **A** and **B** Distension of the distal stomach secondary to afferent limb obstruction at the Roux-en-Y anastomosis. Bleeding from the gastroenterostomy caused obstruction due to large thrombi at the Roux-en-Y anastomosis. Later, pylorospasm resulted in further gastric distension and blowout (see Chapter 6).

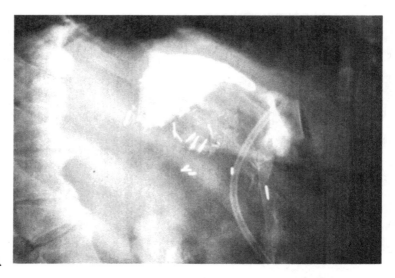

A

FIG. 11-7. **A** Lateral view showing posterosuperior abscess being inadequately drained by small suction catheter and Penrose drain 1 week after open drainage had been established. Several days later abscess drained spontaneously through the drain site, and further surgery was not needed. **B** CT scan on same patient showing abscess (*A*) at the hilum of the spleen (*S*) which would have made a posterior drainage approach extremely hazardous.

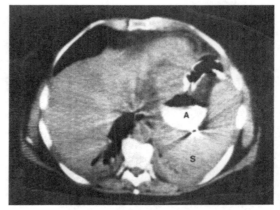

B

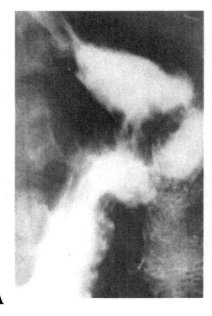

A

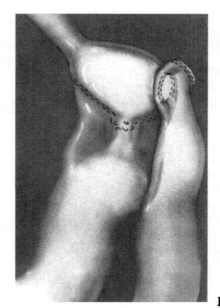

B

FIG. 11-8. Gastric bypass with staple line disruption between the proximal gastric pouch and the distal stomach.

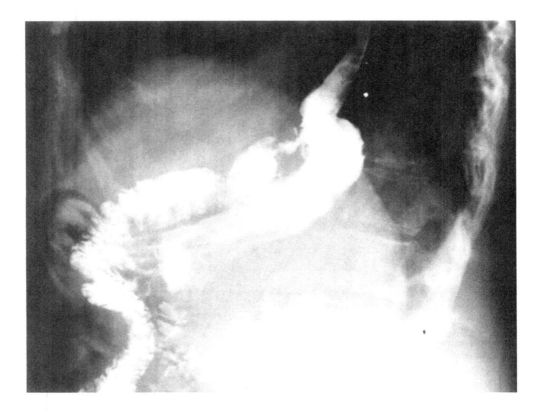

FIG. 11-9. Lateral view showing gastric bypass with staple line disruption and large leak to the distal stomach.

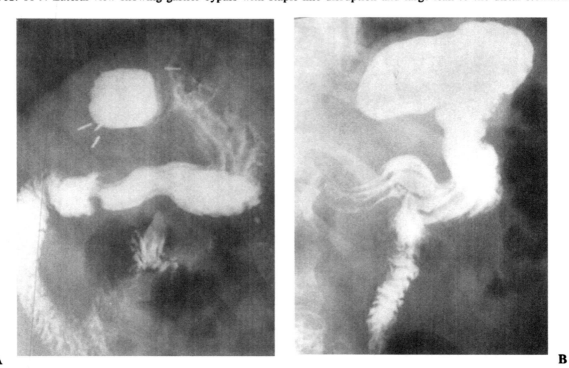

A

B

FIG. 11-10. Increasing pouch size. **A** A normal pouch after gastroplasty. **B** The same patient 1 year later. Note that the pouch has almost doubled in size.

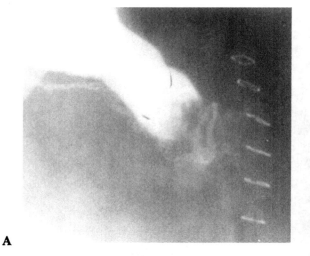

A

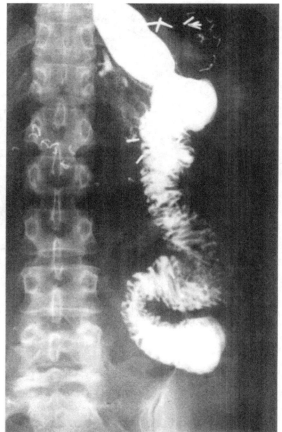

FIG. 11-12. Obstruction at the Roux-en-Y anastomosis.

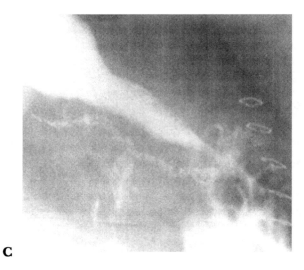

B

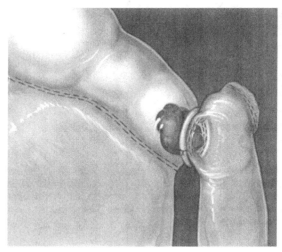

C

FIG. 11-11. **A** and **B** Gastric bypass with meat bolus obstructing anastomosis. **C** Normal channel after meat had been removed endoscopically.

Jejunoileal Bypass Complications

Jejunoileal operations were discontinued at our institution in 1976, and have lost popularity throughout the country because of the long-term morbidity. Only roentgenographic aspects of late complications, and those associated with the take-down or reconstitution of a JIB, which is becoming a much more common procedure, will be considered here.[13]

The most common complications of the JIB include the following:

1. Biliary calculi
2. Urinary calculi
3. Intussusception of proximal end of bypassed limb
4. Liver failure

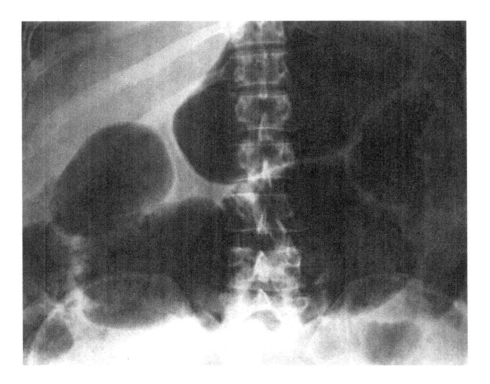

FIG. 11-13. JIB with megacolon. No obstruction is present. Courtesy of Dr. Mathis Frick.

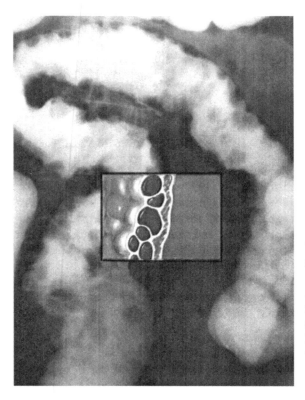

FIG. 11-14. Pneumatosis cystoides intestinalis. When associated with JIB usually seen in excluded small bowel. This was not one of our patients and the involvement here is in the sigmoid colon. The small air cysts are demonstrated nicely.

5. Megacolon with colonic pseudoobstruction
6. Pneumatosis cystoides intestinalis
7. Blind limb reflux
8. Blind limb obstruction
9. Arthritis and dermatitis
10. Osteomalacia

Because these complications are discussed in Chapter 3, only those with diagnostic roentgenographic importance will be included here.

1. *Cholelithiasis* is a common sequel to JIB surgery, and radiologic evaluation of the gallbladder in the late postoperative period is frequently indicated. For the standard cholecystogram, the tablets should be given over a 2-day period as mentioned earlier. Most of these patients have lost weight, and an ultrasound examination for stones is usually of value.[2,15]

2. An IVP, or retrograde pyelogram, may be needed to rule out *nephrolithiasis,* a common complication of JIB. The stones are almost always composed of calcium oxalate, but occasionally uric acid stones are encountered. The incidence of renal lithiasis following JIB is variously reported from 2 to 32% (see Chapter 3). However, these statistics only include those that have exhibited symptoms. The incidence of asymptomatic calculi is unknown, but most likely higher.[16-18]

3. *Intussusception* of the proximal end of the bypassed small intestine is usually a fairly early complication. It is quite difficult to diagnose roentgenographically because it is impossible to visualize the bypassed bowel with oral contrast media. The patient with unexplainable constant mid-abdominal pain should be suspected of having this condition. A flat plate of the abdomen which reveals a diffuse, dense, mid-abdominal mass, oval in shape, is a highly suspicious finding for this condition and is usually an indication for a laparotomy. Ultrasound and CT scan studies are also very helpful in arriving at this tentative diagnosis.[19-21]

4. *Liver failure* is usually determined by liver function tests, and obvious clinical signs and symptoms. A percutaneous liver biopsy is the most direct approach to the diagnosis, but it is an invasive technique with occasional complications.

A noninvasive method of evaluating hepatic functional anatomy is a technetium sulfa colloid liver scan. Characteristically, liver activity is diminished in the diseased (cirrhotic) liver, the spleen is enlarged with increased activity (colloidal shift), and there may be increased activity in the vertebrae reflecting extrahepatic reticuloendothelial proliferation.[22-24]

5. All patients following JIB develop a *megacolon* which in time increases both in length and diameter (Fig. 11-13). Failure to appreciate this normal adaptation to a short small bowel will result in a false diagnosis of chronic colonic obstruction or Hirschsprung's disease. Instead of excessive diarrhea, some of these patients experience pseudoobstruction, and a severe gas-bloat syndrome. Megacolon is apparent on a flat plate of the abdomen or a barium enema examination.[2,25-27]

6. Toxic megacolon and *toxic enteritis* are more serious diseases. They are marked by a distended colon and/or small intestine in a patient who is usually toxic. Pneumatosis cystoides intestinalis

(small cystic defects in the wall of the bowel) can frequently be seen radiographically in these conditions (Fig. 11-14). Pneumatosis intestinalis can be seen with or without toxic enteritis. Feinberg[24] described pneumatosis in 24 of 198 post-JIB patients. Most of these were having no abdominal symptoms at the time of the film and the association of pneumatosis with bypass enteritis seems to be one of chance occurrence. This complication is apparently more frequent when the distal end of the blind small bowel limb is anastomosed to the sigmoid instead of the more proximal colon. Because this has not been the practice at our institution we have not seen this complication following JIB.[12,28-32]

7. *Reflux* from the functional small bowel into the blind limb can be visualized by x ray, and is an occasional cause of failure to lose weight.[33]

8. *Obstruction of the distal blind loop* is a more difficult diagnosis to make, and has no characteristic radiologic findings. It is usually accompanied by progressive abdominal pain and distension and requires a laparotomy for diagnosis.[34]

9. The type of *arthritis* and *dermatitis* that follows JIB is related to absorption of toxic bacterial products or immune bodies (complement–cryoglobulins). Even in the most severe cases, the arthritis seldom results in any permanent joint changes except for fluid occasionally seen in the knee joint. The arthritis improves with broad spectrum antibiotics, and almost always completely disappears with reconstruction of small bowel continuity.[11,35]

10. X-ray evidence of *skeletal decalcification* is seldom seen. Osteomalacia, which does occur in patients with a long-established JIB, is diagnosed by bone biopsy.

Radiography is helpful in diagnosing obstruction at an anastomosis which is one of the most significant postoperative complications. It must be remembered, however, that the functional small bowel—usually the first 10 in of jejunum and the distal 4 to 9 in of ileum—has hypertrophied, and a year or so following the initial JIB procedure usually has a diameter of 5–6 cm. The bypassed small intestine, on the other hand, has a diameter of only 1.5–2 cm. An uniformed radiologist may conclude that an obstruction is present when the discrepancy in size is actually a normally dilated proximal jejunum and a tiny defunctional jejunum distal to the anastomosis. Obstruction at the anastomoses between these disparate bowel lumens oc-

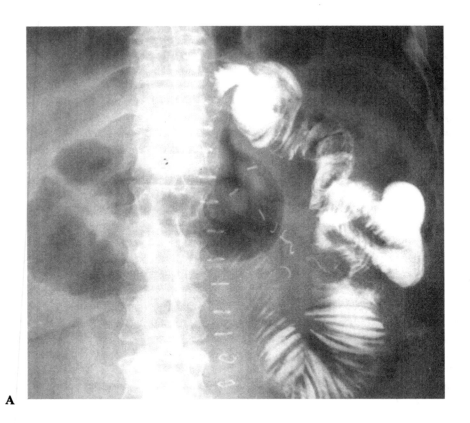

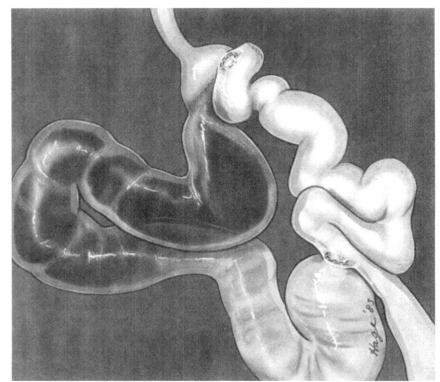

FIG. 11-15. **A** and **B** Site of anastomosis after reconstitution of JIB. Note the great disparity in the size of opposing segments of the jejunojejunal anastomosis. This can be a site of obstruction, but was not in this case.

casionally occurs, however, and this can best be visualized by a flat plate of the abdomen followed by small bowel follow-through examination using water-soluble media (Fig. 11-15). For this reason, a transit time study through the entire small bowel is performed postoperatively, usually on the 8th to 10th day. Contrast medium is instilled into the gastrostomy tube to visualize the distal stomach, duodenum, and jejunum, and by mouth to view the pouch and efferent limb if a GBP has been done. Barium (without added bran) is usually used for this study.

A few of our patients were 10 years past their original JIB when the takedown was performed. In every case, the previously defunctionalized small bowel functioned, but transit times were slow—usually over 4 h and up to 22 h. Gradually, however, the bypassed small bowel function returned to normal.

Summary

Radiographic studies can supply valuable information for morbidly obese patients in the pre- and postoperative periods. An early postoperative upper GI study serves as an essential baseline for later studies. The preliminary scout film visualizes the staple line, and initial fluoroscopy shows the distal esophagus and upper stomach before barium obscures the surgical alteration.

In JIB surgery, radiographic studies are important in the diagnosis of late complications and complications after takedown of a JIB.

References

1. Cohen WN, Mason EE, Blommers TJ: Gastric bypass for morbid obesity. Radiology 122:609–612, 1977.
2. Wade DH, Richards V, Burhenne HJ: Radiographic changes after small bowel bypass for morbid obesity. Radiol Clin North Am 14:493–498, 1976.
3. McNeely F, Macgregor AMC: Distal gastric and duodenal evaluation following gastric bypass by percutaneous transabdominal upper GI series. Scientific Exhibit. Bariatric Surgical Colloquium. Iowa City, June 2–3, 1983.
4. Koehler RE, Halverson JD: Radiographic abnormalities after gastric bypass. Am J Roentgenol 138:267–270, 1982.
5. Backman L: Personal communication. Bariatric Surgery Colloquium, Iowa City, 1981.
6. Moffat RE, Peltier GL, Jewell WR: The radiologic spectrum of gastric bypass complications. Radiology 132:33–36, 1979.
7. Poulos A, Peat K, Lorman JG, Hatfield DR, Griffen WO: Gastric operation for the morbidly obese. Am J Roentgenol 136:867–870, 1981.
8. Bydder GM, Kreel L: Computed tomography in the diagnosis of abdominal abscess. CT 4:132–145, 1980.
9. Van Sonenberg E, Ferucci JT, Mueller PR, Wittenberg J, Simeone JF: Percutaneous drainage of abscesses and fluid collections: technique, results, and applications. Radiology 142:1–10, 1982.
10. Haaga JR, Weinstein AJ: CT-guided percutaneous aspiration and drainage of abscesses. Am J Roentgenol 135:1187–1194, 1980.
11. Shagrin JW, Frame B, Duncan H: Polyarthritis in obese patients with intestinal bypass. Ann Intern Med 75:377–380, 1971.
12. Sicard GA, Vaughan R, Wise L: Pneumatosis cystoides intestinalis: an unusual complication of jejunoileal bypass. Surgery 79:480–483, 1976.
13. Balthazar EJ, Goldfine S: Jejunoileal bypass—roentgenographic observations. Am J Roentgenol 125:138–142, 1975.
14. Peltier G, Hermreck AS, Moffat RE, Hardin CA, Jewell WR: Complications following gastric bypass procedures for morbid obesity. Surgery 86:648–655, 1979.
15. Wise L, Stein T: Biliary and urinary calculi: pathogenesis following small bowel bypass for obesity. Arch Surg 110:1043–1047, 1975.
16. Dickstein SS, Frame B: Urinary tract calculi after intestinal shunt operations for the treatment of obesity. Surg Gynecol Obstet 136:257–260, 1973.
17. Gregory JG, Starkloff EB, Miyai K, Schoenberg HW: Urologic complications of ileal bypass operation for morbid obesity. J Urol 113:521–524, 1975.
18. Vainder M, Kelly J: Renal tubular dysfunction secondary to jejunoileal bypass. JAMA 235:1257–1258, 1970.
19. Starkloff GB, Shively RA, Gregory JG: Jejunal intussusception following small bowel bypass for morbid obesity. Ann Surg 185:386–390, 1977.
20. Tanga MR, Waddell WG, Wellington JL: Jejunal intussusception: a complication of small bowel bypass for intractable obesity. Can J Surg 13:168–169, 1970.
21. Kaufman HJ, Weldon HW: Intussusception—a late complication of small bowel bypass for obesity. JAMA 202:1147–1148, 1967.
22. Andrassy RJ, Haff RC, Lbritz RW: Liver failure after jejunoileal shunt. Arch Surg 110:332–334, 1975.
23. Drenick EJ, Simmons F, Murphy JF: Effect on

hepatic morphology of treatment of obesity by fasting, reducing diets and small bowel bypass. N Engl J Med 282:829–834, 1970.

24. Brown RG, O'Leary JP, Woodward ER: Hepatic effects of jejunoileal bypass for morbid obesity. Am J Surg 127:53–58, 1974.

25. Fikri E, Cassella RR: Jejunoileal bypass for massive obesity: results and complications in 52 patients. Ann Surg 179:460–464, 1974.

26. Barry RE, Benfield JE, Bray GA: Colonic pseudo-obstruction: a new complication of jejunoileal bypass. Clin Res 23:391A, 1975.

27. Moss AA, Goldberg HI, Koehler RE: Radiographic evaluation of complications after jejunoileal bypass surgery. Am J Roentgenol 127:737–741, 1976.

28. Drenick EJ, Ament ME, Finegold SM, Corrodi P, Passaro E: Bypass enteropathy; intestinal and systemic manifestations following small bowel bypass. JAMA 236:269–272, 1976.

29. Wandtke J, Skukas J, Spataro R, Bruneau RJ: Pneumatosis intestinalis as a complication of jejunoileal bypass. Am J Roentgenol 129:601–604, 1977.

30. Ikard RW: Pneumatosis cystoides intestinalis following intestinal bypass. Am Surg 43:467–470, 1977.

31. Feinberg SB, Schwartz MZ, Clifford S, Buchwald H, Varco RL: Significance of pneumatosis cystoides intestinalis after jejunoileal bypass. Am J Surg 133:149–152, 1977.

32. Frick MP, Gedgaudas E: Radiology after intestinal bypass surgery for morbid obesity. In Tepplich JG, Haskin ME: Surgical Radiology. Philadelphia, Saunders, 1981, pp 637–646.

33. Quaade F, Juhl E, Feldt-Rasmussen K, Baden H: Blind-loop reflux in relation to weight loss in obese patients treated with jejunoileal anastomosis. Scand J Gastroenterol 6:537–541, 1971.

34. Harmon JW, Aliapoulos M, Braasch JW: The excluded small-bowel segment. Arch Surg 11:953–954, 1976.

35. Buchanan R, Wilkins R: Arthritis after jejunoileostomy. Arthritis Rheum 15:644–645, 1972.

CHAPTER 12

Body Contour Surgery Following Bypass Surgery

SHERIDAN S. STEVENS AND GEORGE L. PELTIER

Massive weight loss in excess of 40 k or 30% of body weight can result in significant distortion of body contour. Because the control of massive obesity by surgical alteration of the gastrointestinal tract has become accepted and successful, this distortion of body contour is being seen with increasing frequency. These patients change from their obese condition to a thinner, healthier state but they are left with sagging folds of skin and subcutaneous tissues, and displacement of normal anatomic landmarks. With maximum weight loss, the bodily contour deformities stabilize, but do not improve with time. These patients have undergone a major surgical procedure to lose weight and to improve their health and quality of life, but they are left with constant unpleasant reminders of their obese state. They are seldom able to redefine their body image in this new situation. Figure 12-1 illustrates the physical deformities of massive weight loss.

Body Image

Body image is the mental perception that an individual has of his or her body at a given moment in time. Extraneous influences such as clothing, personal opinion, fashion, peer acceptance, and events have a major effect on body image development, and influence body image perception. Planned or accidental changes in the size or shape of the physical body can exert a strong influence on mental–emotional stability. Patients who have sustained massive weight loss by whatever means often have a serious body image distortion and frequently seek the help of a plastic surgeon to improve this image.

While the psychological considerations are more completely discussed elsewhere in this volume, there are two rather disparate groups of patients that can be differentiated by age of onset of obesity. We agree with Goin and Goin that "Someone who is a fat child or adolescent will often have great difficulty in ridding himself of an internal self-portrait as a fat man now regardless of how much weight he has lost subsequently and how long he has been thin." [1] The patient who has been obese most of his life, after surgical control of his obesity, frequently chooses not to have any body contour surgery or only an abdominal panniculectomy.

In contrast, the patient who did not become obese until adulthood and then sustained weight loss through surgery will often seek correction of multiple areas of deformity. This type of patient will be more demanding and critical of the result. It does help in the care of these patients to recognize this difference early, and be prepared to deal with different types of problems. This second type of individual may have an unrealistic body image that may be difficult or impossible to achieve surgically. Without careful preoperative education the final result may fall short of his or her expectation, and the scars will be difficult to accept. The location and appearance of the scars throughout the healing process should be thoroughly discussed with all patients preoperatively to maximize patient satisfaction and avoid unpleasant confrontations. Even the most thorough preoperative discussion does not totally prepare all patients, and the surgeon must plan to spend whatever time is required to understand what the patient is trying to achieve and to try to adjust these expectations to the surgical realities.

This area of surgery is deeply involved in dealing with the patient's psyche and body image, and it is not always possible for the surgeon to understand what the patient is trying to accomplish. Patience, sympathy, and careful preoperative education are essential elements in the successful outcome of body contour surgery for these morbidly obese patients who have sustained a substantial weight loss, and who present to the plastic surgeon with their reduced body covered with ugly folds of hanging skin. Supportive postoperative care until healing is complete is also an essential element in achieving optimal results.

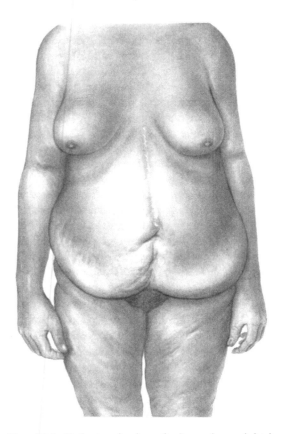

FIG. 12-1. Patients who have had massive weight loss are left with sagging folds of skin and subcutaneous tissue, and displacement of anatomic landmarks.

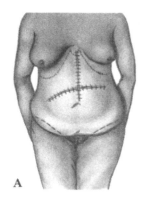 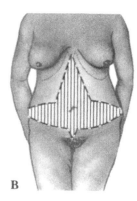

FIG. 12-2. **A** Postoperative incisions from gastric and intestinal bypass procedures. **B** Standard method of lipectomy with shaded area resected. **C** Belt lipectomy. **D** Procedures for midline skin and scar resection. **E** Method of Pitanguy[4] **F** Original method of Kelly.

Indications and Contraindications for Surgery

Indications for body contour surgery are relatively simple. The patient must be strongly self-motivated to have corrective surgery and must have achieved desired weight loss and have been stable at that weight for at least 1 year. The patient who stabilizes his weight at some point above ideal or goal weight can occasionally be benefited by a body contour operation that would improve body image and renew interest in further weight reduction. Generally, goal weight should be reached first. Body contour surgery should rarely, if ever, be combined with elective revision of the gastrointestinal bypass because of the increased risk of wound infection.

Contraindications to surgery are the usual contraindications to an elective operative procedure. Mild hypertension or adult onset diabetes under control are not contraindications to surgery. There are no particular age limitations, and generally these patients fall into the same category as that established for the gastric bypass operation, i.e., approximately 17 to 60 years of age.

Abdominoplasty Procedures

Abdominoplasty procedures were first performed late in the 19th century. Since Kelly's first report, a large number of modifications of the original

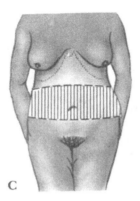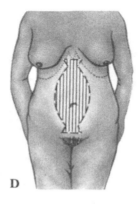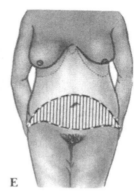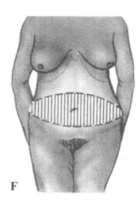

surgical principles have been described.[2] Historically various levels and patterns for transverse excisions, various patterns of midline vertical excisions, and combinations of both transverse and vertical excisions have been advocated. Figure 12-2 shows the various incisions that have been proposed. Limited undermining and short incisions have given way to a more extensive undermining with careful placement of lengthy incisions that can be hidden under clothes and swimwear. Application of the usual body contour techniques is generally not possible without some major modification.

Gastric bypass patients will usually have a midline vertical upper abdominal scar, and those with an intestinal bypass will have a transverse scar above the umbilicus which requires an abdominoplasty incision that will avoid vascular compromise and necrosis of the flaps. The major consideration should be that any scars from prior surgical procedures be removed so they do not compromise the blood supply in the skin flaps. The level of the transverse excision can be low "bikini line," mid-abdominal, as in a "belt lipectomy," or even upper abdominal if the safety of the skin flaps dictates this method (Fig. 12-3). Although midline is best for the vertical excision scar, this can be moved to either side to allow removal of a scar that may compromise skin flaps. The sagging and redundancy in these patients is more extensive than in patients who seek abdominal tightening for postpregnancy redundancy. When massive weight loss patients already have extensive surgical scars, as do the bypass patients, the addition of abdominoplasty scars is less significant than in the postpartum patient with no scars.

Placement of the incision and appearance of the scar are thoroughly discussed with the patient and occasionally adjustments in their location can be made to accommodate his desires.[3] These patients usually have more than one anatomic area

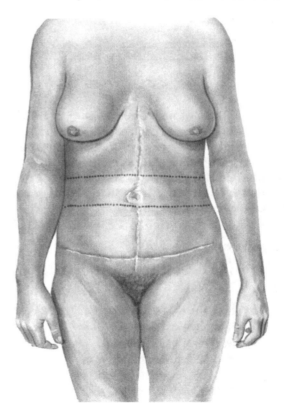

FIG. 12-3. The level of the surgical incision for abdominoplasty can be adjusted from bikini line, to mid-abdomen, or to the belt line. Vertical incisions may be moved right or left of the midline to remove previous surgical scars.

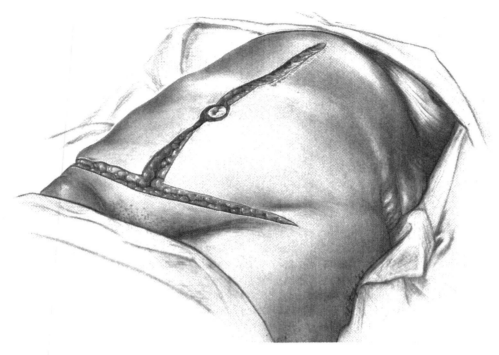

FIG. 12-4. The gastric bypass scar is removed. A circular incision is made around the umbilicus. Dissection is carried down to the external oblique fascia.

that would benefit from corrective surgery which necessitates, in selected patients, combined reduction involving one or more of the following anatomic areas: upper arms, breast, thighs, and/or buttocks. Careful planning is required to provide the most efficient use of operative time in these extensive combined operations.

Indications

Indications for abdominoplasty include the following:

1. Stretching and pain caused by the sheer weight of the panniculus
2. Aggravation of back pain
3. Intertrigo, ulceration, bleeding, and secondary infection in the underlying crease
4. Sexual dysfunction related to the size and weight of the panniculus or to related psychological inhibitions

Additional indications are the ugly appearance of many bypass scars which may be wide, depressed, and fixed to the underlying fascia; diasta-sis recti; abdominal wall laxity; or ventral hernias; all of which should be repaired with an abdominoplasty.

Technique of Abdominoplasty

The procedure found most satisfactory in our practice is a combination of vertical midline excision and bikini line transverse excision, unless old scars would compromise vascularity, in which case modification in level or type of incisions can be made.[4]

1. The patient is placed in a supine position over the central hinge of the operating table, and anesthetized with general endotracheal technique. Standard electrocautery equipment is employed. The genitalia and other involved skin areas are shaved immediately prior to surgery, and a urinary catheter is inserted. Preoperative skin preparation is completed with a suitable skin prep from the nipples to the symphysis pubis with continuation to the level of the operating table laterally.

2. A No. 1 silk suture is secured at the xiphoid process and extended to the pubic hair line where

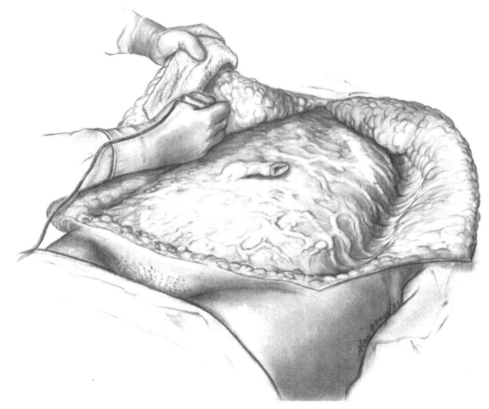

FIG. 12-5. Dissection is carried to the anterior axillary line and to the costal margins. A thick areolar layer is left on the external oblique fascia.

a mark is made. Using the suture and the marking pen, a curvilinear arch is extended laterally from the pubic hair line following the natural skin lines to the vertical projection of the iliac spines.

3. Lateral extensions of the incision may be modified according to current bathing suit fashion.

4. The midline incision is drawn from the xiphoid to the transverse marking incorporating the gastric bypass scar for removal. The midline incision is made from xiphoid to pubis and carried down to the fascia.

5. A small circular incision is made around the umbilicus and the umbilical stalk is preserved. The dissection is carried downward in a conical direction to the fascia, leaving slightly more tissue deep than superficial.[5] The incision is illustrated in Fig. 12-4.

6. The lower transverse skin line incision is also extended to the fascia. Bleeding is controlled by electrocautery, and cutting cautery is used for the majority of the subcutaneous dissection.

7. Undermining of the flaps is carried out to the level of the xiphoid from mid-axillary line to mid-axillary line and only to the anterior axillary line above the costal margin so as not to compromise blood supply. A thin areolar layer is left on the fascia to aid in flap adhesion and prevent seroma formation. Undermining is illustrated in Fig. 12-5.

8. An attempt should be made at this time to remove any subcostal scar that may be present from previous surgery. Tissue inferior to a subcostal scar can undergo necrosis which could seriously compromise the result. Also any nonabsorbable suture from previous surgery should be removed so that it will not be palpable under the skin flaps.

9. After the skin flaps have been maximally developed, interrupted figure-of-eight braided nonabsorbable sutures with the knots buried are used to plicate the rectus abdominus fascia from either side, eliminating diastasis recti and creating some tension across the anterior abdomen, resulting in

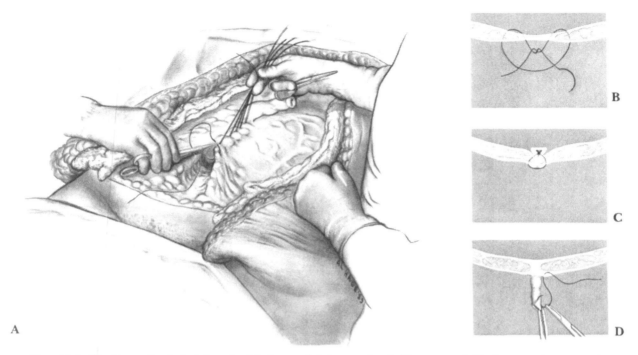

FIG. 12-6. The linea alba is imbricated with figure-of-eight nonabsorbable suture. **A** Each successive suture is placed at regular intervals progressing to the symphisis pubis. **B** and **C** The midline area of the abdomen is then imbricated with nonabsorbable suture. The sutures are tied down folding the tissue inward. **D** The umbilicus is secured to the midline fascia with absorbable suture.

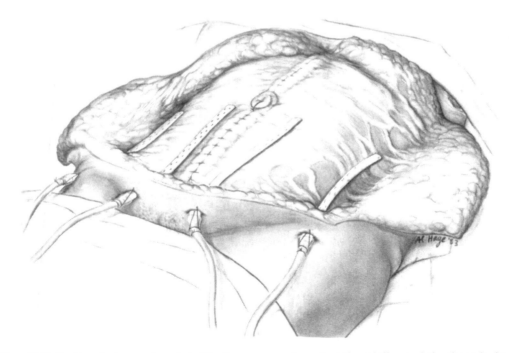

FIG. 12-7. Suction drains are inserted. The flaps are overlapped at the midline and the tissue is drawn inferiorly with the table flexed 30°. The tissue to be excised is marked and checked.

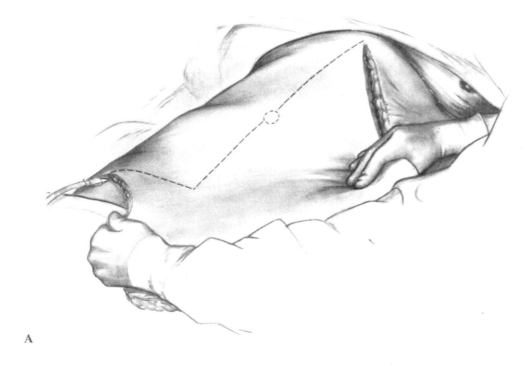

A

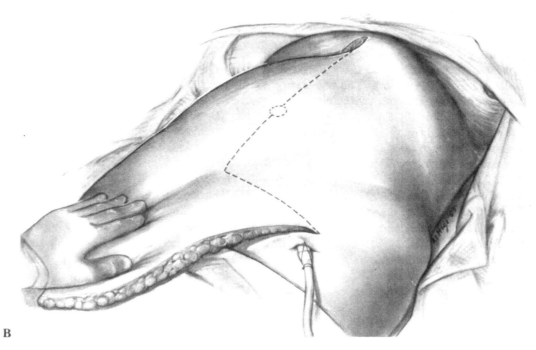

B

FIG. 12-8. **A** The flaps are overlapped at the midline and drawn inferiorly. **B** Tissue is excised along the dotted line. Similar excisions are done on both flaps.

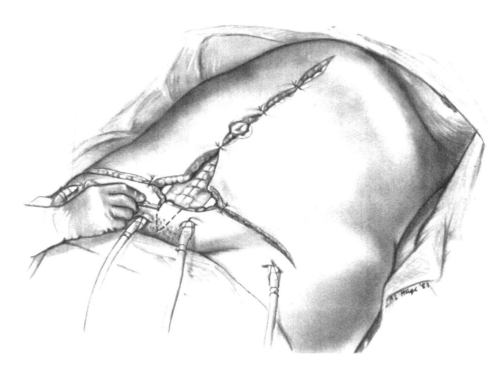

FIG. 12-9. A small triangle of skin is removed from the mons pubis. The wound is reapproximated loosely prior to fine closure.

additional abdominal support and greater definition of the patient's waist. Any umbilical hernia or midline hernias can be repaired at this point in the procedure. Each successive suture is placed at regular intervals progressing to the symphisis pubis as illustrated in Fig. 12-6A. The two steps in placement of the imbricate suture are illustrated in Fig. 12-6B and C. Initially the suture is placed to fold the linea alba inward and the suture is cinched down. The umbilicus is sutured to the new fascia midline with absorbable suture as illustrated in Fig. 12-6D.

10. In an extremely flaccid abdomen an occasional lateral plication of the external oblique fascia on either side can be made in a similar fashion to the midline imbrication.

11. Ten-millimeter suction drains are inserted laterally and medially as in Fig. 12-7.

12. Preparatory to resecting the excess skin flaps, the table is flexed acutely to 30°. The flaps are overlapped at the midline and drawn inferiorly over the pubic incision. Estimations of tissue removal are marked and checked to ensure that too much tissue is not removed, as in Fig. 12-8A.

13. A sharp blade is then used to remove the panniculus. A slight amount of tension is placed on the abdominal flap. The majority of the tension should be lateral to the mons pubis to prevent pulling of the pubic hair onto the abdominal wall, as in Fig. 12-8B. The wound is inspected for sources of bleeding.

14. The wound is closed with absorbable sutures in Scarpa's fascia and in the dermis.

15. The skin is closed with running subcuticular absorbable sutures. The skin is then secured with Steri-strips.

16. The umbilicus, attached in its usual location, is brought out through a short midline transverse incision.[6] This is then secured in place with absorbable sutures as in Fig. 12-9. This transverse incision should be no longer than 1.5 cm or the umbilicus will become too large postoperatively.

17. A mildly compressive dressing using absorbent pads and a Velcro abdominal binder is applied. Figure 12-10A and B shows a patient with a large panniculus prior to surgery. The patient's abdomen 6 months following surgery is illustrated in Fig. 12-10C and D.

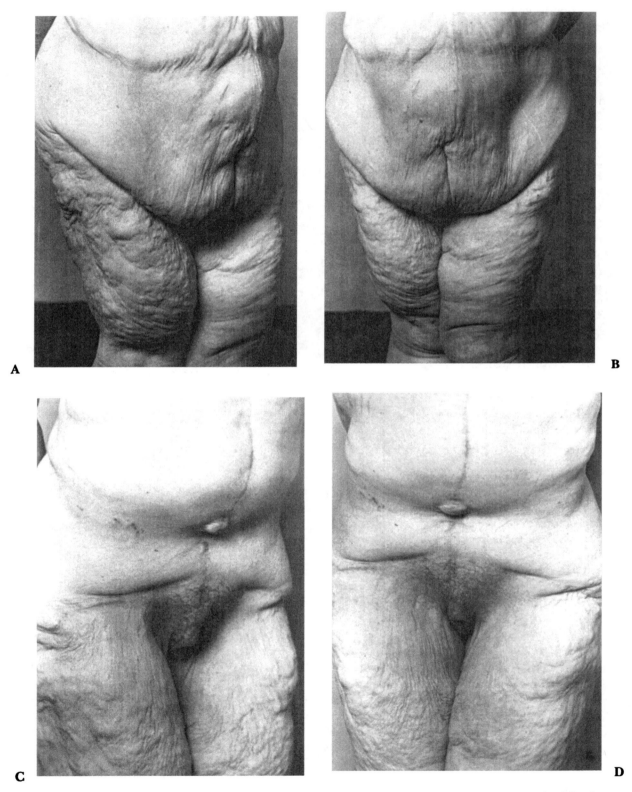

FIG. 12-10. **A** and **B** A patient just prior to abdominoplasty. **C** and **D** The same patient 6 months following abdominoplasty.

Postoperative Care

In the postoperative period the patient is managed with intravenous fluids and a course of perioperative antibiotics. Patients wear thigh-high TED hose when possible to the operating room and are encouraged to begin moving feet and legs as soon as they awaken. Ambulation is begun the next morning. Oral intake is begun as tolerated; pain medication is used as needed. The catheter and intravenous fluids are usually stopped when oral intake and ambulation are progressing satisfactorily. The drains are removed when each drains less than 30 ml per 24 h or 10 ml per 8-h period. Once the drains are removed the patient may remove the binder to shower and cleanse incisions. Steri-strips are replaced as necessary and maintained for 3 weeks. The binder or some sort of mild compression is advised for 6 weeks.

Complications

Complications include pulmonary insufficiency, atelectasis, or pneumonitis related at least in part to the tightness of the skin closure. Pulmonary complications usually cause an exacerbation of abdominal wound problems. Thrombophlebitis and pulmonary embolism have been reported and prevention is attempted with supportive stockings during and after surgery and early ambulation.

Occasionally, small areas of necrosis develop in the flap, but these can be managed with careful topical care. They are allowed to heal by contracture and scar epithelialization to be revised 1 year later if needed. A seroma in the potential space left beneath the flaps is the most common problem and is managed with frequent aspiration until it does not reform.

Later Management

Sports and heavy lifting are not recommended for the first 6 weeks. A gradual resumption of normal activities is recommended at this time. Patients may resume driving a car at 2 weeks. They may resume sexual activity when they feel sufficiently comfortable. Skin will be numb following surgery. This usually resolves within weeks, except in the area above the pubis where it may be permanent. Patients should be informed of this preoperatively.

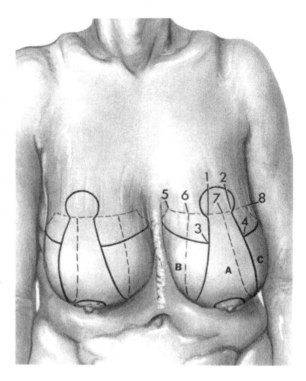

FIG. 12-11. Marking and planning for surgery is completed with the patient in the upright position. The keyhole pattern is applied at the point designated for new nipple position. The vertical pedicle (*A*) and the inframammary line (5–6–7–&8) are marked clearly. Areas for resection are delineated (*B* and *C*).

Breasts

Patients who have had massive weight loss with resulting breast deformity have several problems. These patients have intertrigo beneath the breasts, which becomes worse in warm weather. They have pain from stretching of the skin, and cervical, thoracic, and interscapular pain from the weight of the breasts. Previous spine disease may be aggravated by the weight of the breasts. Patients who still have large ptotic breasts with these symptoms following massive weight loss are candidates for reduction mammoplasty. Patients with ptosis, but with none of the above symptoms, may be candidates for a mastopexy, and those who have a loss of breast volume without ptosis may have augmentation mammoplasty to fill out their breast shape.

Reduction mammoplasty is performed using the McKissock technique employing a vertical dermal flap labeled as area *A* in Fig. 12-11.[7] The patient is admitted to the hospital prior to surgery

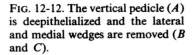

FIG. 12-12. The vertical pedicle (*A*) is deepithelialized and the lateral and medial wedges are removed (*B* and *C*).

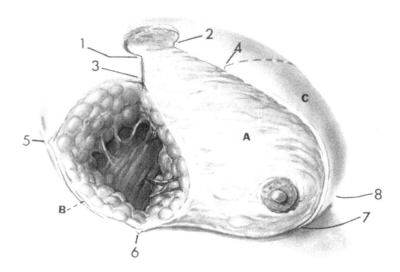

and routine laboratory work and radiography are completed. With the patient seated on the edge of the operating table the measurements and markings of the McKissock technique are drawn on the patient's breasts with a marking pen. In Fig. 12-11, numbers 5–8 are points on the inframammary fold. Points 3 and 4 are on the anterior breast and their location is aided by a commercially available wire frame. These points will eventually be on the new inframammary fold. The area marked *A* is the vertical dermal flap. The areas marked *B* and *C* will be resected. The new nipple location is marked at the level of the old inframammary fold in the midline of the breast using obstetric calipers. The distance from the new inframammary fold to the new nipple is marked at 5–6 cm, depending on the height of the patient. The new nipple is made 37 mm in diameter.

General endotracheal anesthesia is then established with the patient supine on the operating table. A urinary catheter is inserted. The chest is prepped and draped in a standard manner from lower neck to just above the umbilicus. Preparation is carried to the level of the table on both sides of the chest. The vertical dermal flap, area *A*, is deepithelialized as seen in Fig. 12-12. Large lateral and medial wedges of skin and breast labeled *B* and *C* are removed down to the pectoralis major muscle, as in Fig. 12-13. The deep portion

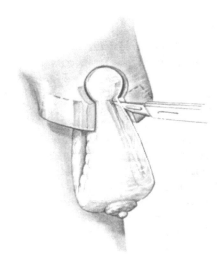

FIG. 12-13. The tissue under the keyhole is removed creating the vertical dermal flap and the flap is separated from the remaining breast tissue.

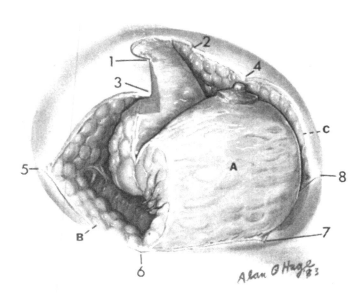

of the breast is then cored out to create the flap. The vertical dermal flap is then folded inward, bringing the nipple to its new location where it is secured with suture, as in Fig. 12-14. The lateral breast flaps are reapproximated in the midline and the nipple is secured in place using nonabsorbable suture as in Fig. 12-15. The skin closures are reinforced with Steri-strips. Suction drains are inserted laterally and remain for 2–3 days. The patient is discharged with a supportive bra to be worn at all times for 6 weeks. Patients are usually immediately relieved of the preoperative symptoms. Scars migrate from the inframammary line up onto the breast. The periareolar and vertical scars remain relatively unobtrusive as in Fig. 12-16. Complications are usually limited to the wound where there is occasional fat necrosis with short-term wound drainage.[8] Symmetry is usually not exact and ptosis may still progress following this procedure. Patients are cautioned to continue to support their breasts with a good quality brassiere. Figure 12-17A and B demonstrates a patient's breasts prior to reduction. Figure 12-17C and D demonstrates the same patient postoperatively.

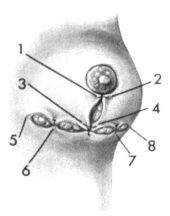

FIG. 12-15. The new breast flaps are placed in their new locations using buried suture. The areas between the points are closed with buried absorbable suture.

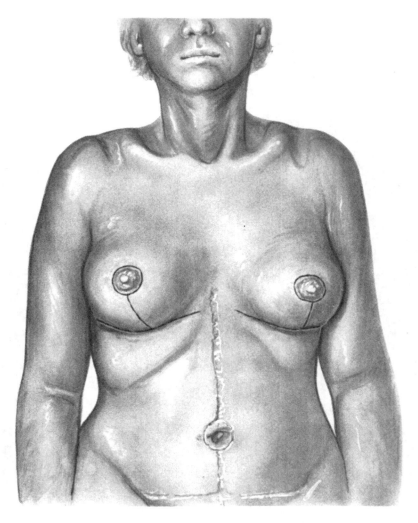

FIG. 12-16. Scars in the inframammary line may migrate up onto the breast. Periareolar scars remain narrow and largely unobtrusive.

Ptosis of the breasts without hypertrophy in the massive weight loss patient is usually severe. Preoperative and operative preparation is similar to that of the reduction mammoplasty.[9] Techniques for the nipple and inframammary fold location are identical to that used in the McKissock technique. The vertical dermal flap is deepithelialized and the lateral incisions are carried only into the subcutaneous layer. The nipple and skin flaps are then secured to their future position using absorbable suture. The redundant inferior, medial, and lateral wedges are then excised. The wound is closed with subcuticular absorbable suture and Steri-strips. The patient is not drained and the postoperative dressing is a supportive brassiere.[10]

The augmentation mammoplasty may be performed on those patients with distinct loss of breast volume without ptosis. There are many techniques for the augmentation mammoplasty and use of a saline- or silicone-filled prosthesis is standard. Most of these patients can be managed in an outpatient surgical facility. Frequently, this procedure is combined with another body contouring operation. Methods and techniques of augmentation mammoplasty will not be discussed in this book.

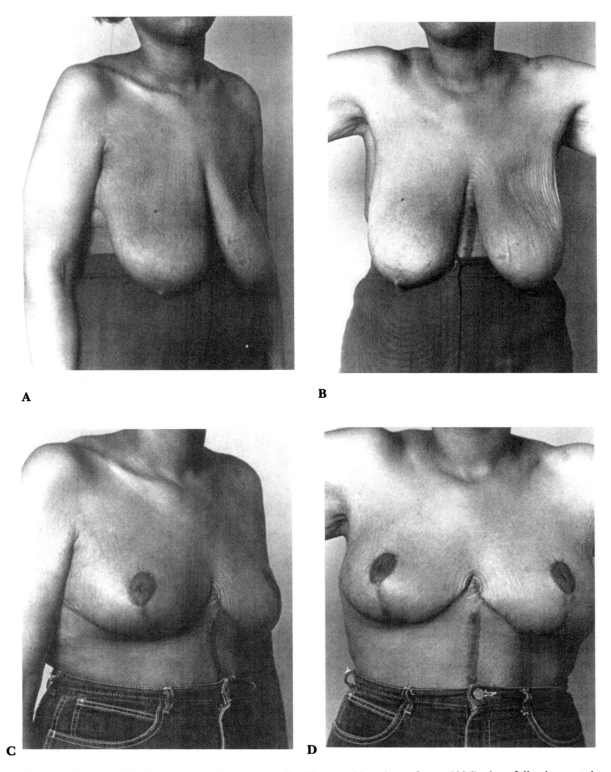

FIG. 12-17. **A** and **B** Preoperative photographs of a 20-year-old patient after a 100-lb. loss following gastric bypass. **C** and **D** Photographs following reduction of the breast and skin envelope. Six hundred forty grams of tissue was removed from the left breast and 680 g was removed from the right breast.

Thigh and Buttock Plasty

Patients with massive weight loss may develop rather marked folds and sagging of buttocks and thigh skin. Symptoms from the folds and sagging are intertrigo, discomfort from elastic or tight-fitting clothing, and difficulty finding suitable swimwear, sportswear, and underwear. Correction of thigh and buttocks is usually simultaneous.[11]

Incisions

Placement of incision lines with these procedures is crucial because the scars on buttocks and thighs descend quite markedly with healing. A scar originally placed low on the buttocks will be drawn down onto the upper posterior thigh. The thigh resection is usually limited to an upper medial excision, leaving the scar in the crural fold. Resection down onto the thigh may be necessary and this occasionally will extend to the knee. In these patients an attempt is made to place the scar in the midline of the medial aspect of the thigh. Undermining in these procedures is much more lim-

ited than in the abdominoplasty because the potential for disastrous wound sloughs is quite great. Excessively tense closure can result in wide, depressed scars.

As shown in Figs. 12-18 and 12-19, the patient is marked in a standing position and the estimates of the amount of tissue to be removed must be definitively marked. Any tendency to remove more tissue than was defined with the patient standing must be vigorously resisted, because it will lead to an excessive skin resection. The upper limb of the buttock wedge excision should be well up on the prominence of the buttock, so that the scar will not descend into the posterior thigh with healing (Fig. 12-20). The medial thigh upper limb incision is at the upper edge of the crural fold. No undermining is done on the superior aspect of the buttock or thigh incision in an effort to prevent downward migration of the scars. During the procedure, it is necessary to change the patient's position. An estimation is made during the planning stage whether any dog-ear that remains with the closure should be removed from the anterolateral or posterolateral end of the excision. If the best

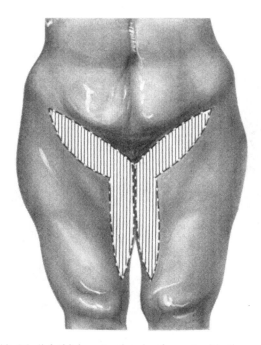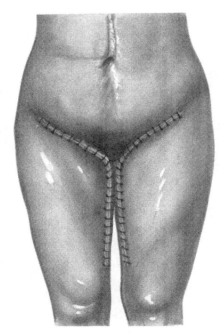

FIG. 12-18. Medial thigh reduction is planned with the patient standing. Medial thigh extension is frequently necessary to reduce the thigh skin envelope. Extreme tension and undermining are avoided to prevent skin slough.

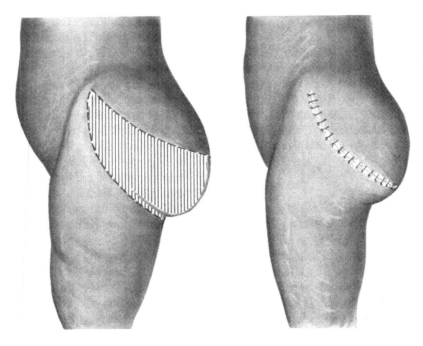

FIG. 12-19. No undermining is done superiorly in the buttock incision to avoid excessive scar migration downward. The patient must be repositioned during surgery to facilitate exposure.

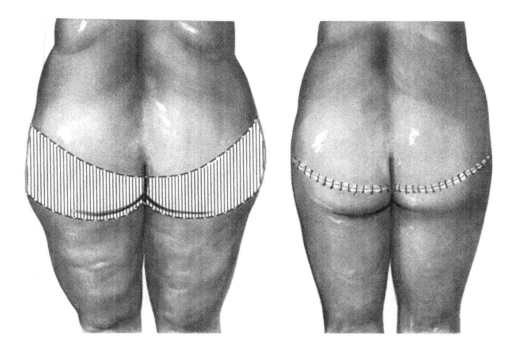

FIG. 12-20. Scars resulting from buttock lipectomy tend to migrate toward the leg after several months. Therefore the incisions are placed high on the buttock.

contour would be obtained by removing the dog-ear anteriorly and laterally, the patient is anesthetized in a supine position and then turned prone onto the operating table. The posterior excision and closure on the medial aspect of the thighs is carried out as far forward as technically possible, and the patient is repositioned to a supine position on the operating table to carry out the anterior excision and closure. If the dog-ear must be removed posteriorly and laterally, the anterior and medial excisions are closed first. Of course, one must have adequate help and be extremely careful in turning an anesthetized patient. This procedure is very demanding and should *not* be combined with any other body contour surgery.

Both procedures are commonly wedge excisions to the underlying muscle fascia. Limited undermining inferiorly is carried out to allow advancement and closure in layers with absorbable suture. Drains are usually not used. Pressure dressings are applied. If medial thigh excisions are necessary to provide satisfactory contour improvement, the excision is a vertical wedge excision with the apex of the wedge toward the knee. Limited undermining anteriorly and posteriorly is used to facilitate closure, again with absorbable suture, and no drains are used. Drawings of the planned excisions and closures are shown in Fig. 12-19 and 12-20.

Postoperative Care

The postoperative recovery from this procedure is the most difficult of the body contour procedures because of the location of the scars in the area of weight bearing when sitting. The patient is usually unable to sit for 2–3 weeks following the procedure. Routine voiding must now be performed in a standing position, which can be difficult and untidy for the patient. For this reason, hospitalization is commonly 10–14 days. A Foley catheter is left in place until the patient can comfortably move from lying flat to a standing position without hip flexion. No hip flexion is recommended for 2 weeks; then patients may slowly start to flex hips in an attempt to resume sitting. Sitting becomes comfortable 6–8 weeks following surgery. Because of the tendency of thigh and buttock scars to widen and become prominent, Steri-strip support is continued for 6–8 weeks. Showering can begin when the patient is able to get in and out of bed easily. Perioperative antibiotics are used. Blood loss should be carefully monitored and appropriate blood replacement should be ready for use. Hip flexion or wide thigh abduction may be uncomfortable for 2–3 months, but resolves as the skin tension relaxes. Full return to normal activity is not recommended for 6–8 weeks. Preoperative and postoperative views are seen in Fig. 12-21.

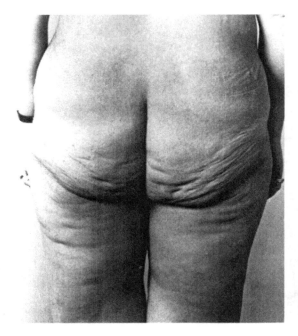
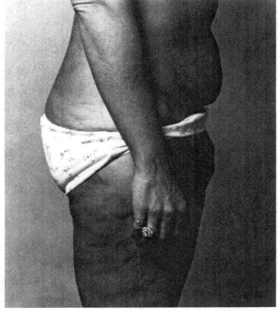

A   **B**

FIG. 12-21. A–C Preoperative views of 32-year-old patient who lost 140 lb. (*Continued*)

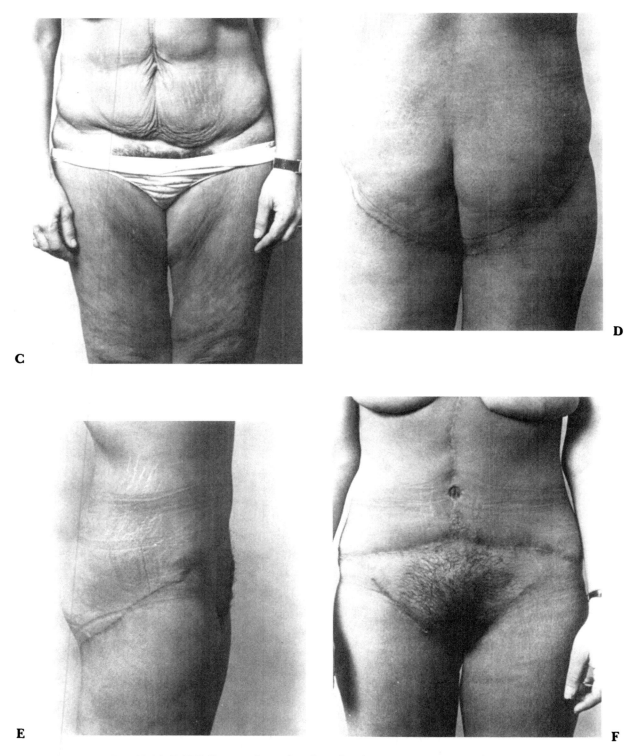

C

D

E

F

FIG. 12-21. D–F Follow-up views after abdominoplasty, thigh, and buttock plasty.

Arm Plasty

Some flaccidity and redundancy of the skin of the arms is common in these patients, and causes discomfort with tight clothing and an inability to wear short-sleeved clothing. There is no way to correct this deformity without leaving a scar that may be visible. The scar should follow the groove of the medial posterior border of the biceps muscle to just above the medial epicondyle of the humerus, and then curve posteriorly onto the poste-rior aspect of the elbow if necessary to remove a dog-ear. This procedure is commonly combined with breast reduction, breast repositioning, or breast enlargement, and excision of lateral upper chest wall flaccidity. For these combined procedures, the scar line then crosses the axilla and extends down the lateral chest wall between the posterior axillary fold and the mid-axillary line to the level of the inframammary fold, where it joins the scar of the incisions of the breast procedures. A straight line scar in the axilla would result

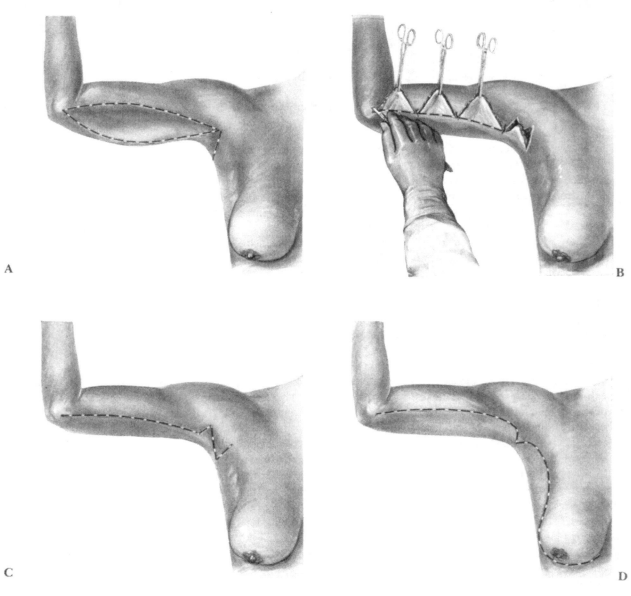

A

B

C

D

FIG. 12-22. **A** Planning incisions for the resection of upper arm skin. **B** Method for skin excision with a Z-plasty in the axilla to prevent linear contracture. **C** Resection of skin with Z-plasty marking in the axilla. **D** Plan for resection of skin if breast reduction is done simultaneously.

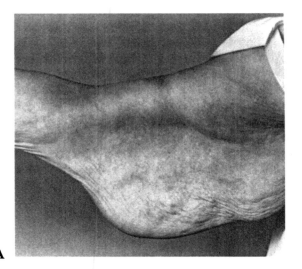
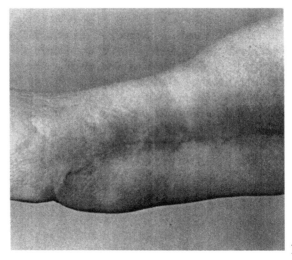

A   B

FIG. 12-23. A Patient shown in Fig. 12-21 prior to arm skin resection. B Patient following surgery.

in a scar contracture across the axilla, so this should be broken up either with a Z-plasty or a marked posterior V-curve in the incision line. Incision designs are shown in Fig. 12-22.

This surgery is done, as are the others, under general anesthesia, and is commonly combined with an abdominoplasty if both are to be done, or with breast-modifying procedures. The extent of undermining in this procedure is somewhat more extensive than with the thigh and buttocks. Undermining is carried out anteriorly for 1–2 cn. Posteriorly the incision is deepened directly to the fascia of the muscle with undermining at the level of the fascia. The undermining is carried out posteriorly as far as is necessary to provide a satisfactory contour restoration. Some skin numbness is to be expected around and distal to the incisions. The posterior skin and subcutaneous tissue is advanced over the anterior edge of the incision, and the posterior flap is incised to the level of the anterior edge of the incision at three or four levels and basting sutures are applied. The redundancy is then excised. If the lateral chest wall is to be done it is performed in a similar manner. Closure is accomplished with absorbable suture to the subcutaneous layer and absorbable subcuticular closure is reinforced with Steri-strips. No drains are used, but pressure dressings are gently applied with Ace wraps. Pre- and postoperative views are shown in Fig. 12-23.

Perioperative antibiotics are routinely used for 2–5 days. Patients should not use the arms for anything strenuous or in a rapid manner for 4 weeks. The arm plasty alone is usually done on an outpatient basis. Patients may shower over Steri-stripped incisions at 48 h and should wear elastic support for 4 weeks.

Wound healing is generally uncomplicated in the absence of excessive tension which can produce wound disruption or widened scars. Patients are allowed to return to normal activity at 4 weeks. Steri-strip support of the wound is continued for 4 weeks.

Summary

Massive weight loss in excess of 40 kg can result in significant distortion of body contour. These patients seek surgical correction of their deformities in an effort to relieve their physiologic and psychological symptoms.

Abdominoplasty is employed to remove a large redundant panniculus, extensive abdominal scarring, and to correct hernias and diastasis recti. This procedure leaves a low transverse incision and a vertical midline incision. Sagging of the buttocks and thighs is corrected by excising redundant tissue while carefully designing the incisions so they will remain in inconspicuous locations. Batwing deformity of the arms is corrected frequently in conjunction with mammoplasty by excising redundant tissue and skin. The surgical incisions are designed to remain on the medial arm. Reduction mammoplasty, augmentation mammoplasty, and mammary repositioning are used to correct the various types of breast deformity, which result from massive weight loss. Massive weight loss patients are able to tolerate corrections of their physical form and the resulting scars with minimal complications.

References

1. Goin JM, Goin MK: Changing the Body—Psychological Effects of Plastic Surgery. Philadelphia, Williams & Wilkins, 1981, p 66.
2. Kelly HA: Report of gynecologic cases (excessive growth of fat). Bull Johns Hopkins Hosp 10:197, 1889.
3. Grazier FM, Klingbeil JR: Body Image, A Surgical Perspective, St. Louis, Mosby, 1980.
4. Pitanguy I: Dermolipectomy of the abdominal wall, thigh, buttocks, and upper extremity. In Converse J (ed): Reconstructive Plastic Surgery. Philadelphia, Saunders, 1977, pp 3800–3823.
5. Gonzalez-Ulloa M: Abdominal wall disfigurement. Ann Plastic Surg 4:357, 1980.
6. Dubou R, Oesterhart DK: Placement of the umbilicus in an abdominoplasty. Plastic Reconstruct Surg 61:291–293, 1978.
7. McKissock PK: Reduction mammoplasty with a vertical dermal flap. Plastic Reconstruct Surg 49:245, 1972.
8. Shons AR: Plastic reconstruction after bypass surgery and massive weight loss. Surg Clin North Am 59:1139–1152, 1979.
9. Goulian D: Dermal mastopexy. Plastic Reconstruct Surg 47:105–110, 1971.
10. Owsley JQ, Peterson RA: Symposium of Aesthetic Surgery of the Breast. St. Louis, Mosby, 1978, pp 3–108.
11. Lewis JR: Aesthetic surgery of the trunk and extremities. Clin Plastic Surg 2:457–503, 1975.

Conclusion

JOHN H. LINNER

Surgery for morbid obesity is more than a particular operation or a refinement of technique. It is a comprehensive approach to patient management from preoperative education to continuing care through the postoperative period, and ideally, for the patient's lifetime. Without this type of commitment, results will not be optimal, and the incidence of failure excessive.

The choice of operation cannot be categorically recommended as of this writing, and may perhaps not be clearly established for many years. As is true for the surgical management of intractable duodenal ulcer, several different procedures may prove satisfactory, and no one operation clearly superior.

In our hands the Roux-en-Y gastric bypass has been so definitely superior to the horizontal gastroplasty that we currently prefer it over all other operations for obesity. It is a somewhat more demanding operation technically than gastroplasty, but for reasons outlined in the text it is more effective. If after a 3- to 5-year follow-up the vertical banded gastroplasty or some variant appears to be as effective and safer, we would adopt its use. It is imperative that surgeons undertaking bariatric surgery keep up with the current literature, but do not embrace new or novel techniques until there has been a suitable follow-up period. It may be that the ultimate role of the Roux-en-Y gastric bypass operation will be as a staged procedure in the management of the most recalcitrant obese patients, or in those situations where one of the simpler gastroplasty or banding type procedures have failed.

Although we do not necessarily believe that bariatric surgery need be limited to large centers, it is vital that facilities and personnel be available for good pulmonary function studies, superior anesthetic management, and safe postoperative mechanical ventilatory assistance. Adequate lighting, effective retracting devices, and suitable instrumentation are also essential for the safe conduct of surgery on these huge patients. Unless these minimum requirements can be met bariatric surgery should not be undertaken in any setting.

The other necessary ingredient for success is a serious and continuing interest in the field of bariatric surgery on the part of the surgeon and other involved personnel. It does not have to be to the exclusion of all other types of general surgery, but it cannot be a casual commitment. When the surgical management of obesity is properly executed, the satisfaction of being instrumental in providing a whole new dimension of living to this compromised segment of the population is extremely great.

It is to the advancement of this end that this book was written.

Patient Questionnaire

Date _____

Social Security No. _____ Name _____

Birthdate _____ Address _____

City, State, Zip Code _____

Phone No. _____ Sex _____ Height (Inches) _____

Marital Status (S) (M) (D) (W) _____

Were you heavy as a child? _____

Do you snack between meals? _____

Do you eat large meals? _____

Do you eat a lot of sweets? _____

Do you smoke? _____ How many pks/day? _____

Do you drink alcohol? _____ Number of drinks or beers/week _____

_____

Are you chemically dependent? _____

Have you ever had psychiatric care? _____

Your usual occupation _____

Currently employed? _____

Do you have any of the following conditions listed below? If Yes, please check where appropriate.

(1) Diabetes _____   (7) Ulcer _____

(2) High blood pressure _____   (8) Kidney disease _____

(3) Heart disease _____   (9) Arthritis _____

(4) Lung problems _____   (10) Gout _____

(5) Liver disease _____   (11) Neurologic problem _____

(6) Gallbladder disease _____

Please list any previous surgery _____

_____

Any allergies? _____

Which weight reduction organizations have you joined? _____

_____

What symptoms have you had that you believe are due to obesity? _____

_____

_____

Name of physician who sent you: _____

Pamphlet of Preoperative Information

JOHN H. LINNER AND RAYMOND L. DREW

This brochure was designed to help answer some of the many questions you may have about an operation for your obesity. Obviously you are concerned about being overweight and have probably tried many different methods to lose weight, all of them unsuccessful on a long-term basis.

To be eligible for an operation to help correct your obesity, you must be 100 lb. over or double your ideal weight as determined by the Metropolitan Life Insurance Company weight tables. Our currently accepted criteria for surgery for obesity are as follows:

1. Two times the ideal weight or more than 100 lb. over ideal weight as mentioned above
2. Failure of conventional weight reduction methods
3. Patient's willingness to cooperate with follow-up program
4. Absence of severe psychoemotional or medical problems that would make surgery unsuccessful
5. Absence of "glandular" causes of obesity (very rare)
6. Patient should not be drug or alcohol dependent unless well into a good treatment program with 1 year of sobriety
7. Smoking must be discontinued 3 weeks prior to surgery
8. The patient must understand that the surgical operation is only a part of the total treatment program for his or her obesity

In making a decision regarding surgical treatment for obesity, you must weigh the risks of the operation against the risk of being massively obese. Surgery should be considered as a last resort after conservative methods have been given a good honest try.

The Danger of Being Massively Obese

There is considerable evidence that massive obesity definitely shortens life and is associated with many other diseases. Some of these are as follows:

1. Diabetes mellitus
2. Hypertension (high blood pressure)
3. Coronary heart disease
4. Stroke
5. Congestive heart failure
6. Restrictive lung disease
7. Pickwickian syndrome (falling asleep while sitting up)
8. Degenerative arthritis of the lower extremity joints and spine
9. Gallbladder disease
10. Infertility
11. Possible increase of cancer of the breast and uterus
12. Varicose veins and stasis ulcer
13. Psychosocial incapacity (group acceptance, getting a job, and so on)

Morbid obesity is not only a medical disease, but is also a serious economic, social, and psychologic disability. No one is more aware of this than you are, the obese person.

The Risks of Surgery

In making a decision regarding surgery you must also be aware of the possible risks of surgery, even though with a team approach mortality and serious complications have been uncommon. The team is made up of our office staff, the hospital personnel including anesthesiologists and their nurses, operating room nurses and other personnel, intensive care nurses, respiratory care specialists, dieticians, and floor nurses with experience in the pre- and postoperative care of obese patients.

The immediate risks of the operation are quite similar to those of any major operation, most of which are listed below. The list is not complete because it is impossible to include every possible event that could happen in every surgical setting and still keep the size of the brochure within reason. You will be discussing all of these complications and expected results from surgery with the surgeon and usually some other member of the team, and will have an opportunity to ask additional questions. We want you to understand as thoroughly as possible what to expect from the surgery and the potential risks so you can make a better judgment with respect to whether you want to have the surgery and also to help you obtain a good result.

Early Complications

1. *Thrombophlebitis or blood clots in the legs with pulmonary embolism.* With the use of prophylactic heparin anticoagulation therapy, early walking, and elastic leg support stockings, this complication has become very rare.

2. *Atelectasis (lung collapse) and/or pneumonia.* These are fairly common complications and can be largely prevented by discontinuance of cigarettes 3 weeks preoperatively, breathing exercises, and coughing postoperatively. The patient receives breathing exercises every 2 hours for the first 24 hours after surgery to help prevent lung complications.

3. *Wound infection and wound separation.* Fortunately this is also rare and has occurred in less than 1% of our series.

4. *Peritonitis following leakage from the stomach pouch or adjacent intestine.* This is an unusual complication and has occurred in less than 2% of our patients. It is a serious complication and usually requires a secondary operation to correct it and to drain the resulting abscess.

5. *Obstruction of the new stomach pouch outlet.* This also is unusual and normally gets better with time. It has been necessary in a few instances to dilate a tight opening with a gastroscope, or if this proves unsuccessful to reoperate and enlarge the opening. All the channels or anastomoses from the small pouch into the lower stomach or adjacent intestine are made around a standard-sized dilator with a purse-string suture or a Silastic tube around the outside to prevent later enlargement and failure to lose weight. In the first week or two some patients develop edema or swelling of this anastomosis, making it difficult or impossible for them to take anything more than a clear or full liquid diet. It might be necessary to prepare foods in a blender for a period of several weeks to several months before the outlet opens to its full capacity. Very rarely a patient requires hospital admission for intravenous feeding. Only when all these methods fail would additional surgery be required. This has been necessary in less than 2% of our patients.

6. *Enlargement of the pouch and/or enlargement of the channel.* The small pouch which holds between 12 and 15 cc of fluid will gradually stretch over a period of time, increasing its capacity and preventing you from losing weight indefinitely. In our early experience some of the pouches were too large and a revision to a smaller pouch was necessary. Because our current gastric pouches and outlets have been made much smaller this type of failure is now rarely seen. It should be noted, however, that any of these operations can be defeated if you consume caloric liquids such as soda, beer, milk (except skim milk), ice cream, soft puddings, and snack foods. These will go through any pouch regardless of its size and will result in a poor weight loss.

7. *Staple line disruption or breakdown.* This has become quite rare since we have been reinforcing the staple line with interrupted stitches.

8. *Small bowel obstruction from adhesions.* This is unusual and if it does happen may require an operation for correction.

9. *Spleen injury and possible splenectomy.* Splenectomy (removal of the spleen) has been necessary in less than 1% of our patients and these did not experience any ill effects. Some patients develop an increased vulnerability to infection such as pneumonia following splenectomy, and certain precautions must be taken in these cases.

10. *Death.* Any operation carries with it the

possibility of a postoperative death. In our experience with over 500 gastric stapling operations our mortality rate is less than 1%. The average mortality nationwide for this operation is between 2 and 3%.

11. *Skin sag.* In many very obese people, especially over the age of 40, the skin of the abdomen, and sometimes the breasts, underarms, legs, and buttocks, can sag quite a bit after they have lost a considerable amount of weight. Although much of this improves with time, in a few instances the patient feels better having this excess skin removed. Although we as general surgeons can correct the sagging abdominal skin, we usually refer the patient to a plastic surgeon for this and all other aspects of body contour surgery.

12. *Psychosocial adjustments.* Losing weight usually is beneficial from the point of view of emotional and social adjustments, but occasionally some people require additional counseling to adjust to their new body image. Arrangements can be made for this kind of help through our office.

Long-term Effects of Surgery

Our follow-up after gastric bypass surgery has been up to 7 years, and we have found that loss of weight has improved the quality of life considerably for most patients.

Long-term Complications

1. *Polyneuritis.* This can happen from vitamin B_1 deficiency but shouldn't if you take vitamins and eat a balanced diet (one multivitamin pill daily).
2. *Anemia.* Iron deficiency anemia or anemia due to B_{12} and/or folic acid deficiency can be detected by having your blood checked on an annual basis. Anemia due to a bleeding ulcer can occur, but is rare (less than 1%) and diagnosed by x ray or gastroscopy.
3. *Stomal ulcer.* Incidence is less than 1%.
4. *Staple line disruption.* This was discussed earlier, but can occur as a late complication as well.

Tolerance to the small pouch and outlet usually occurs after a few years, and you will regain weight if you don't get exercise and avoid overeating.

Don't try to push in the maximum amount of food, because this tends to stretch the pouch.

How Much Weight Will I Lose?

It is impossible to predict how much you will lose following your operation. The average weight loss after 1 year in our group of patients has been approximately 30% of their preoperative weight, which for a 300-lb. person would be 100 lb. Additional loss is experienced at a slower rate the second year, and usually there are no losses after the second year unless you work at it with exercise and some dieting. Most people reach within 20 to 30 lb. of their *ideal weight.* We have advised patients to select a *goal weight* which is between 10 and 40 lb. over their ideal weight as the end point for their weight loss. This is more realistic and just as healthy as trying to reach an ideal weight. The operation will do 75% of the job for you, but 25% is your responsibility which includes restricting caloric fluids and snacking. If you are a heavy soda or beer drinker you must prove to yourself you can control this habit before surgery, because if you cannot stop drinking soda or beer you will not achieve a good result. You would then be wise not to have the operation at all. Compulsive eaters who cannot control snacking on high sugar foods, caloric liquids, or junk-type foods should become actively involved through a counselor or a support group, or join O.A. (Overeaters Anonymous) for additional help.

When you feel strong enough, usually in about 6 to 8 weeks, you must start on a graduated exercise program such as walking, swimming, or bicycling to get your body in good condition. Sustained physical exertion of any type will help you lose additional weight and give you a feeling of well being. Remember, you must increase your exercise tolerance slowly, but make it a way of life.

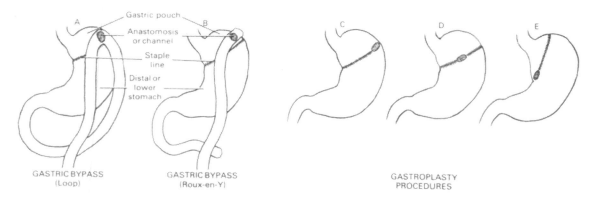

CHOICE OF OPERATION

GASTRIC BYPASS
(Loop)

GASTRIC BYPASS
(Roux-en-Y)

GASTROPLASTY
PROCEDURES

Choice of Operation

Above are diagrams of the more commonly used gastric stapling operations, and the decision as to which to use depends on your particular type of eating habits, your initial weight, and other factors that would have to be discussed separately. It should be noted that with the Roux-en-Y gastric bypass, an ordinary upper GI x ray would not reveal the bypassed stomach. The bypassed stomach can be viewed postoperatively with the gastroplasty procedure. Average weight losses have been better with the *gastric bypass* than the *gastroplasty* in our experience.

Intestinal Bypass

We no longer perform the jejunoileal bypass (intestinal bypass) and have converted approximately 35% of these operations to the gastric bypass. Careful follow-up is essential.

Some Tips on Postoperative Diet and Eating Habits

It is important to eat three meals a day and to take only small amounts of fluids with the meals. Most of your fluids should be consumed between meals and these should be low-calorie fluids, such as water, skim milk, coffee, tea, and not over one bottle of diet soda daily. Alcohol should be avoided until your goal weight has been reached and then taken in modest, well-diluted quantities. Food should be cut small, chewed well, and if necessary,

prepared in a blender. You should stop eating as soon as you feel full. The primary foods to avoid are apple skins, orange pulp, raw coconut, grape peelings, and raw carrots as these can plug up the small opening.

During the first 6 months raw fruits and vegetables should be eaten especially carefully. The diet should consist mostly of *protein* foods and to a lesser extent carbohydrate and fat. Good sources of protein are fish, cottage cheese, eggs, peanut butter, and of course the various meats. Some meats are tolerated better than others and you simply have to find out which ones work best for you.

In addition to the low-calorie but balanced diet, it is important to take one multivitamin tablet with minerals (or liquid vitamin) on a daily basis. Occasionally some patients require additional iron and/ or vitamin B_{12} or folic acid. These deficiencies usually do not occur until after the first or second year.

Activity and Exercise

Gradually increase activity as you get stronger. Walking is a good form of exercise and you should eventually try to walk at least 2 to 3 miles a day. In the winter, shopping centers and skyways are good places to walk. Most people can drive their car within 3 weeks. Don't sit too long (over one-half hour) with your legs cramped; you could get blood clots. Light housework and lifting up to 35 lb. is permissible during the first 6 weeks after surgery. After 6 weeks, the wound should be well healed, and you can start a graduated program of sports, exercise, physical work, and sex as tolerated. Every person has a different exercise tolerance.

The length of absence from work varies, depending on occupation and rate of recovery. This has to be determined on an individual basis.

Follow-up

It is important to be examined in our office every 3 months the first year, and then at 6-month intervals the second year, and once a year thereafter. If you should move out of town or are unable to come into our office for some reason, we would appreciate hearing from you at least on an annual basis to keep track of your progress and help you if there are any problems. After the first year your hemoglobin should be checked at least annually. If you are anemic, additional blood studies to determine whether you are deficient either in iron, vitamin B_{12}, or folic acid should be done.

You will not have as many bowel movements as you did before surgery because you will be eating much less food. You may wish to use a stool softener or bulk-producing laxative such as Colace, Dialose Plus, or Metamucil.

You undoubtedly have many additional questions which cannot be covered completely in this outline. Remember the dietician will go over your diet and mode of eating with you postoperatively, and we will discuss this with you at some length at your initial visit. We do want to see you 3 weeks after discharge from the hospital and then at 3-month intervals the first year, and 6-month intervals the second year. We keep very careful records on all patients we have operated upon and feel we have a lifetime commitment to our patients who undergo this kind of surgery.

Be sure to check with our office secretaries regarding your insurance coverage and whether a letter will be necessary to your insurance company to document the medical necessity for your gastric stapling operation.

It is necessary to make an appointment to have your photograph taken before surgery. This will be done in our office, at no cost to you. Follow-up photographs when you have lost your maximum weight are also required. We would like your permission to show these occasionally to medical groups. Please sign a slip to okay this.

Ask our secretaries for the names and phone numbers of patients who have had the operation so you can talk to them about their experience.

You will need a complete medical evaluation prior to surgery which could either be done by your own doctor or a physician we would recommend. We have a list of the preoperative work-up procedures to give your doctor.

Some patients will require a psychiatric evaluation and an MMPI (Minnesota Multiphasic Personality Inventory), and a letter of approval for surgery from the psychiatrist.

Please ask any questions you have which were not covered in the brochure. Discuss it with your family so that you will have their support and understanding, and they can help you with your objectives. We want you to have an excellent result from your surgery, and achieve your goal of better health and quality of life through significant weight reduction.

Bypass Follow-up

1. Weight _____

2. Weight loss. _____

3. How are you doing? _____

_____

4. Any specific problems? _____

_____

5. How do you rate your surgery? Check one of each group listed below.

ACCEPTANCE: ☐ 1. "Poor" (not very pleased; kindly state reasons)

                          ☐ 2. "Fair"

                          ☐ 3. "Good"

                          ☐ 4. "Excellent"

SATIETY: ☐ 1. 0–2 hours

                          ☐ 2. 2–3 hours

                          ☐ 3. 3–4 hours

                          ☐ 4. 4+ hours

DUMPING: ☐ 1. 0—none

                          ☐ 2. Mild—up to 1 oz. milk, some sweets.

                          ☐ 3. Moderate—all sweets.

                          ☐ 4. Severe—all foods.

DYSPHAGIA: ☐ 1. None—can eat anything.

(Food Sticks)   ☐ 2. Mild—all but two meats and/or bread.

                          ☐ 3. Moderate—only ground or soft foods.

                          ☐ 4. Severe—only liquids.

DIARRHEA: ☐ 1. 0–2 BMs/day.

                          ☐ 2. 3–4 BMs/day.

                          ☐ 3. 5–7 BMs/day.

                          ☐ 4. 8+ BMs/day.

Dietary Instructions for Post–Gastric Bypass Surgery*

Gastric bypass surgery was developed as a means to lose weight. However, there are some behavior patterns which must be modified simultaneously to achieve desired weight loss and to maintain the lower weight. This appendix contains some information which has been helpful to those people who have made their surgery successful.

Eating Methods After Surgery

After surgery, you will find you need to make changes in your eating pattern, not only to prevent pain and vomiting, but also for desired weight reduction. Perhaps even more important is development of appropriate eating habits to prevent disruption of the staple line and obstruction of the stoma (opening leaving the upper stomach). Changes considered to be important are outlined in the following paragraphs.

Eat Slowly and Chew Food Until It Is of a Mushy Consistency

Swallowing food in chunks may block the opening and prevent food from passing into the gastrointestinal tract. Hints to help you eat more slowly are the following:

1. Set aside 30 to 45 minutes to eat each meal.
2. Actually count the number of times you chew each bite. Aim for 30.

* Adapted with permission from the Dietary Department, The University of Iowa Hospitals and Clinics, Iowa City, Iowa.

3. Make a sign EAT SLOWLY and place it on the table in front of you.
4. Explain to family members why you must eat slowly so they will not urge you to eat faster.
5. Take small bites of food. You may want to try eating with a baby spoon.
6. Pay attention to taste. Learn to savor each bite, noticing its flavor, texture, and consistency.
7. Chew well. Ground or very soft foods will be necessary if you have dentures.

Stop Eating as Soon as You Are Full

Besides causing you to vomit, extra food over a period of time may stretch your stomach or pouch. At first, you may be eating only one-quarter cup of solid food (2 to 3 teaspoons of each item sent on your tray).

Indications of fullness may be as follows:

1. You may notice a feeling of pressure or fullness in the center just below your rib cage.
2. You may have feelings of nausea.
3. You may experience pain in your shoulder area or upper chest.

Set Aside Three Meal Times per Day and Eat Solid Foods Only at These Times

It is important to eat nourishing foods and not to get into the habit of snacking. If you eat often throughout the day, you may not lose weight because you can take in enough calories to maintain your weight. Individuals who continuously munch on crackers, potato chips, or other foods not only have failed to lose but have even gained weight.

Drink Four to Six Cups of Liquid per Day Between Meals

Liquids are needed to replace normal body water losses and thus prevent dehydration. Recommended beverages are skim milk, water, low-calorie beverages, tea, and coffee. The following are hints for drinking beverages:

1. Do not drink beverages for 30 or 45 minutes before or after meals. (There is not enough room in your stomach pouch for both food and liquids.)
2. Sip beverages slowly. One way to begin this is by taking sips of beverages from a medicine cup or shot glass instead of drinking from a regular glass.
3. Eliminate high-calorie drinks such as milkshakes, soda, beer, and other alcoholic beverages from your diet. By sipping high-calorie liquids throughout the day, many calories can be consumed without the effect of fullness. This will result in a poor weight loss record.

	Calories
Alcoholic beverages	
(1.5 oz. gin, vodka, whiskey)	100–125
Beer (12-oz. can)	150
Milkshake	840
Soda (12-oz. can)	120
Whole milk (8 oz.)	160

Eat a Balanced Diet

Since the quantity of food you can consume at a meal is reduced, it is important that what you do eat be of good nutritional value.

Eating foods from each of the four food groups will provide adequate amounts of protein, vitamins, and minerals for your needs.

Progression of the Diet During Hospitalization

As you begin to eat again after surgery, in addition to water you will first be offered clear liquids. Clear liquids include jello, clear juice, and broth. Remember, for each meal you will be able to eat only a couple of small spoonfuls of each item sent on your tray. It is better to eat some of all items rather than all of just one item.

After a short period of time you will be advanced to a soft or chopped diet. We serve this type of soft food to you because chunks of food can obstruct the outlet of your stomach, causing you to vomit and experience pain. You may be tempted to drink only liquids but that could prevent you from developing the habit of chewing your food well, and result in poor nutrition after a time.

Sometimes specific food items may cause discomfort or vomiting. However, because there are many reasons one may vomit, you should be careful not to avoid a food just because you vomited once after eating it. You may wait awhile, but then try that same food again.

The Diet at Home

For a total of 4 weeks after surgery, continue to eat soft foods. For protein you may eat cottage cheese, yogurt, sliced cheese, cheese dishes, eggs and egg dishes, and fish. You may carefully eat meats that are ground or very thinly sliced after cooking. You may also eat canned fruits and vegetables, baked potatoes (without the skin), mashed potatoes, rice, macaroni, noodles, crackers, and cooked or ready-to-eat nonbran cereals.

If you are tolerating the foods listed above during the first 4 weeks after your first checkup, you may begin to experiment more with foods. Well-cooked meats, raw fruits, raw vegetables, and salads may be tried. When starting a new food, eat only a bite or two the first time. Remember to chew well. Never swallow anything that isn't chewed completely—spit it out if it can't be completely chewed.

Vitamins

A small solid tablet, chewable, or liquid multivitamin supplement is recommended. Consult your local pharmacist regarding a specific brand.

Certain Foods May Be Difficult to Tolerate

Since toleration of foods varies from individual to individual, use your own discretion as to whether to include them in your diet. Through trial and error you may find that you are able to tolerate some of these foods, but there may be others which your digestive system cannot handle as well. These foods include the following:

Tough meats, especially hamburger. (Even after grinding, the gristle in hamburger is difficult to digest.) Meat tenderizer often helps.

Membranes of oranges or grapefruits.

Cores, seeds, or skins of fruits or vegetables.

Fibrous vegetables such as stringy celery or sweet potatoes.

Breads, especially if fresh and soft. (May remain in a ball even after a lot of chewing.)

Chili or other highly spiced foods.

Fried foods.

Milk. (Milk is an important part of your diet, supplying much needed protein and calcium. If you are unable to tolerate it as a beverage, it should be incorporated into the diet through foods such as soups, yogurt, or cheese.)

Sweets, especially if concentrated or liquid, such as ice cream. ("Dumping" is the unpleasant effect of concentrated sugars emptying too quickly into the small intestine. Symptoms include weakness, breaking into a sweat, and a heavy feeling in the abdomen about 10 minutes after eating. In severe cases there may be diarrhea half an hour later—this acts as a useful deterrent to eating sweet foods.)

REMEMBER !

For successful weight loss after gastric bypass surgery, a change in your eating habits is necessary. The operation alone is not a cure—it is not magical. You will not be able to lose as much weight as you would like if you either eat continuously all day, or if you stretch your stomach by eating large amounts of food at one time. You will lose the weight you want only if you are willing to control what you eat, and the way in which you eat it.

IT IS IMPORTANT TO:

Eat slowly.

Chew food well.

Stop eating when you are full.

Eat three meals; avoid snacking.

Sip low-calorie beverages between meals.

Select a balanced diet.

Exercise regularly.

Basic Food Groups

Recommended Number of Servings/Day	Food Group	Comments
2	Milk Group 1 cup skim milk 1 cup yogurt (plain) 1.5 slices cheese	These foods are high in protein and calcium. Protein is needed for wound healing and renewal of body cells. Calcium is needed for bones.
3	Meat Group 1 oz. cooked lean meat, fish, or poultry 1 egg One-quarter cup cottage cheese One-quarter cup liverwurst	These foods are high in protein and iron. Iron is needed to prevent anemia and increase resistance to infection.
3	Fruit and Vegetable Group One-half cup cooked fruit or vegetable One-half cup fruit or vegetable juice	This group provides vitamins and minerals needed to regulate body processes, prevent nutritional deficiencies, and increase resistance to infection.
2	Grain Group One-half cup cooked cereal One-half cup ready-to-eat cereal 1 rusk 4 saltines One-half cup rice, noodles, or macaroni One-half slice toast	These foods are needed for proper amounts of iron, B-vitamins, and carbohydrate, and as bulk for better bowel habits.

Index

Understanding the Science and Practice of Public Health

Understanding the Science and Practice of Public Health

Richard Crosby

Good Samaritan Endowed Professor
College of Public Health
University of Kentucky

JB JOSSEY-BASS™
A Wiley Brand

Library of Congress Cataloging-in-Publication Data applied for:

9781119860921 (Paperback); 9781119860945 (Adobe PDF); 9781119860938 (ePub)

Cover and Author Image: Courtesy of Richard Crosby
Cover design: Wiley

SKY10045073_032823